The ECT Handbook

Third Edition

Edit

Colle
Appr   2
Due f

RCPsych Publications

© The Royal College of Psychiatrists 2013
Reprinted 2014

RCPsych Publications is an imprint of the Royal College of Psychiatrists,
17 Belgrave Square, London SW1X 8PG
http://www.rcpsych.ac.uk

British Library Cataloguing-in-Publication Data.
A catalogue record for this book is available from the British Library.
ISBN 978-1-908020-58-1

Distributed in North America by Publishers Storage and Shipping Company.

The views presented in this book do not necessarily reflect those of the Royal College of
Psychiatrists, and the publishers are not responsible for any error of omission or fact.

The Royal College of Psychiatrists is a charity registered in England and Wales (228636)
and in Scotland (SC038369).

Printed by Bell & Bain Limited, Glasgow, UK.

Contents

Abbreviations

BPRS	Brief Psychiatric Rating Scale
CONECTS	Committee of Nurses at ECT in Scotland
ECG	electrocardiogram, electrocardiograph
ECTAS	ECT Accreditation Service
EEG	electorencephalogram, electroencephalography
GABA	gamma-aminobutyric acid
MAOI	monoamine oxidase inhibitor
MMSE	Mini-Mental State Examination
NALNECT	National Association of Lead Nurses in ECT
NICE	National Institute for Health and Clinical Excellence
rTMS	repetitive transcranial magnetic stimulation
SEAN	Scottish ECT Accreditation Network
SSRI	selective serotonin reuptake inhibitor

List of figures, tables and boxes

List of contributors

Professor Ian M. Anderson, Honorary Consultant Psychiatrist, Manchester Mental Health and Social Care Trust, and Professor of Psychiatry, Neuroscience and Psychiatry Unit, University of Manchester

Dr Richard Barnes, Consultant in Old Age Psychiatry, Mossley Hill Hospital, Liverpool

Professor Susan M. Benbow, Director, Older Mind Matters Ltd, and Visiting Professor of Mental Health and Ageing, Staffordshire University

Dr Daniel M. Bennett, Consultant Forensic Psychiatrist, NHS Tayside, and Honorary Senior Lecturer in Psychiatry, University of Aberdeen

Dr C. John Bowley, retired Consultant Anaesthetist, Nottingham University Hospitals

Dr Sarah Browne, Research Technician, Division of Neuroscience, University of Dundee, Ninewells Hospital and Medical School, Dundee

Dr David Christmas, Consultant Psychiatrist, Advanced Interventions Service, Ninewells Hospital and Medical School, Dundee

Ms Joanne Cresswell, ECTAS Programme Manager, ECTAS, Centre for Quality Improvement, Royal College of Psychiatrists

Mrs Linda Cullen, National Clinical Coordinator, Scottish ECT Audit Network

Dr Peter Cutajar, Consultant Psychiatrist, Learning Disabilities, Nottinghamshire Healthcare NHS Trust

Dr Michael Dixon, Lead Pharmacist for Research & Development, Medicines Information, Leeds and York Partnership NHS Foundation Trust, Leeds

Dr Ross A. Dunne, Academic Clinical Fellow, Specialty Registrar in Old Age Psychiatry, Fulbourn Hospital, Cambridgeshire and Peterborough NHS Foundation Trust, Cambridge

Dr Andrew Easton, Consultant Forensic Psychiatrist, Seacroft Hospital, Leeds Partnership NHS Foundation Trust

Dr M. Sam Eljamel, Consultant Neurosurgeon, Advanced Interventions Service, Ninewells Hospital and Medical School, Dundee

Dr Christopher F. Fear, Consultant Psychiatrist, 2gether NHS Foundation Trust, Gloucester

Dr Grace M. Fergusson, Consultant Psychiatrist, Argyll and Bute Hospital, Lochgilphead

Professor I. Nicol Ferrier, Professor of Psychiatry, School of Neurology, Neurobiology and Psychiatry, University of Newcastle, Newcastle upon Tyne

Mr Stephen Finch, Lead ECT Nurse, Greater Manchester West Mental Health NHS Foundation Trust, Bolton Mental Health Directorate

Professor Chris P. Freeman, Regional Consultant for Eating Disorders, Royal Edinburgh Hospital, and The Old Pencaitland Farmhouse, East Lothian

Mr Eamonn Heaney, Formerly Lead Nurse for ECT, Parkwood Clinic, Blackpool, Lancashire Care NHS Foundation Trust

Dr Jo Jones, Consultant Psychiatrist, Learning Disabilities, Nottinghamshire Healthcare NHS Trust

Professor Ennapadam S. Krishnamoorthy, TS Srinivasan Chair, TS Srinivasan Institute of Neurosciences, VHS Hospital, Chennai, India

Dr Heinrich C. Lamprecht, Consultant Psychiatrist, Mental Health Services for Older People, Guiborough, Tees, Esk & Wear Valleys NHS Foundation Trust

Dr Donald Lyons, Mental Welfare Commission for Scotland

Dr Denis Martin, BChD, LDS (Leeds), Specialty Doctor, ECT Service, Wooton Lawn Hospital, Gloucester

Professor Keith Matthews, Professor of Psychiatry and Honorary Consultant Psychiatrist, Division of Neuroscience, University of Dundee, Ninewells Hospital and Medical School, Dundee

Professor Declan M. McLoughlin, Research Professor of Psychiatry, Trinity College Institute of Neuroscience, Trinity College Dublin, and St Patrick's University Hospital, Dublin, Ireland

Dr Walter J. Muir (deceased), formerly Reader in the Psychiatry of Learning Disability, Division of Psychiatry, University of Edinburgh

Dr Angelica Santiago, Consultant Psychiatrist, Bradford & Airedale Early Intervention, Culture Fusion, Bradford

Dr Allan I. F. Scott, Consultant Psychiatrist, Royal Edinburgh Hospital

Dr Hugh Series, Consultant Psychiatrist, Oxford Health NHS Foundation Trust

Dr Douglas Steele, Professor of Neuroimaging and Honorary Consultant Psychiatrist, Advanced Interventions Service, Ninewells Hospital and Medical School, Dundee

Dr Alan G. Swann, Consultant Psychiatrist in Old Age Psychiatry, Newcastle General Hospital, Newcastle upon Tyne

Dr Jonathan Waite, Consultant Psychiatrist, Nottinghamshire Healthcare NHS Trust

Dr Heather A. C. Walker, retired Consultant Anaesthetist, North Manchester General Hospital

Dr Simon C. Walker, Consultant Anaesthetist, William Harvey Hospital, Ashford, Kent

Dr Andrew M. Whitehouse, Emeritus Consultant Psychiatrist, Nottinghamshire Healthcare NHS Trust

Preface

Jonathan Waite and Andrew Easton

Since the last edition of *The ECT Handbook* was published there have been three important developments: the implementation of accreditation services for ECT clinics, revision of the mental health legislation and the publication of the National Institute for Health and Clinical Excellence (NICE) guidance on the management of depression that significantly amends the recommendations on the use of ECT in depressive disorders.

The ECT Accreditation Service (ECTAS) and the Scottish ECT Accreditation Network (SEAN) had been planned at the time of the last handbook; they are now firmly established as a means of ensuring enhancing the standards of clinical practice in ECT in member clinics. Participating in the accreditation process has led nurses working in ECT to develop their own networks: the Committee of Nurses at ECT in Scotland (CONECTS) and the National Association of Lead Nurses in ECT (NALNECT) in other parts of the UK. Progressive cycles of ECTAS peer review have been successful in improving levels of performance by member clinics.

In Britain, the 2007 amendments of the Mental Health Act 1983 and the Mental Health (Care and Treatment) Act (Scotland) 2003 have changed the legal framework for patients who do not or cannot consent to ECT; patients with capacity who refuse ECT may not be given the treatment contrary to their objections. There is also new legislation on mental health treatment in Ireland (Mental Health Commission, 2009*a,b*) and the law in Northern Ireland in being revised.

The NICE (2009) guidelines for the treatment and management of depression in adults include revised recommendations of the use of ECT in depressive illness. The Royal College of Psychiatrists' Special Committee on ECT welcomes and endorses this new guidance.

The Special Committee on ECT and Related Treatments, like NICE, has reversed its previous recommendation in favour of routine adoption of unilateral electrode placement. New evidence from an adequately powered, methodologically sound study (Kellner *et al*, 2010) has allowed reconsideration of the balance between maximising the benefit of ECT and minimising adverse cognitive effects. The Committee now feels that for most patients receiving ECT in Britain, treatment should start with bitemporal electrode placement.

This edition of the *Handbook* is the fourth report of the Special Committee on ECT and Related Treatments. It contains new chapters on possible mechanisms of ECT action, dental aspects, non-ECT brain stimulation techniques and patient perspectives; the other chapters have been updated. The College's courses for ECT practitioners, prescribers and team members have continued to prove popular and will continue to be held annually.

The editors would like to thank all the contributors, and particularly Candace Gillies-Wright, who have supported their work, and that of the College's Special Committee on ECT and Related Treatments.

References

Kellner, C. H., Knapp, R., Husain, M. M., *et al* (2010) Bifrontal, bitemporal and right unilateral electrode placement in ECT: randomised trial. *British Journal of Psychiatry*, **196**, 226–234.

Mental Health Commission (2009a) *Code of Practice: Code of Practice on the Use of Electro-Convulsive Therapy for Voluntary Patients*. Mental Health Commission.

Mental Health Commission (2009b) *Rules: Rules Governing the Use of Electro-Convulsive Therapy*. Mental Health Commission.

National Institute for Health and Clinical Excellence (2009) *Depression: The Treatment and Management of Depression in Adults (Update)* (Clinical Guideline CG90). NICE.

Introduction: the role ECT in contemporary psychiatry

Royal College of Psychiatrists' Special Committee on ECT and Related Treatments

The previous edition of *The ECT Handbook* was produced in 2005, shortly after the publication of the National Institute for Health and Clinical Excellence (NICE) Technology Appraisal *Guidance on the Use of Electroconvulsive Therapy* (TA59; National Institute for Health and Clinical Excellence, 2003). There was concern within the Royal College of Psychiatrists' Special Committee on ECT (now Special Committee on ECT and Related Treatments) about the contents of the NICE recommendations. A Consensus Group was convened to consider the College's response to NICE. The opening chapter of the second edition of *The ECT Handbook* set out the areas of divergence between the College and NICE.

No full review of TA59 has been undertaken; the NICE guidance on the use of ECT for conditions other than depression remains unaltered. However, in October 2009 NICE published a clinical guideline on depression (CG90), which includes recommendations on the use of ECT in the treatment of depression. There are significant changes in this advice from that which was contained in TA59. The Special Committee welcomes and endorses the revised guidance contained in CG90. There are now no substantial differences between the College's views and those of NICE on the place of ECT in the treatment of depression. The Special Committee's views are also in line with those of the British Association for Psychopharmacology (Anderson *et al*, 2008).

Depression

The National Institute for Health and Clinical Excellence (2009) states that ECT should be considered for severe depression that is life-threatening, or where a rapid response is required or where other treatments have failed. Electroconvulsive therapy should not be used routinely in moderate depression but should be considered if there has been no response to multiple drug treatments and psychological treatment. If patients have not responded well to ECT in the past, ECT should only be considered again after review of the adequacy of previous treatment, a consideration of other options and after discussion with the patient and their advocates or carers if appropriate.

There is advice on the process of consent and compliance with mental health legislation. The choice of electrode placement and stimulus dose should balance efficacy against the risk of cognitive impairment. Bilateral ECT is more effective than unilateral ECT but may cause more cognitive impairment; with unilateral ECT, a higher stimulus dose is associated with greater efficacy, but also increased cognitive impairment compared with a lower stimulus dose.

Progress should be assessed after each treatment using a formal valid outcome measure, and treatment should be stopped when remission has been achieved or sooner if adverse effects outweigh benefits. Cognitive functioning should be assessed before the start of the course, and monitored at least every three to four treatments, and at the end of the course. Cognitive assessment should include orientation and time to re-orientation after each treatment. Measurement of new learning, retrograde amnesia and subjective memory impairment should be carried out at least 24 h after a treatment.

If at any stage there is evidence of significant cognitive impairment, consideration should be given to changing from bilateral to unilateral electrode placement, reducing the stimulus dose or stopping treatment. This will depend on the balance of risks and benefits and should be discussed with the person with depression.

If treatment is successful, measures should be initiated to try to prevent a relapse, such as starting antidepressant medication. Lithium augmentation of antidepressants may be helpful.

This advice is now consistent with the 2005 Consensus Group's view. Electroconvulsive therapy in the treatment of depression is considered in Chapter 14.

Mania

The 2003 NICE guidance recognised that ECT could be considered for treatment of a prolonged or severe manic episode. The NICE clinical guideline on bipolar disorder (CG38; National Institute for Health and Clinical Excellence, 2006) makes no changes to the recommendations of TA59 except to advise stopping or reducing lithium or benzodiazepines before giving ECT, monitoring the length of fits carefully if the patient is taking anticonvulsants and monitoring mental state carefully for evidence of switching to the opposite pole.

In 2005, the Consensus Group's view was that the treatment of choice for mania is a mood-stabilising drug plus an antipsychotic drug. Electroconvulsive therapy could be considered for severe mania associated with life-threatening physical exhaustion or treatment resistance. There is no change in the Special Committee's view. Chapter 15 reviews ECT in the treatment of mania.

Catatonia

In 2005, the Consensus Group concluded:

> 'Catatonia is a syndrome that may complicate several psychiatric and medical conditions. The treatment of choice is a benzodiazepine drug; most experience is with lorazepam. ECT may be indicated when treatment with lorazepam has been ineffective.' (Scott, 2005: p. 54)

There is no change in the guidance of NICE and the Special Committee does not wish to change the views previously expressed. Electroconvulsive therapy in the treatment of schizophrenia and catatonia is discussed in Chapter 16.

Acute schizophrenia

The NICE ECT Technology Appraisal did not recommend ECT for the treatment of schizophrenia; in 2005 the Consensus Group concluded that ECT should be considered as a fourth-line option for patients with schizophrenia for whom clozapine has already been proven ineffective or intolerable (Scott, 2005).

No new evidence has been published which has caused the committee to modify its previous guidance.

ECT technique

There are no definitive data on how frequently ECT is now used in Britain. The Department of Health no longer collects national data. Figures from the Care Quality Commission (2010) on referrals for second opinion appointed doctors to review the use of ECT in detained patients in England and Wales point to a continuing reduction in use following the survey conducted in 2006 (Bickerton et al, 2009). Audit data from the Scottish ECT Accreditation Network (SEAN) (2012) suggest that there has been little change in the amount of ECT given from 2008 to 2011.

In Britain, it is likely that ECT is only used in severe or treatment-resistant illness or in patients who have previously responded well to the treatment. The choice of ECT is based on the balance between adverse cognitive effects, maximising the effectiveness of treatment and the need to provide rapidly effective remission of symptoms.

The evidence for maximal efficacy has been collected from studies using bitemporal electrode placement with a charge of 1.5–2.5 times seizure threshold with a pulse width of 0.8–1.5 ms. There is, as yet, no convincing evidence that briefer pulses of electricity are equally effective or that ultra-brief ECT causes any less cognitive impairment. Where minimising cognitive side-effects is important, use of right unilateral ECT at 6 times seizure threshold is likely to be therapeutically effective.

In 2005 the Consensus Group stated that: 'The cognitive adverse effects of ECT can be substantially reduced by the use of unilateral electrode placement' (Scott, 2005: p. 7). As a result of new research on the efficacy and adverse effects of ECT using bitemporal, bifrontal and right unilateral electrode placements (Kellner et al, 2010), NICE have amended their previous guidance that unilateral electrode placement is preferable. They now advise that the choice of electrode placement and stimulus dose should balance efficacy against the risk of cognitive impairment, bearing in mind that bilateral ECT is more effective than unilateral ECT but may cause more cognitive impairment, whereas with unilateral ECT, a higher stimulus dose is associated with greater efficacy, but also increased cognitive impairment compared with a lower stimulus dose. The Special Committee concurs with this advice.

The 2005 Consensus Group stated that cognitive adverse effects could also be reduced by the avoidance of substantially suprathreshold electrical doses. The Handbook gave guidance on stimulus dosing and dose titration schedules.

The Special Committee still believes that it is good practice to use dose titration; guidelines on the selection of electrical dose are given in Chapter 4.

ECT and detained patients

The 2007 amendments to the Mental Health Act 1983 define a new class of practitioner – the responsible clinician, who is in charge of the treatment of a detained patient. Responsible clinicians do not have to be registered medical practitioners, but may be psychologists, nurses, social workers or occupational therapists. The Special Committee believes that only responsible clinicians who are medical practitioners should refer patients for ECT.

References

Anderson, I. M., Ferrier, I. N., Baldwin, R. C., et al (2008) Evidence based guidelines for treating depressive disorders with antidepressants: a revision of the 2000 British Association for Psychopharmacology guidelines. Journal of Psychopharmacology, 22, 343–396.

Bickerton, D., Worrall, A. & Chaplin, R. (2009) Trends in the administration of electroconvulsive therapy in England. Psychiatric Bulletin, 33, 61–63.

Care Quality Commission (2010) Monitoring the use of the Mental Health Act in 2009/10. CQC.

Kellner, C. H., Knapp, R., Husain, M. M., et al (2010) Bifrontal, bitemporal and right unilateral electrode placement in ECT: randomised trial. British Journal of Psychiatry, 196, 226-234.

National Institute for Health and Clinical Excellence (2003) Guidance on the Use of Electroconvulsive Therapy (Technology Appraisal TA59). NICE.

National Institute for Health and Clinical Excellence (2006) Bipolar Disorder: The Management of Bipolar Disorder in Adults, Children and Adolescents, in Primary and Secondary Care (Clinical Guideline CG38). NICE.

National Institute for Health and Clinical Excellence (2009) *Depression: The Treatment and Management of Depression in Adults* (Clinical Guideline CG90). NICE.

Scott, A. I. F. (ed.) (2005) *The ECT Handbook: The Third Report of the Royal College of Psychiatrists' Special Committee on ECT* (2nd edn) (Council Report CR128). Royal College of Psychiatrists.

Scottish ECT Audit Network (2012) *Scottish ECT Accreditation Network Annual Report 2012: A Summary of ECT in Scotland for 2011*. NHS National Services Scotland.

CHAPTER 1

Mechanism of action of ECT

Ian M. Anderson and Grace M. Fergusson

Seventy-five years after its introduction, ECT remains the most effective treatment for severe depressive disorder (UK ECT Review Group, 2003). Nevertheless, ECT is relatively underresearched compared with other forms of treatment for mental disorders; in particular there has been a relative lack of research using newer brain imaging techniques. Possible factors for the neglect of ECT include its adverse public image, funding priorities, the interests of researchers and the practical and ethical difficulties in studying this group of severely ill patients. Here, we briefly review some of the important neurobiological effects of ECT, concentrating on those related to its use in treating affective disorders, its principal indication. For more detailed information, see the reviews by Nobler & Sackeim (2008), Pigot *et al* (2008), Kato (2009), Merkl *et al* (2009) and Scott (2011).

A frequent criticism of ECT is that its mode of action is not understood. This is scarcely surprising given that the same can be said of other biological treatments in psychiatry. For example, although we understand much about the pharmacology of antidepressant and antipsychotic drug treatments, we still do not know how these pharmacological effects bring about improvement in mood or psychosis. Similarly for ECT, we know that both the generalised seizure and the dose of electricity used are important in bringing about its therapeutic effects, and that it has multiple, varied and lasting effects on the central nervous system (Merkl *et al*, 2009; Scott, 2011). Nevertheless, how these are translated into clinical effects remains obscure.

In recent years, advances in neuroscience have led to the development of various models of psychiatric disorders, particularly mood disorders, which encompass biological, psychological, social and developmental aspects (Mayberg, 2002; Seminowicz *et al*, 2004; Ebmeier *et al*, 2006; Beck, 2008; Akil *et al*, 2010). A common feature of these models is that psychiatric disorders are the result of disruptions of neural circuits, the functional networks of neurons that mediate thought, feelings and behaviour. Key areas concerned with networks involved in mood disorders include the hippocampus and amygdala, cingulate cortex (especially sub- and pregenual regions) and other areas of the prefrontal cortex. Underlying these networks are the structural and functional attributes of neurons and their connections. It is at this level that biological treatments are thought to exert their effects. There is good evidence that ECT has important effects on the function, and possibly structure, of neurons in these networks.

Putative mechanisms of ECT

Changes in brain structure, function and neural connectivity

Depression is associated with reduction in volume of the hippocampus (Arnone *et al*, 2012*a*) and excessive levels of circulating corticosteroids may play a causal role (Goodyer *et al*, 2010). Successful short-term antidepressant drug treatment has recently been shown to increase hippocampal grey matter in patients with depression (Arnone *et al*, 2012*b*). Although previous research has not found that ECT causes structural brain changes (UK ECT Review Group, 2003; Nobler & Sackeim, 2008), one study found that ECT caused an increase in bilateral hippocampal volume (Nordanskog *et al*, 2010). An earlier study, using magnetic resonance spectroscopy, found increased hippocampal choline concentrations, a putative measure of membrane turnover after ECT (Ende *et al*, 2000). This suggests that ECT may affect the structure of the hippocampus, a key component of neural circuitry involved in mood. The effects of ECT on the hippocampus may also underlie its effects on cognition, particularly memory (Gregory-Roberts *et al*, 2010).

As discussed above, prefrontal and medial temporal cortex have all been implicated in the genesis of depression; studies of the effect of ECT on regional cerebral blood flow (rCBF) and cerebral metabolic rate (rCMR) have however produced inconsistent results. Reviews have concluded that the most consistent finding is reduced anterior cingulate/prefrontal cortex rCBF or rCMR, possibly with some relationship with adverse cognitive effects (Nobler & Sackeim, 2008; Schmidt *et al*, 2008; Scott, 2011). However, other studies have found increased anterior cingulate and hippocampal rCMR correlating with improvement in symptoms (McCormick *et al*, 2007), as well as normalisation of reduced anterior cingulate theta wave activity (McCormick *et al*, 2009).

In summary, although there is evidence that ECT alters the function and the structure of important brain areas, especially the frontotemporal circuits involved in mood, methodological factors such as small and heterogeneous samples mean that a consistent picture has yet to emerge.

Effects on neurotransmitters

Monoamines

The monoamine theory of depression and antidepressant action goes back to the development of the first antidepressants and has been influential in driving the development of virtually all currently available antidepressant medications. More recent theories of antidepressant action emphasise adaptive changes in receptors and post-receptor mechanisms (e.g. Blier & Abbott, 2001). Preclinical studies investigating the effects of electroconvulsive shock (ECS), the animal equivalent of ECT, have found enhanced postsynaptic serotonergic (5-hydroxytryptamine, 5-HT) receptor sensitivity, downregulation of 5-HT$_2$ receptors, α_2- and β-adrenoceptors and increased striatal dopamine and dopamine receptors (Lisanby & Belmaker, 2000; Dremencov et al, 2003; Merkl et al, 2009). A human positron emission tomography (PET) study reported decreased anterior cingulate dopamine-D$_2$ receptor binding after ECT (Saijo et al, 2009), while in a non-human primate PET study, ECS decreased cortical 5-HT$_2$ receptor binding (Strome et al, 2005).

In support of the importance of monoamines in the effect of ECT, functional polymorphisms of the dopamine D$_2$ receptor which regulate postsynaptic effects, and the COMT gene which metabolises noradrenaline and dopamine have been associated with differential response to ECT (Merkl et al, 2009). However, neither using tryptophan depletion to decrease 5-HT function nor using α-methyl-para-tyrosine to reduce dopamine and noradrenaline function has been associated with symptomatic relapse after ECT (Cassidy et al, 1997, 2009). This suggests that increased levels of serotonin or catecholamines are not necessary to maintain improvement immediately after a course of ECT.

Other neurotransmitters and neuromodulators

An early model of the mechanism of action of ECT linked its anticonvulsant and antidepressant properties through common effects on gamma-aminobutyric acid (GABA), the major inhibitory neurotransmitter (Kato, 2009; Merkl et al, 2009). One theory has proposed that GABA-ergic inhibition may be restored by ECS as a result of upregulation of immediate early gene production modulating ion channel function (Kato, 2009). There has also been considerable interest in the role of glutamate in depression and its treatment (Mitchell et al, 2010). Electroconvulsive shock has been shown to alter modulate glutamate receptor expression or function (Naylor et al, 1996; Dong et al, 2010; Mitchell & Baker, 2010). In humans receiving ECT, pre-treatment low glutamate plus glutamine/glutamate concentrations have been found in dorsolateral prefrontal cortex (Michael et al, 2003) and anterior cingulate cortex (Pfleiderer et al, 2003; Merkl et al, 2011), which either normalised after ECT (Michael et al, 2003; Pfleiderer et al, 2003) or predicted treatment response (Merkl et al, 2011). In addition, it has been proposed that the adverse cognitive effects of ECT are mediated through indiscriminate activation of glutamate receptors in the hippocampus at the time of the seizure (Gregory-Roberts et al, 2010). Electroconvulsive therapy also has effects on peptide neuromodulators; for example, as with other antidepressant treatments, ECT increases brain and cerebrospinal neuropeptide Y concentrations (Mathe et al, 2007).

In summary, ECT has a variety of actions on neurotransmitter systems involved in neuronal functioning and these are likely to contribute to both its therapeutic and adverse effects.

Endocrine effects

There is a long history of interest in endocrine mechanisms in depression, most notably the hypothalamic–pituitary–adrenal (HPA) axis; hypercortisolaemia in Cushing's disease has long been known to be associated with depression. Hypothalamic–pituitary–adrenal axis abnormalities, including cortisol hypersecretion and impaired central cortisol feedback, are found in severe depression (de Kloet *et al*, 2007). Electroconvulsive therapy normalises HPA axis dysfunction, including restoring dexamethasone suppression of cortisol (Merkl *et al*, 2009). It is possible that central effects of ECT on neural systems involving corticosteroid receptors in structures such as the hippocampus may be important in its action. Acutely, ECT treatment is also associated with surges in plasma catecholamines and other hormones, which are important in its cardiovascular effects (see Chapter 21), but these have not been found to be associated with efficacy.

Gene expression, neurogenesis and synaptic plasticity

In animals, ECS induces widespread changes in gene expression. These include changes in proteins associated with neurotransmitters, neuropeptides and neuroprotective factors as well as those associated with synaptic plasticity (e.g. increased production of the immediate early gene product Homer1a) and neurogenesis (e.g. increased brain derived neurotrophic factor, BDNF) (Kato, 2009). Electroconvulsive shock has been shown to increase cell proliferation in areas such as the hippocampus in common with other antidepressant treatments (Kato, 2009; Merkl *et al*, 2009). Neurogenesis and alterations in synaptic plasticity have been proposed as a common mechanism underlying antidepressant activity (Racagni & Popoli, 2008), which would influence neuronal function and connectivity between brain structures relevant to mood and cognition.

Conclusions

We now have considerable evidence for the effects of ECT on brain function, although a comprehensive picture has still to emerge. The challenge remains to integrate the findings from different approaches and from mechanisms acting at different levels into a coherent model. It seems likely that multiple neurobiological effects modulating brain circuits associated with mood contribute to ECT's action and that these also interact with, or are dependent on, individual anatomical, biochemical, physiological and psychological variables.

The hope for the future is that a better understanding of the mechanisms underlying the action of ECT will allow refinement in its application as well as progress in the treatment of those mental (and some physical) disorders helped by ECT. This is important in order to address the two Achilles' heels of ECT: the high rates of relapse after successful treatment and the adverse cognitive effects. It should be possible to address both issues when we have a better understanding of how ECT works. The lack of research into ECT is concerning and may prove a major obstacle to progress.

Key points

- Electroconvulsive therapy does not just cause a general non-specific disruption of brain function and there is no evidence it produces brain damage.
- Electroconvulsive therapy produces diverse changes in brain functional and structural components, including cerebral blood flow and metabolism, gene expression, neurogenesis and synaptic plasticity, with resultant effects on neurotransmitter pathways and endocrine systems.
- The effects of ECT, as with other biological treatments, are likely to be acting to normalise abnormal brain function underlying the illness state.
- It is not yet clear which changes are responsible for improvement and which may cause adverse effects.

References

Akil, H., Brenner, S., Kandel, E., *et al* (2010) The future of psychiatric research: genomes and neural circuits. *Science*, **327**, 1580–1581.

Arnone, D., McIntosh, A. M., Ebmeier, K. P., *et al* (2012a) Magnetic resonance imaging studies in unipolar depression: systematic review and meta-regression analyses. *European Neuropsychopharmacology*, **22**, 1–16.

Arnone, D., McKie, S., Elliott, R., *et al* (2012b) State-dependent changes in hippocampal grey matter in depression. *Molecular Psychiatry*, 6 Nov, doi: 10.1038/mp.2012.150. (Epub ahead of print.)

Beck, A. T. (2008) The evolution of the cognitive model of depression and its neurobiological correlates. *American Journal of Psychiatry*, **165**, 969–977.

Blier, P. & Abbott, F. V. (2001) Putative mechanisms of action of antidepressant drugs in affective and anxiety disorders and pain. *Journal of Psychiatry and Neuroscience*, **26**, 37–43.

Cassidy, F., Murry, E., Weiner, R. D., *et al* (1997) Lack of relapse with tryptophan depletion following successful treatment with ECT. *American Journal of Psychiatry*, **154**, 1151–1152.

Cassidy, F., Murry, E., Weiner, R. D., *et al* (2009) Antidepressant response to electroconvulsive therapy is sustained after catecholamine depletion. *Progress in Neuropsychopharmacology and Biological Psychiatry*, **33**, 872–874.

de Kloet, E. R., Derijk, R. H. & Meijer, O. C. (2007) Therapy insight: is there an imbalanced response of mineralocorticoid and glucocorticoid receptors in depression? *Nature Reviews Endocrinology*, **3**, 168–179.

Dong, J., Min, S., Wei, K., *et al* (2010) Effects of electroconvulsive therapy and propofol on spatial memory and glutamatergic system in hippocampus of depressed rats. *Journal of ECT*, **26**, 126–130.

Dremencov, E., Gu, E., Lerer, B., *et al* (2003) Effects of chronic antidepressants and electroconvulsive shock on serotonergic neurotransmission in the rat hippocampus. *Progress in Neuropsychopharmacology and Biological Psychiatry*, **27**, 729–739.

Ebmeier, K. P., Donaghey, C. & Steele, J. D. (2006) Recent developments and controversies in depression. *Lancet*, **367**, 153–167.

Ende, G., Braus, D. F., Walter, S., *et al* (2000) The hippocampus in patients treated with electroconvulsive therapy: a proton magnetic resonance spectroscopic imaging study. *Archives of General Psychiatry*, **57**, 937–943.

Goodyer, I. M., Croudace, T., Dudbridge, F., *et al* (2010) Polymorphisms in BDNF (Val66Met) and 5-HTTLPR, morning cortisol and subsequent depression in at-risk adolescents. *British Journal of Psychiatry*, **197**, 365–371.

Gregory-Roberts, E. M., Naismith, S. L., Cullen, K. M., *et al* (2010) Electroconvulsive therapy-induced persistent retrograde amnesia: could it be minimised by ketamine or other pharmacological approaches? *Journal of Affective Disorders*, **126**, 39–45.

Kato, N. (2009) Neurophysiological mechanisms of electroconvulsive therapy for depression. *Neuroscience Research*, **64**, 3–11.

Lisanby, S. H. & Belmaker, R. H. (2000) Animal models of the mechanisms of action of repetitive transcranial magnetic stimulation (RTMS): comparisons with electroconvulsive shock (ECS). *Depression and Anxiety*, **12**, 178–187.

Mathe, A. A., Husum, V., El Khoury, A., *et al* (2007) Search for biological correlates of depression and mechanisms of action of antidepressant treatment modalities. Do neuropeptides play a role? *Physiology and Behaviour*, **92**, 226–231.

Mayberg, H. S. (2002) Modulating limbic-cortical circuits in depression: targets of antidepressant treatments. *Seminars in Clinical Neuropsychiatry*, **7**, 255–268.

McCormick, L. M., Boles Ponto, L. L., Pierson, R. K., *et al* (2007) Metabolic correlates of antidepressant and antipsychotic response in patients with psychotic depression undergoing electroconvulsive therapy. *Journal of ECT*, **23**, 265–273.

McCormick, L. M., Yamada, T., Yeh, M., *et al* (2009) Antipsychotic effect of electroconvulsive therapy is related to normalization of subgenual cingulate theta activity in psychotic depression. *Journal of Psychiatric Research*, **43**, 553–560.

Merkl, A., Heuser, I. & Bajbouj, M. (2009) Antidepressant electroconvulsive therapy: mechanism of action, recent advances and limitations. *Experimental Neurology*, **219**, 20–26.

Merkl, A., Schubert, F., Quante, A., *et al* (2011) Abnormal cingulate and prefrontal cortical neurochemistry in major depression after electroconvulsive therapy. *Biological Psychiatry*, **69**, 772–779.

Michael, N., Erfurth, A., Ohrmann, P., *et al* (2003) Metabolic changes within the left dorsolateral prefrontal cortex occurring with electroconvulsive therapy in patients with treatment resistant unipolar depression. *Psychological Medicine*, **33**, 1277–1284.

Mitchell, N. D. & Baker, G. B. (2010) An update on the role of glutamate in the pathophysiology of depression. *Acta Psychiatrica Scandinavica*, **122**, 192–210.

Naylor, P., Stewart, C. A., Wright, S. R., *et al* (1996) Repeated ECS induces GluR1 mRNA but not NMDAR1A-G mRNA in the rat hippocampus. *Brain Research: Molecular Brain Research*, **35**, 349–353,

Nobler, M. & Sackeim, H. (2008) Neurobiological correlates of the cognitive side effects of electroconvulsive therapy. *Journal of ECT*, **24**, 40–45.

Nordanskog, P., Dahlstrand, U., Larsson, M. R., *et al* (2010) Increase in hippocampal volume after electroconvulsive therapy in patients with depression: a volumetric magnetic resonance imaging study. *Journal of ECT*, **26**, 62–67.

Pfleiderer, B., Michael, N., Erfurth, A., *et al* (2003) Effective electroconvulsive therapy reverses glutamate/glutamine deficit in the left anterior cingulum of unipolar depressed patients. *Psychiatry Research*, **122**, 185–192.

Pigot, M., Andrade, C. & Loo, C. (2008) Pharmacological attenuation of electroconvulsive therapy-induced cognitive deficits: theoretical background and clinical findings. *Journal of ECT*, **24**, 57–67.

Racagni, G. & Popoli, M. (2008) Cellular and molecular mechanisms in the long-term action of antidepressants. *Dialogues in Clinical Neuroscience*, **10**, 385–400.

Saijo, T., Takano, A., Suhara, T., *et al* (2009) Electroconvulsive therapy decreases dopamine D(2) receptor binding in the anterior cingulate in patients with depression: a controlled study using positron emission tomography with radioligand [11C]FLB 457. *Journal of Clinical Psychiatry*, **71**, 793–799.

Schmidt, E. Z., Reininghaus, B., Enzinger, C., *et al* (2008) Changes in brain metabolism after ECT-positron emission tomography in the assessment of changes in glucose metabolism subsequent to electroconvulsive therapy – lessons, limitations and future applications. *Journal of Affective Disorders*, **106**, 203–208.

Scott, A. I. F. (2011) Mode of action of electroconvulsive therapy: an update. *Advances in Psychiatric Treatment*, **17**, 15–22.

Seminowicz, D. A., Mayberg, H. S. , McIntosh, A. R., *et al* (2004) Limbic-frontal circuitry in major depression: a path modelling metanalysis. *Neuroimage*, **22**, 409–418.

Strome, E. M, Clark, C. M., Zis, A. P., *et al* (2005) Electroconvulsive shock decreases binding to 5-HT2 receptors in nonhuman primates: an in vivo positron emission tomography study with [18F]setoperone. *Biological Psychiatry*, **57**, 1004–1010.

UK ECT Review Group (2003) Efficacy and safety of electro-convulsive therapy in depressive disorders: a systematic review and meta-analysis. *Lancet*, **361**, 799–808.

CHAPTER 2

The ECT suite

Chris P. Freeman and Grace M. Fergusson

There should ideally be a designated area for ECT within each general psychiatry unit; this is recommended on the basis of patient convenience and economy of nurse staffing. However, it is recognised that with the numbers of patients undergoing ECT falling, there is an increasing trend for psychiatric services to share one facility in an attempt to maintain standards of anaesthetic and psychiatric practice within the confines of a National Health Service budget.

Suite layout

The design of the ECT suite will depend on the type of service provided. The minimum requirement for a local unit with small patient numbers is two rooms: a treatment room and a recovery room. An ECT unit where patients would be required to wait before treatment will need a waiting room in addition. A suite providing ECT to neighbouring psychiatric units should ideally include an ECT office and a final post-ECT waiting area.

The waiting room should be a comfortable, relaxing and informal environment, with a range of distractions, for example an outside window, pictures and magazines, and toilet facilities should be available. Patients' arrival should be booked to provide a smooth throughput with the minimum amount of waiting time. Patients waiting for ECT should not be able to see into the treatment area while the treatment is taking place, and patients waiting for treatment should not be in the same room as patients who have completed their treatment.

The treatment room should be accessible from the waiting area. In the treatment area the patient is assisted onto a trolley or bed and prepared for treatment. This room should be well lit and contain all the equipment necessary for routine and emergency treatment. It should be big enough to allow unrestricted staff movements. Adequate work surfaces and a sink with hot and cold water should be available. There should be a clock with a second hand. If nitrous oxide and/or anaesthetic inhalation agents are ever used, the treatment room should be equipped with scavenging equipment and agent monitoring. There should be good sound-proofing between the waiting area and treatment room.

The recovery area must be large enough to accommodate easily the trolleys and associated monitors of all the patients who are regaining consciousness, and there should be enough room for recovery nursing staff to work in. The size will therefore vary according to the activity levels of the ECT suite and should be calculated on the basis of the maximum number of unconscious patients expected at any one session, bearing in mind that the average time for recovery varies from 5 to 30 min.

There should be a direct link between the treatment and recovery areas, through a doorway wide enough to admit a trolley or bed easily, that will allow ready access for the anaesthetic team and emergency equipment if necessary. Telephone access should be provided in case of the need to summon help. Patients should remain in this primary recovery area until they are able to walk and are reoriented.

From the recovery area the patients may be escorted to the post-ECT waiting area, where refreshments can be provided, to await transport back to their base unit. This room should be designed to accommodate all patients and escorting nurses in a relaxed environment.

A separate office is required for the administration of a busy ECT clinic or one serving neighbouring psychiatric units. The office should have a computer with internet and intranet access and a telephone.

Regionalisation of ECT services

A Department of Health review in England & Wales and the National Audit of ECT in Scotland (Freeman *et al*, 2000; Department of Health, 2003; Fergusson *et al*, 2004) have both confirmed a significant fall over the past 10 years in the number of patients who receive ECT. This, together with an anaesthetic requirement for increased staffing and monitoring, has resulted in a move towards regional centres serving several catchment populations. There are certain advantages and disadvantages inherent in this development.

Advantages

- Expensive anaesthetic monitoring and ECT equipment are shared.
- Suitably trained personnel – anaesthetist, operating department personnel, psychiatrist – are similarly shared.
- Regional centres can give a sufficient number of treatments to allow staff to maintain their skills.
- They provide adequate training opportunities for all sectors of staff.

Disadvantages

- They may be inconvenient to reach for some patients.
- Trained nurse escorts are required in satellite units when patients are transferred for ECT.

- Problems of clearly assigning clinical responsibility and ensuring the safe transport of patients to and from the ECT clinic.
- There is a need to consider the transfer of care for very frail or physically sick patients.

Staffing

Nursing staff

The number of nursing staff required at any ECT session will depend on the number of patients undergoing treatment and the type of service provided. In any case, the following conditions apply:

- there must be one trained nurse, with managerial responsibility, in overall charge of the ECT session
- one trained nurse should be in charge at each stage of the treatment process
- there should be one trained nurse, known to the patient, accompanying them throughout
- there should be one person, trained in cardiopulmonary resuscitation, with each unconscious patient; the number of staff in the recovery area should exceed the number of unconscious patients by one
- additional nurses should be available to help in the recovery areas of a busy clinic or if required for backup.

All clinical staff present during a treatment session should be trained in basic life support. There must be one life support provider (in addition to the anaesthetist) trained to at least immediate level present during the treatment session (see also Chapter 11).

Medical staff

The following are required:

- a senior psychiatrist
- a senior anaesthetist (see Chapter 3)
- operating department personnel or equivalent, whose sole role is to assist the anaesthetist.

There should be one life support provider with competence at advanced level present during the treatment session.

Equipment for the ECT suite

The following are required.

ECT machine

A brief-pulse, constant-current ECT machine is required with a wide output range and a facility for two-channel electroencephalography (EEG). The machine should be capable of providing stimuli according to the guidelines in Chapter 4. It should be possible to alter stimulus settings easily and quickly.

It is important that there is a backup arrangement in case the ECT machine develops a fault. This might be with a medical physics department or a neighbouring ECT service, to provide an ECT machine which staff are competent to use before the next treatment day. Appropriate electrodes and conducting gel or solution will also be required.

Trolley or bed with firm base

This should have braked wheels and cot sides. It must comfortably accommodate a reclining adult and should be capable of rapid tilting to a head down position. One trolley/bed per patient until recovery is required.

There should be moving and handling equipment, including a sheet to help to turn the patient.

Oxygen

This should be delivered by intermittent positive pressure ventilation via a mask and self-inflating bag from either a cylinder with a reserve or an anaesthetic machine, with appropriate circuits for supply and scavenging. There should be one face mask per patient.

Suction

Suction machine plus backup, tubing and catheters must be available.

Sundries

These will include disposable gloves, mouth gags, airways, syringes, needles, intravenous cannulae, tape, scissors, swabs, skin cleanser/degreaser and weighing scales.

Disposal

Appropriate disposal facilities are required for sharps and clinical waste.

Monitoring

For the purposes of monitoring the patient during the administration of ECT, the following will be required:

- a logbook of patients receiving ECT
- a blood glucose testing kit
- a stopwatch or clock with second hand plus EEG for determining seizure length
- a manual or automatic sphygmomanometer for measuring blood pressure

- an electrocardiograph (ECG) monitor with electrodes
- a pulse oximeter to determine oxygen saturation
- a capnograph to measure end-tidal carbon dioxide levels.

Anaesthetic drugs

These will be as agreed by local protocol in consultation with the anaesthetist. (Chapter 3 considers the anaesthetic equipment and procedures in more detail.)

Emergency drugs and equipment

These are detailed under a separate section below.

Recovery room

The following are required:

- a pulse oximeter for monitoring each unconscious patient
- a blood pressure monitor, as above
- an oxygen source (see p. 11)
- suction equipment (see p. 11)
- emergency drugs and equipment (see below).

Chapter 3 gives further information on the recovery room, in relation to anaesthesia.

Emergency drugs and equipment

Emergency drugs and equipment should be available in the treatment room and easily accessible to all other ECT areas during treatment sessions. These should be agreed with the local pharmacy or resuscitation committee, and will normally include:

- a cardiac defibrillator
- a laryngoscope, plus a backup, as well as laryngeal mask airways, endotracheal tubes and associated connectors; there must be means to establish an emergency surgical airway (e.g. an emergency cricothyroidotomy kit)
- intravenous infusion sets, fluids, stand and associated sundries
- a stethoscope
- a thermometer
- ice packs
- an emergency drug box, the contents of which will have been agreed by local protocol
- dantrolene plus sterile water should be stored within 5 min of the clinic – if this is not within the clinic, there must be a protocol for where it is stored.

Maintenance

An agreement should be in place for the regular maintenance of all equipment, either with the machine manufacturer or with the medical physics department.

Standards for ECT clinics

Comprehensive standards have been produced for ECT clinics (Cresswell *et al*, 2011; Scottish ECT Accreditation Network, 2011) and these are regularly updated.

References

Cresswell, J., Doncaster, E. & Murphy, G. (eds) (2011) *The ECT Accreditation Service (ECTAS): Standards for the Administration of ECT* (9th edn). Royal College of Psychiatrists' Centre of Quality Improvement.

Department of Health (2003) *Electroconvulsive Therapy: Survey Covering the Period from January 2002 to March 2002, England*. Department of Health.

Fergusson, G. M., Cullen, L. A., Freeman, C. P. L., *et al* (2004) Electroconvulsive therapy in Scottish clinical practice: a national audit of demographics, standards and outcome. *Journal of ECT*, **20**, 166–173.

Freeman, C. P. L., Hendry, J. & Fergusson, G. (2000) *National Audit of Electroconvulsive Therapy (ECT) in Scotland. Final Report*. Scottish Executive (http://www.sean.org.uk/AuditReport/Contents.html).

Scottish ECT Accreditation Network (2011) *Annual Report 2011: Summary of ECT in Scotland for 2012*. NHS National Services Scotland.

Anaesthesia for ECT

Simon C. Walker, C. John Bowley and Heather A. C. Walker

The anaesthetic team

Anaesthesia for ECT must be given by an experienced anaesthetist, capable of managing potential complications at a site that is usually isolated from theatres and often remote from the main hospital. Assistance is provided by a suitably trained operating department practitioner or anaesthetic nurse, and patients must be recovered by staff who have received appropriate theoretical and practical training (Royal College of Anaesthetists, 2009). Each department involved in ECT should allocate the responsibility for providing this service to a lead consultant anaesthetist (Cresswell *et al*, 2012) whose duties should include:

- ensuring suitable training, guidance and support is provided for those giving anaesthesia for ECT
- supervising and advising on the assessment of patients and their preparation for general anaesthesia
- ensuring the provision of suitable anaesthetic and monitoring equipment, appropriately trained anaesthetic assistants and recovery staff
- drawing up and reviewing of guidelines, regular audit against national standards, and reviewing of critical incidents
- liaising with other members of the ECT team, including regular multidisciplinary team meetings.

Equipment in the ECT suite (see also Chapter 2)

The main treatment area should be of adequate size, well lit and be equipped with tilting trolleys with cot sides that can be padded. This will be used for treatment and recovery until the patient can sit in a chair. Consideration should be given to equipment to facilitate the moving and handling of an unconscious patient. A secure drug storage cupboard, a small fridge and hand-washing facilities should be immediately available, and the room should have a clock with a second hand.

A full anaesthetic machine is not necessarily required but there must be a flow-controlled oxygen supply, either by pipeline or cylinder (plus reserve), with a Bain or Waters circuit to support ventilation. Airway circuits should be checked for function and patency prior to use. Suction of sufficient power must be available with Yankauer ends and soft suction catheters.

The recovery area should be immediately accessible from the treatment area and each first-stage recovery bay should be equipped with suitable lighting, an oxygen supply and suction.

Drugs

In addition to a variety of anaesthetic agents and muscle relaxants, there should be suitable drugs to treat unwanted effects of ECT (e.g. autonomic responses, prolonged and tardive seizures), anaesthetic/medical emergencies (e.g. anaphylaxis, resuscitation and peri-arrest conditions, malignant hyperthermia) and post-anaesthetic side-effects (e.g. headaches, nausea, vomiting). A list of appropriate drugs should be agreed by the anaesthetist with the ECT team and pharmacy, and a system for ensuring stock levels are checked and resupplied must be in place.

Monitoring

During anaesthesia, non-invasive blood pressure, ECG, pulse oximetry and end-tidal carbon dioxide monitoring are mandatory, and a peripheral nerve stimulator and means of measuring temperature and blood glucose should be immediately available. Each patient in recovery must have pulse oximetry and non-invasive blood pressure with immediate access to ECG, a nerve stimulator and capnography (Association of Anaesthetists of Great Britain and Ireland, 2007).

Emergency equipment

Emergency/resuscitation equipment should include a selection of airways, laryngoscopes, a range of endotracheal tubes, a bougie and laryngeal masks. Means for establishing an emergency surgical airway should be considered and other difficult airway devices may be helpful (Royal College of Anaesthetists, 2009; Cresswell et al, 2012). A selection of intravenous fluids, giving sets, a pressure infuser and a drip stand should be available.

Cardiac arrest drugs and other emergency anaesthetic drugs should be available according to guidelines agreed locally with the resuscitation committee and the anaesthetic department, with a fully equipped resuscitation trolley. The defibrillator should be checked (and recorded) before each session. Guidelines for resuscitation and other anaesthetic emergencies should be prominently displayed and periodic emergency resuscitation 'drills' practised.

The range and quantity of drugs and equipment needs to be assessed in context of the degree of isolation of the ECT suite and the time required to obtain drugs and equipment in an emergency. Consideration should be made for the equipment necessary for the emergency transport of an anaesthetised patient, with suitable monitoring and ventilation.

Pre-ECT assessment

Initial assessment can be performed by the psychiatrist or a suitably trained and supported senior ECT nurse or nurse practitioner. Guidelines drawn up with the help of the lead anaesthetist will help identify potential problems requiring early anaesthetic assessment or further investigation.

Medical history should be complete and highlight items which may have an impact on anaesthesia, in particular cardiorespiratory disease such as ischaemic heart disease, hypertension, chronic obstructive airway disease, cerebrovascular disease, diabetes, hiatus hernia/gastro-oesophageal reflux, liver disease, adverse reactions to previous anaesthetics or a family history of reaction to anaesthetics.

A full drug history including allergies and adverse reactions is essential. Early advice from the anaesthetist should be sought for patients taking diabetes medication, long-term or high-dose steroids or monoamine oxidase inhibitors (MAOIs). For possible interactions between ECT and psychotropic medication, refer to Chapter 5.

Physical examination should expose any evidence of cardiac failure, severe valvular heart disease, poorly controlled hypertension, significant infection, poor dentition, obesity, marked cachexia or factors that might prejudice airway management such as arthritis of the neck or jaw or poor mouth opening. The patient's vital signs and weight should be recorded.

Investigations

Guidelines for investigations required as part of the pre-anaesthetic assessment should be agreed. These might include the following (National Institute for Health and Clinical Excellence, 2003):

- Full blood count: for all patients over 60, and patients with cardiorespiratory disease, renal disease or diabetes.
- Sickle test: for all patients of African, Caribbean, Middle Eastern, Mediterranean or Asian ethnic extraction.
- Urea and electrolytes: as per full blood count, and patients taking lithium (recent lithium levels may be advisable).
- Liver function tests: for patients with cachexia, a history of liver disease or recent overdose.
- International normalised ratio (INR): for patients taking warfarin and coumarin anticoagulants.
- Glycated haemoglobin (HbA1c): for patients with diabetes.

- Pregnancy test: for females of childbearing age who cannot rule out pregnancy.
- Electrocardiogram: for all patients over 60 and patients with known cardiorespiratory or renal disease, diabetes, irregular pulse or heart murmur.
- Chest X-ray only after discussion with anaesthetist, for example new-onset or recent exacerbation of cardiopulmonary symptoms (chest pain, cough, shortness of breath).
- Lung function tests: only after discussion with anaesthetist, for example severe chronic obstructive airways disease or shortness of breath at rest.

All history, examination and test results must be available in the notes for full anaesthetic assessment prior to commencing a course of ECT.

Fitness for ECT/general anaesthesia

Patients whose condition or results give cause for concern should be referred promptly for anaesthetic assessment. Local guidelines should be agreed for specific medical conditions, drugs or functional capacity that should trigger referral. Such guidelines should include a clear pathway to ensure a timely response. This will facilitate any further investigation or referral required and minimise the risk of last-minute cancellations.

There are very few absolute contraindications to anaesthesia for ECT but some serious medical conditions require detailed evaluation and discussion of the balance between the risks and benefits (American Psychiatric Association, 2001). For example:

- recent myocardial infarction or unstable angina
- recent cerebrovascular events
- raised intracranial pressure/untreated cerebral aneurysm
- unstable major fracture/cervical spine injury
- phaeochromocytoma
- uncontrolled cardiac failure or severe valvular disease
- deep venous thrombosis.

It may be possible to reduce the risks with stabilisation and optimisation of the condition, and expert help should be sought early.

The presence of a cochlear or other brain implant may make ECT impossible; in these instances, discussion with experts familiar with the specific implant is essential. Patients with implanted pacemakers can receive ECT (MacPherson *et al*, 2006), although implantable cardioverter defibrillators should have defibrillation and antitachycardia functions deactivated prior to ECT and reactivated immediately after.

Electroconvulsive therapy is probably relatively safe in pregnancy (American Psychiatric Association, 2001). In the second trimester, consideration must be given to the risks of aorto-caval compression and oesophageal reflux that may require lateral tilt while supine and pre-treatment with antisecretory drugs, sodium citrate and endotracheal intubation (Miller, 1994). Treatment should be planned in consultation with the patient's obstetrician, and consideration of methods of fetal monitoring and whether the presence of a midwife would be appropriate.

In cases that are assessed to be high risk, consideration should be given to transferring the patient to an environment where closer monitoring and greater availability of emergency equipment and support are available, such as a theatre suite or its recovery area. Should such treatment prove uneventful, then it may be possible to continue the course of treatment in the ECT suite with the agreement of the ECT team.

Preparation of the patient for ECT

Patients should not have solids or drinks containing milk or particulates (cloudy) for 6h prior to treatment. They may drink clear fluids (e.g. water, black tea) until 2h before treatment. Chewing gum counts as clear fluid (Royal College of Nursing, 2005).

Unless specifically stated, all regular medications, with the exception of insulin, should be taken, not less than 2h prior to treatment. Patients with diabetes requiring insulin should attend early on the list and restart their usual regimen after recovery with their first food. Patients taking steroids equivalent to prednisolone 10mg/day or more may need peri-operative supplementation.

A checklist should be completed for all patients to verify:

- identity (patients should be provided with a name band, including hospital number)
- legal status/details of consent
- fasting state
- presence/removal of dentures/jewellery/hearing aids/contact lenses
- details of any pre-medication
- transport requirements
- date of last ECT/general anaesthetic.

Prescription charts and, if applicable, fluid charts should be available.

Patients should be given the opportunity to pass urine. Blood pressure, pulse, temperature and weight should be recorded. For patients with known diabetes, a blood glucose estimate should be performed immediately prior to each treatment.

Checklists must be signed and dated by the ECT suite staff.

Before their first treatment, day care patients and their carers should agree to and sign a declaration (Appendix I) that the patient will not:

- drive a car (if otherwise allowed)/ride a bicycle
- drink alcohol
- operate machinery (including kitchen equipment)

- avoid taking important decisions/signing documents for at least 24 h after their anaesthetic.

The patient must be escorted home by private transport and have responsible adult supervision for the 24 h after each treatment. Any written advice on the post-treatment period should be given to both the patient and escort (Association of Anaesthetics of Great Britain and Ireland, 2005).

Conduct of anaesthesia

Anaesthesia for ECT not only enables the procedure but also may have a significant influence on its efficacy. Patients frequently present for several anaesthetics within a short period of time and patients with comorbid medical conditions may be poorly treated due to difficulties obtaining accurate histories and/or failure by the patient to appropriately access community medical services.

The objective of anaesthesia is to provide the shortest period of unconsciousness necessary to cover muscle relaxation, the electrical stimulus and resultant seizure. A rapid return to full consciousness and orientation is desirable.

After introducing the team, the patient is asked to lie on the trolley and the ECG, pulse oximeter and non-invasive blood pressure monitor are attached; initial readings are recorded and intravenous access secured. Any short-acting agents needed to modify the anticipated autonomic response to ECT may be administered at this point and pre-oxygenation commenced.

Induction agents

Initially the dose of induction agent is usually titrated against the patient's response but subsequent doses or agent may be modified in the light of the clinical response, seizure threshold or haemodynamic responses. Any proposed change should be discussed with the ECT team. Brain function monitoring has been used to both ensure adequate anaesthesia and avoid excessive dosing of induction agent (Hanss *et al*, 2006; Sartorius *et al*, 2006) but may be unreliable at predicting emergence from anaesthesia due to post-ictal suppression of the EEG (Umeda *et al*, 2004).

Propofol

Propofol (0.75–2.0 mg/kg) is widely used. Advantages include familiarity, ease of use and pleasant induction. It may also reduce early cognitive impairment (Fredman *et al*, 1994a; Butterfield *et al*, 2004) and nausea and vomiting (Bailine *et al*, 2003). Seizure duration may be reduced compared with other agents but this does not alter seizure quality indicators (Geretsegger *et al*, 1998; Gazdag *et al*, 2004), it does not affect efficacy (Fear *et al*, 1994; Malsch *et al*, 1994; Martensson *et al*, 1994; Bauer *et al*, 2009) and it may be useful in the presence of prolonged seizures.

Thiopental

Thiopental (1.5–2.5 mg/kg) is successfully used despite concern about its anticonvulsant properties, which have not been substantiated in clinical trials. It has the disadvantage of having to be reconstituted into solution and haemodynamic response may be less well attenuated when compared with propofol (Kadoi et al, 2003). Its recovery characteristics may not be as good as shorter-acting agents such as propofol, remifentanil or sevoflurane.

Etomidate

Etomidate (0.15–0.3 mg/kg) tends to produces longer seizures than other agents (Avramov et al, 1995; Saffer & Berk, 1998; Tan & Lee, 2009). It has proved effective in patients in whom it has been found to be difficult to produce any seizure activity or who demonstrate brief or abortive seizures (Avramov et al, 1995; Khalid et al, 2006) and may lead to shorter courses of ECT (Patel et al, 2006). The haemodynamic responses tend to be greater in comparison with other agents and the incidence of pain on injection, slower recovery and abnormal movements can be problematic (Griffeth & Mehta, 2007; Freeman, 2009).

Ketamine

Ketamine is generally considered unsuitable for routine use due to its potential emergence phenomena, long recovery period and tendency to produce hypertension (Rasmussen et al, 1996). However, it has been used successfully where it has proved particularly difficult to produce any seizure activity despite maximal stimulus energy (Krystal et al, 2003). Its use may reduce memory impairment (McDaniel et al, 2006).

Methohexital

Methohexital (0.5–1.5 mg/kg) was for a long time the gold standard for anaesthetic agents for ECT and remains the standard for comparison. Problems with supply and its unlicensed status in the UK present practical difficulties to those who wish to use it and are the most significant disadvantages to its use.

Alfentanil, remifentanil and fentanyl

Alfentanil and remifentanil can be used to increase seizure duration and reduce haemodynamic response (Akcaboy et al, 2005; Hooten & Rasmussen, 2008; Nasseri et al, 2009). Alfentanil (10μg/kg) may prolong the duration of apnoea (van den Broek et al, 2004). Remifentanil (1μg/kg) is effective without any alteration in recovery characteristics and has been used in higher doses as a sole agent in patients who are refractory to seizure induction (Sullivan et al, 2004; Hossain & Sullivan, 2008). It is not clear whether the increased duration of seizures is due to a sparing effect on the anaesthetic agent or an inherent property of the opiate.

Fentanyl may shorten the duration of the seizure (Weinger *et al*, 1991).

Sevoflurane

Inhalational induction is possible if gas scavenging and appropriate monitoring are available. Sevoflurane has been used successfully with comparable effects to intravenous agents (Hodgson *et al*, 2004; Loughnan *et al*, 2004; Rasmussen *et al*, 2007). Its use has been reported in the third trimester of pregnancy to attenuate uterine contraction following ECT (Ishikawa *et al*, 2001).

Muscle relaxants

Muscle relaxants are used to modify the muscle activity during stimulation and the subsequent seizure, and reduce the risk of injury. In most cases it is not necessary to ablate all visible signs of muscle activity and this may be a useful indicator of generalised seizure activity in case of inadequate EEG signal. Some conditions may make complete paralysis preferable (e.g. severe osteoporosis, pre-existing fractures, deep vein thrombosis, spinal disease or surgery). As with the induction agent, subsequent doses should be continually reviewed in the light of the patient's changing response. A true rapid-sequence induction with cricoid pressure and endotracheal intubation may be indicated when regurgitation of stomach contents remains a real risk despite the protective measures of antacid therapy and appropriate fasting.

Suxamethonium

Suxamethonium (0.5–1.5 mg/kg) remains the relaxant of choice due to its rapid onset and short duration. The electrical stimulus should be applied only after fasciculation has ceased as the relaxant effect on relatively poorly perfused skeletal muscle may be considerably slower than on the larynx, especially in patients with a reduced cardiac index (Matsumoto *et al*, 2009). Myalgia is common but usually mild, although it can be more troubling in younger patients and with the first treatment (Dinwiddie *et al*, 2010).

Pseudocholinesterase deficiency, neuromuscular disease, hyperkalaemia, the presence of cholinesterase inhibitors, a history of malignant hyperthermia, neuroleptic malignant syndrome, catatonia or major burns may preclude its use and suggest conversion to a non-depolarising agent.

Atracurium, mivacurium and rocuronium

Atracurium (0.3–0.5 mg/kg), mivacurium (0.08–0.2 mg/kg) or rocuronium (0.3–0.6 mg/kg) may be acceptable alternatives, although their relatively prolonged action will need continued anaesthesia and/or active reversal after treatment. Sufficient time must be allowed for the onset of a non-depolarising block (Fredman *et al*, 1994*b*).

Dental issues

The initial contraction of the masseter and other muscles of mastication is due to the direct effect of the ECT stimulus and should not be mistaken for inadequate muscle relaxation. The supraphysiological bite produced presents a significant danger to the patients' dentition and demands the prior positioning of a suitable bite block in all patients (see Chapter 9). To reduce the risk of damage to dentition, the lower jaw can be held closed as the stimulus is applied.

Ventilation

A period of hyperventilation (approximately 20 breaths) immediately before the application of the electrical stimulus has been shown to enhance seizure duration (Sawayama *et al*, 2008). During the clonic phase of the seizure, manual ventilation with 100% oxygen is quite easily achieved in most patients, and the measured oxygen saturation should never fall below 90%.

Drugs used to modify the autonomic effects of ECT

During the electrical stimulus there is a significant increase in parasympathetic activity leading to sinus bradycardia and frequent asystoles (Hase *et al*, 2005), which can be prolonged (Tang & Ungvari, 2001). This may be exacerbated by the effects of suxamethonium and may be greater with subconvulsive stimuli. Severe bradycardia can usually, but not invariably, be prevented by pre-treatment with anticholinergic agents, glycopyrrolate (100–600 μg) having a theoretical advantage over atropine (300–600 μg) as it does not cross the blood–brain barrier. Sometimes higher doses or avoidance of suxamethonium are required (Robinson & Lighthall, 2004; Birkenhäger *et al*, 2010).

This is followed by a sympathetic surge during the seizure, causing a significant rise in heart rate and blood pressure (Swartz & Shen, 2007), which return towards baseline over 10–20 min. It is important to ensure that coexisting cardiovascular disease is optimally treated and that any regular medication is taken prior to treatment. If additional control is needed, remifentanil supplementation of the induction agent can be considered or an antihypertensive agent such as esmolol (1.0–4.5 mg/kg bolus (Castelli *et al*, 1995) or 0.5 mg/kg and 0.1–0.3 mg/kg/min infusion (Howie *et al*, 1992)), labetalol (0.05–0.4 mg/kg) (Castelli *et al*, 1995) or verapamil (0.1 mg/kg) (Wajima *et al*, 2002). Labetalol and higher doses of esmolol may shorten the duration of the seizure (Kovac *et al*, 1991; Weinger *et al*, 1991).

Missed or inadequate seizures

Missed seizures may be due to insufficient stimulus intensity, excess dynamic impedance, premature stimulus termination, hypercarbia, dehydration or the effects of other treatment (e.g. benzodiazepines). After checking the electrode position, restimulation at a higher energy is possible but a delay of at least 20 s should be incorporated to allow for the development of any delayed seizure. Manual ventilation during this period will help maintain hyperoxia and hypocarbia. A third stimulus may be required, especially during the first treatment session while stimulus energy is being titrated; this may sometimes necessitate small additional doses of suxamethonium, particularly if there has been a slow onset or any other delay after induction. Future treatments should also consider a decreasing dosage or change in the anaesthetic agent, hyperventilation and ensuring adequate hydration.

Prolonged or tardive seizures

A prolonged seizure (duration greater than 2–3 min) and a tardive seizure (late return of seizure activity) are later complications, with the latter likely to occur in recovery. The principles of treatment are to maintain oxygenation, monitor EEG activity and be prepared to abort the seizure with further doses of anaesthetic agents or benzodiazepines.

A local protocol for missed, prolonged or tardive seizures should be agreed.

Recovery

The need to maintain an adequate patient to staff ratio of 1:1(+1) in the immediate recovery area means that the throughput of patients from the treatment area may need to be controlled. Post-treatment oxygen supplementation should be continued until pulse oximetry indicates that the patient can maintain a satisfactory oxygen saturation on air. Vital signs should be observed and blood pressure and pulse oximeter readings should be continued. A continuous record should be kept, including observations of level of consciousness, heart rate, blood pressure, respiratory rate, oxygen therapy and saturation, any symptoms such as pain or sickness and any drugs given.

The patient may be transferred to a second-stage recovery once conscious and communicating, reliably maintaining their airway and physiologically stable.

Patients should remain in the second-stage recovery area until they are oriented and able to appropriately mobilise. The availability of something to eat and drink will usually be welcomed and allows time for the patient to further recover from the effects of the ECT and anaesthesia. The presence of the escort with whom the patient is familiar can be very reassuring during the later stages of recovery, and can free the recovery staff to attend to subsequent patients.

Explicit criteria for discharge from first- and second-stage recovery should be agreed by the ECT team and written instructions covering the post-treatment period should be provided to new out-patients and their escort (Cresswell *et al*, 2012). The anaesthetist must remain immediately available until the last patient is deemed fit for discharge.

Record-keeping and organisation

An anaesthetic record should be kept, including a full anaesthetic assessment, a record of anaesthetic consent, airway equipment and monitoring used, the doses of all anaesthetic agents used, the patient's response, and monitor recordings before and immediately after treatment and in recovery (Royal College of Anaesthetists, 2006). Information pertinent to future treatments such as suggested alteration in anaesthetic agent, muscle relaxant or treatment of autonomic effects should also be noted.

Regular audit should be carried out against local protocols and national standards such as those suggested by the Royal College of Anaesthetists (2009, 2012) and ECTAS (Cresswell *et al*, 2012), and regular review of morbidity and critical incidents must be carried out.

References

Akcaboy, Z. N., Akcaboy, E. Y., Yigitbasl, B., *et al* (2005) Effects of remifentanil and alfentanil on seizure duration, stimulus amplitudes and recovery parameters during ECT. *Acta Anaesthesiologica Scandinavica*, **49**, 1068–1071.

American Psychiatric Association (2001) *American Psychiatric Association Committee on ECT: Electroconvulsive Therapy: Recommendations for Treatment, Training, and Privileging* (2nd edn). American Psychiatric Press.

Association of Anaesthetists of Great Britain and Ireland (2005) *Day Case and Short Stay Surgery: 2*. AAGBI.

Association of Anaesthetists of Great Britain and Ireland (2007) *Recommendations for Standards of Monitoring during Anaesthesia and Recovery* (4th edn). AAGBI.

Avramov, M. N., Husain, M. M. & White, P. F. (1995) The comparative effects of methohexital, propofol, and etomidate for electroconvulsive therapy. *Anesthesia and Analgesia*, **81**, 596–602.

Bailine, S. H., Petrides, G., Doft, M., *et al* (2003) Indications for the use of propofol in electroconvulsive therapy. *Journal of ECT*, **19**,129–132.

Bauer, J., Hageman, I., Dam, H., *et al* (2009) Comparison of propofol and thiopental as anesthetic agents for electroconvulsive therapy: a randomized, blinded comparison of seizure duration, stimulus charge, clinical effect, and cognitive side effects. *Journal of ECT*, **25**, 85–90.

Birkenhäger, T. K., Pluijms, E. M., Groenland, T. H., *et al* (2010) Severe bradycardia after anesthesia before electroconvulsive therapy. *Journal of ECT*, **26**, 53–54.

Butterfield, N. N., Graf, P., Macleod, B. A., *et al* (2004) Propofol reduces cognitive impairment after electroconvulsive therapy. *Journal of ECT*, **20**, 3–9.

Castelli, I., Steiner, L. A., Kaufmann, M. A., *et al* (1995) Comparative effects of esmolol and labetalol to attenuate hyperdynamic states after electroconvulsive therapy. *Anesthesia and Analgesia*, **80**, 557–561.

Cresswell, J., Murphy, G. & Hodge, S. (2012) *The ECT Accreditation Service (ECTAS): Standards for the Administration of ECT* (10th edn). Royal College of Psychiatrists' Centre for Quality Improvement.

Dinwiddie, S. H., Huo, D. & Gottlieb, O. (2010) The course of myalgia and headache after electroconvulsive therapy. *Journal of ECT*, **26**, 116–120.

Fear, C. F., Littlejohns, C. S., Rouse, E., *et al* (1994) Propofol anaesthesia in electroconvulsive therapy. Reduced seizure duration may not be relevant. *British Journal of Psychiatry*, **165**, 506–509.

Fredman, B., d'Etienne, J., Smith, I., *et al* (1994*a*) Anesthesia for electroconvulsive therapy: effects of propofol and methohexital on seizure activity and recovery. *Anesthesia and Analgesia*, **79**, 75–79.

Fredman, B., Smith, I., d'Etienne, J., *et al* (1994*b*) Use of muscle relaxants for electroconvulsive therapy: how much is enough? *Anesthesia and Analgesia*, **78**, 195–196.

Freeman, S. A. (2009) Post-electroconvulsive therapy agitation with etomidate. *Journal of ECT*, **25**, 133–134.

Gazdag, G., Kocsis, N., Tolna, J., *et al* (2004) Etomidate versus propofol for electroconvulsive therapy in patients with schizophrenia. *Journal of ECT*, **20**, 225–229.

Geretsegger, C., Rochowanski, E., Kartnig, C., *et al* (1998) Propofol and methohexital as anesthetic agents for electroconvulsive therapy (ECT): a comparison of seizure-quality measures and vital signs. *Journal of ECT*, **14**, 28–35.

Griffeth, B. T. & Mehra, A. (2007) Etomidate and unpredicted seizures during electroconvulsive therapy. *Journal of ECT*, **23**, 177–178.

Hanss, R., Bauer, M., Bein, B., *et al* (2006) Bispectral index-controlled anaesthesia for electroconvulsive therapy. *European Journal of Anaesthesiology*, **23**, 202–207.

Hase, K., Yoshioka, H., Nakamura, T., *et al* (2005) Asystole during electroconvulsive therapy. *Masui*, **54**, 1268–1272.

Hodgson, R. E., Dawson, P., Hold, A. R., *et al* (2004) Anaesthesia for electroconvulsive therapy: a comparison of sevoflurane with propofol. *Anaesthesia and Intensive Care*, **32**, 241–246.

Hooten, W. M. & Rasmussen Jr, K. G. (2008) Effects of general anesthetic agents in adults receiving electroconvulsive therapy: a systematic review. *Journal of ECT*, **24**, 208–223.

Hossain, A. & Sullivan, P. (2008) The effects of age and sex on electroconvulsive therapy using remifentanil as the sole anesthetic agent. *Journal of ECT*, **24**, 232–235.

Howie, M. B., Hiestand, D. C., Zvara, D. A., *et al* (1992) Defining the dose range for esmolol used in electroconvulsive therapy hemodynamic attenuation. *Anesthesia and Analgesia*, **75**, 805–810.

Ishikawa, T., Kawahara, S., Saito, T., *et al* (2001) Anesthesia for electroconvulsive therapy during pregnancy – a case report. *Masui*, **50**, 991–997.

Kadoi, Y., Saito, S., Ide, M., *et al* (2003) The comparative effects of propofol versus thiopentone on left ventricular function during electroconvulsive therapy. *Anaesthesia and Intensive Care*, **31**, 172–175.

Khalid, N., Atkins, M. & Kirov, G. (2006) The effects of etomidate on seizure duration and electrical stimulus dose in seizure-resistant patients during electroconvulsive therapy. *Journal of ECT*, **22**, 184–188.

Kovac, A. L., Goto, H., Pardo, M. P., *et al* (1991) Comparison of two esmolol bolus doses on the haemodynamic response and seizure duration during electroconvulsive therapy. *Canadian Journal of Anaesthesia*, **38**, 204–209.

Krystal, A. D., Weiner, R. D., Dean, M. D., *et al* (2003) Comparison of seizure duration, ictal EEG, and cognitive effects of ketamine and methohexital anesthesia with ECT. *Journal of Neuropsychiatry and Clinical Neuroscience*, **15**, 27–34.

Loughnan, T., McKenzie, G. & Leong, S. (2004) Sevoflurane versus propofol for induction of anaesthesia for electroconvulsive therapy: a randomized crossover trial. *Anaesthesia and Intensive Care*, **32**, 236–241.

MacPherson, R. D., Loo, C. K. & Barrett, N. (2006) Electroconvulsive therapy in patients with cardiac pacemakers. *Anaesthesia and Intensive Care*, **34**, 470.

Malsch, E., Gratz, I., Mani, S., *et al* (1994) Efficacy of electroconvulsive therapy after propofol and methohexital anesthesia. *Convulsive Therapy*, **10**, 212–219.

Martensson, B., Bartfai, A., Hallen, B., *et al* (1994) A comparison of propofol and methohexital as anesthetic agents for ECT: effects on seizure duration, therapeutic outcome, and memory. *Biological Psychiatry*, **35**, 179–189.

Matsumoto, N., Tomioka, A., Sato, T., *et al* (2009) Relationship between cardiac output and onset of succinylcholine chloride action in electroconvulsive therapy patients. *Journal of ECT*, **25**, 246–249.

McDaniel, W. W., Sahota, A. K., Vyas, B. V., *et al* (2006) Ketamine appears associated with better word recall than etomidate after a course of 6 electroconvulsive therapies. *Journal of ECT*, **22**, 103–106.

Miller, L. J. (1994) Use of electroconvulsive therapy during pregnancy. *Hospital Community Psychiatry*, **45**, 444–450.

Nasseri, K., Arasteh, M. T., Maroufi, A., *et al* (2009) Effects of remifentanil on convulsion duration and hemodynamic responses during electroconvulsive therapy: a double-blind, randomized clinical trial. *Journal of ECT*, **25**, 170–173.

National Institute for Health and Clinical Excellence (2003) *The Use of Routine Preoperative Tests for Elective Surgery* (Clinical Guideline CG3). NICE.

Patel, A. S., Gorst-Unsworth, C., Venn, R. M., *et al* (2006) Anesthesia and electroconvulsive therapy: a retrospective study comparing etomidate and propofol. *Journal of ECT*, **22**, 179–183.

Rasmussen, K. G., Jarvis, M. R. & Zorumski, C. F. (1996) Ketamine anesthesia in electroconvulsive therapy. *Convulsive Therapy*, **12**, 217–223.

Rasmussen, K. G., Laurila, D. R., Brady, B. M., *et al* (2007) Anesthesia outcomes in a randomized double-blind trial of sevoflurane and thiopental for induction of general anesthesia in electroconvulsive therapy. *Journal of ECT*, **23**, 236–238.

Robinson, M. & Lighthall, G. (2004) Asystole during successive electroconvulsive therapy sessions: a report of two cases. *Journal of Clinical Anesthesia*, **16**, 210–213.

Royal College of Anaesthetists (2006) *The Good Practice Guide: A Guide for Departments of Anaesthesia, Critical Care and Pain Management* (3rd edn). Royal College of Anaesthetists.

Royal College of Anaesthetists (2009) *Guidelines for the Provision of Anaesthetic Services*. Royal College of Anaesthetists.

Royal College of Anaesthetists (2012) *Raising the Standard: A Compendium of Audit Recipes* (3rd edn). Royal College of Anaesthetists.

Royal College of Nursing (2005) *Perioperative Fasting in Adults and Children*. RCN.

Saffer, S. & Berk, M. (1998) Anesthetic induction for ECT with etomidate is associated with longer seizure duration than thiopentone. *Journal of ECT*, **14**, 89–93.

Sartorius, A., Muñoz-Canales, E. M., Krumm, B., *et al* (2006) ECT anesthesia: the lighter the better? *Pharmacopsychiatry*, **39**, 201–204.

Sawayama, E., Takahashi, M., Inoue, A., *et al* (2008) Moderate hyperventilation prolongs electroencephalogram seizure duration of the first electroconvulsive therapy. *Journal of ECT*, **24**, 195–198.

Sullivan, P. M., Sinz, E. H., Gunel, E., *et al* (2004) A retrospective comparison of remifentanil versus methohexital for anesthesia in electroconvulsive therapy. *Journal of ECT*, **20**, 219–224.

Swartz, C. M. & Shen, W. W. (2007) ECT generalized seizure drives heart rate above treadmill stress test maximum. *Journal of ECT*, **23**, 71–74.

Tan, H. L. & Lee, C. Y. (2009) Comparison between the effects of propofol and etomidate on motor and electroencephalogram seizure duration during electroconvulsive therapy. *Anaesthesia and Intensive Care*, **37**, 807–814.

Tang, W. K. & Ungvari, G. S. (2001) Asystole during electroconvulsive therapy: a case report. *Australian and New Zealand Journal of Psychiatry*, **35**, 382–385.

Umeda, E., Nakai, T. & Satoh, T. (2004) Bispectral index monitoring during anesthesia with propofol for electroconvulsive therapy. *Masui*, **53**, 810–812.

van den Broek, W. W., Groenland, T. H., Kusuma, A., *et al* (2004) Double-blind placebo controlled study of the effects of etomidate-alfentanil anesthesia in electroconvulsive therapy. *Journal of ECT*, **20**, 107–111.

Wajima, Z., Yoshikawa, T., Ogura, A., *et al* (2002) Intravenous verapamil blunts hyperdynamic responses during electroconvulsive therapy without altering seizure activity. *Anesthesia and Analgesia*, **95**, 400–402.

Weinger, M. B., Partridge, B. L., Hauger, R., *et al* (1991) Prevention of the cardiovascular and neuroendocrine response to electroconvulsive therapy: I. Effectiveness of pre-treatment regimens on hemodynamics. *Anesthesia and Analgesia*, **73**, 556–562.

CHAPTER 4

ECT prescribing and practice

Ross A. Dunne and Declan M. McLoughlin

Prescribing ECT

When should the course of ECT finish?

The aim of ECT should be remission of symptoms with a minimum of side-effects. Remission rates for those with severe, usually treatment-resistant depression are approximately 60–80% (Husain *et al*, 2004; Eranti *et al*, 2007). In a multicentre US study of thrice-weekly bitemporal ECT (*n*=253), a 30% decrease in symptoms after six treatments was found to predict final remission (Fig. 4.1) (Husain *et al*, 2004). The majority of these remissions occurred before the ninth treatment. However, 40% of patients who had not responded after six treatments went on to remission. So no definitive recommendation can be given to stop treatment in those who have failed to respond after six treatments. However, if after six satisfactory treatments there has been no clinical response whatsoever, clinicians may wish to reassess the need for ECT and consult with the patient, based on the decreased predicted response and remission rate for subsequent treatment (e.g. 40% *v.* 70% in the above study). If patients are failing to respond or are responding slowly, ECT teams should liaise further with referring clinicians regarding ECT dosing, medications, side-effects and any other reasons for modifying or stopping the treatment course. A patient who has had no response within 12 treatments is unlikely to have a sustained response to ECT.

How often should ECT be prescribed?

In addition to electrode placement, stimulus intensity and waveform (discussed later), the effectiveness of ECT is influenced by frequency of administration. Electroconvulsive therapy is usually given twice weekly in the UK, Ireland and several other European countries, whereas in the USA, thrice-weekly treatment is common practice. The UK ECT Review Group (2003) meta-analysis failed to find statistically significant differences between twice- and thrice-weekly bitemporal ECT with a fixed number of

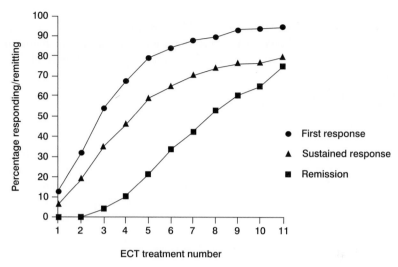

Fig. 4.1 Cumulative response and remission rates to bilateral ECT. First response is defined in this study as the first time a 50% decrease in Hamilton Rating Scale for Depression (HRSD) score was measured. Sustained response is the first time a 50% decrease in score was measured, which was sustained to end of treatment. Remission is defined as two consecutive HRSD scores <10. Adapted from Husain *et al* (2004).

treatments (Kellner *et al*, 1992; Gangadhar *et al*, 1993; Lerer *et al*, 1995; Janakiramaiah *et al*, 1998; Shapira *et al*, 1998; Vieweg, 1998; UK ECT Review Group, 2003). There were trends showing thrice-weekly ECT to be no more effective than twice-weekly treatment but to have more cognitive side-effects. The clinical and cognitive outcomes of clinical trials in which patients are treated thrice weekly may not be fully applicable to routine UK practice.

One open study suggested that unilateral ECT delivered more often could be as effective as bitemporal ECT given twice weekly (Stromgren, 1975; Stromgren *et al*, 1976). However, more recent studies found no advantage for more intensive scheduling (McAllister *et al*, 1987).

Some clinicians may wish to decrease the frequency of ECT in order to avoid the anterograde memory difficulties and disorientation that are more common in their elderly patients. However, this risks decreasing the efficacy of ECT. There is a much more robust evidence base for the effects of stimulus intensity and electrode placement on both cognitive side-effects and clinical efficacy than there is for the effects of frequency of treatment (Semkovska *et al*, 2011). For patients with marked cognitive side-effects due to twice-weekly bitemporal ECT, it is worth considering changing to unilateral treatment or reducing the above-threshold dose to minimise such side-effects while continuing to give effective twice-weekly treatments. Electroconvulsive therapy administered once a week has been shown to be less therapeutically effective and unless there are very marked cognitive side-effects it is probably best avoided (Janakiramaiah *et al*, 1998). Weekly treatment could however be considered for continuation or maintenance ECT as a step-down procedure to longer inter-treatment intervals.

Electrode placement

Bilateral electrode placement

Commonly used electrode placements are shown in Fig. 4.2. Bitemporal placement is the standard form of bilateral ECT and indeed for practical purposes is synonymous with it (Fig. 4.2(a)). The electrodes are placed on both temples 4 cm perpendicularly above the midpoint of a line joining the lateral canthus of the eye and the tragus of the ear. This has been the position in all major research studies on bitemporal ECT. Decisions made on the basis of that evidence will only be valid if electrode placement is similar for the patient.

A less commonly used bilateral placement is bifrontal ECT (Fig. 4.2(b)), which was developed in the early 1970s (Abrams & Taylor, 1973). It was believed to be potentially less cognitively impairing than bitemporal ECT because the electrodes were placed further from the temporal lobes, but also believed to be more effective than low-dose unilateral ECT. In a recent meta-analysis, no advantage for bifrontal ECT regarding antidepressant effect was found but it may have some modest short-term benefits for specific memory domains; however, these need to be better characterised before bifrontal ECT can be recommended for routine clinical use (Dunne & McLoughlin, 2012) .

Unilateral electrode placement

In unilateral ECT, one (flat) electrode is placed at the right temple, using the same position as in bitemporal ECT, and one (usually concave) electrode over the parietal lobe, just to the right of the vertex (Fig. 4.2(c)). The placement of the 'parietal or 'non-temporal' electrode in unilateral ECT varied widely up to 1975 (McAndrew *et al*, 1967; d'Elia, 1970; d'Elia & Widepalm, 1974). Thereafter, most researchers used the d'Elia (1970) placement shown in Fig. 4.2(c). The exact position of the parietal electrode is not vital, although some have noticed increased nausea and ataxia after treatment with more occipital placement (Cannicott, 1962; Martin *et al*, 1965; Impastato & Karliner, 1966). There should be enough distance between the electrodes such that shunting is minimised and therefore seizure threshold adequately assessed. Too short a distance will result in the passage of more charge through skin and subcutaneous tissues and decreased impedance, which may even prevent some machines from discharging. Shunting may be the source of very early accounts of 'missed' seizures with unilateral ECT. Practitioners often worry about the difficulty

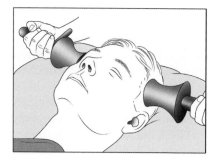

(a) Bitemporal placement was the original electrode placement in electroconvulsive therapy (ECT). It involves placing the electrodes 4 cm above the midpoint of a line joining the outer canthus and the tragus of the ear. Good contact between skin and electrode is important.

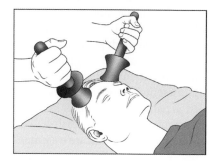

(b) Bifrontal electrodes are placed 5 cm above the lateral angle of each orbit on a line parallel to the sagittal plane (Letemendia *et al*, 1993).

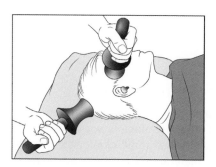

(c) d'Elia placement for right unilateral ECT was developed in 1970 and maximises the inter-electrode distance to prevent shunting. Application of a little electrode gel to the hair and scalp provides contact for the posterior electrode. It is placed 3 cm lateral to the vertex, on the right-hand side. The anterior electrode is placed 4 cm above the midpoint of a line joining the outer canthus and the tragus of the ear.

Fig. 4.2 Electrode placements during ECT: (a) bitemporal, (b) bifrontal and (c) unilateral electrode placements.

with electrical contact through hair during administration of unilateral ECT but this can usually be overcome by ensuring the hair and scalp are clean, using small quantities of a conducting gel and maintaining firm contact. Supportive pressure to the left side of the head can act as a useful counterbalance to ensure good electrode contact. Alternatively, some anaesthetists will care for the patient in the left lateral position, easing access to the correct non-dominant electrode position.

To which side should I apply unilateral ECT?

The very first studies on unilateral ECT placed electrodes on the 'non-dominant' (usually the right) side as researchers presumed this would reduce recovery time and acute memory side-effects. Indeed, concerns were also raised about the possibility of cataracts caused by the electrical charge, although these were never substantiated (Lancaster *et al*, 1958). Left unilateral ECT does cause greater acute effects on verbal function in strongly right-handed patients than right unilateral ECT, but longer-term outcomes are lacking (Fleminger *et al*, 1970). More than 90% of the population are right-handed. The incidence of right-sided language dominance is only 3–4% in right-handed people, but rises to 15% in the ambidextrous and 27% in left-handed people (Geschwind & Levitsky, 1968; Knecht *et al*, 2000). Therefore, routine clinical assessment of handedness is unlikely to usefully inform treatment decisions. Most unilateral ECT is given to the right-hand side. Even in strongly left-handed patients, this will usually be the language non-dominant side. If immediate post-ictal dysphasia emerges, then the treating team is justified in using left-unilateral ECT, not because this dysphasia may be immediately impairing (most such described dysphasia has passed within an hour) but because it may indicate treatment on the language-dominant side and therefore theoretically greater risk of impairment of verbal memory (Pratt *et al*, 1971; Warrington & Pratt, 1973; Annett *et al*, 1974; Squire & Slater, 1978; Svoboda *et al*, 2006).

Stimulus dosing

Is a seizure necessary for ECT to be effective?

The aim of the clinician administering ECT is to induce a therapeutic seizure. It is now clear, however, that a seizure alone is not sufficient for antidepressant effect. For example, generalised tonic–clonic seizures can be reliably induced by low-dose right unilateral ECT but these are no more effective than sham treatment for depression (Lambourn & Gill, 1978; Sackeim *et al*, 1987*a*, 1991). The aim of contemporary 'modified' ECT, using an anaesthetic agent and muscle relaxant, is to reduce the intensity of the motor seizure to avoid physical injury and minimise discomfort. In modified ECT, some patients will have no visible motor seizure or minimal movements. Therefore, seizure adequacy cannot be judged solely by the presence, absence or duration of the motor seizure. Additionally, the EEG seizure duration has been found not to correlate with motor seizure duration in most studies (see p. 36). We do, however, know that to have an antidepressant effect, the applied electrical stimulus dose needs to be an adequate multiple of the seizure threshold.

The seizure threshold is defined as the minimum charge required to induce unequivocal ictal EEG activity (i.e. polyspike followed by 3 Hz spike-and-wave activity). By convention this should last at least 15 s so that a generalised seizure can be clearly documented (see Chapter 6). Seizure threshold can vary up to 40-fold between individuals (Sackeim *et al*, 1987*b*) but for the majority treated with bitemporal ECT it is between 50 and 250 mC, with a three- to fivefold variation between patients. Before the routine use of EEG monitoring, a generalised tonic–clonic motor seizure of 15 s was deemed satisfactory. For bitemporal ECT, a stimulus dose of 1.5 times seizure threshold is therapeutic. In unilateral ECT, the evidence is less clear (see p. 37), but the charge must be several multiples of the seizure threshold to have an adequate antidepressant effect. One-and-a-half times seizure threshold dosing in bilateral ECT is chosen because it is known to be therapeutic. It avoids the missed seizures possible when at-threshold dosing is used in patients whose threshold rises across treatment. Additionally, higher doses (i.e. more than 1.5 times seizure threshold) have not been demonstrated to have significantly greater efficacy. Although they may possibly produce a quicker response, higher doses have been shown to be associated with more cognitive difficulties (Sackeim *et al*, 1993; UK ECT Review Group, 2003).

Electroconvulsive therapy seizure duration provides, at best, a moderate predictor of the efficacy of treatment (Kimball *et al*, 2009). For example, the anaesthetic agent propofol can shorten average seizure duration without diminishing therapeutic efficacy (Simpson *et al*, 1988; Mitchell *et al*, 1991; Fear *et al*, 1994; Caliyurt *et al*, 2004; Hooten & Rasmussen, 2008; Bauer *et al*, 2009; Eranti *et al*, 2009; Eser *et al*, 2009). Seizure duration and therapeutic efficacy are therefore at least partly dissociable. The requirement for an adequate seizure on EEG monitoring reflects the need to avoid missed seizures in those for whom stimulation is at or just above threshold.

How do I establish the seizure threshold?

The seizure threshold is higher with bitemporal than unilateral ECT and often rises during a course of ECT, while seizure duration may fall in parallel. However, it is clear that seizure duration itself does not correlate well with seizure threshold or antidepressant efficacy of ECT, except that subconvulsive stimulation appears to be ineffective (Kales *et al*, 1997; Chung, 2002). The seizure threshold is established by attempting to induce a seizure, first with the lowest dose, then successively higher doses of charge in a procedure called 'stimulus titration'. An example of a stimulus titration protocol is shown in Table 4.1. For the vast majority of patients it is possible to establish the seizure threshold in the first treatment session.

Previous ECT records may help guide treatment and several clinical factors are associated with increased seizure threshold: older age, male gender, anticonvulsant medications (including benzodiazepines), bitemporal electrode placement, pulse width and recent treatment with ECT. These should be taken into account when deciding on the initial stimulus dose. For example, in the protocol in Table 4.1 the initial stimulus level for a young adult female undergoing unilateral ECT would be at the

Table 4.1 Example of an ECT stimulus dosing protocol

Level	Threshold dose (seizure threshold), mC	Treatment dose, mC		
		Bitemporal (1.5 times seizure threshold)	Unilateral (4 times seizure threshold)	Unilateral (6 times seizure threshold)
1	25	50	100	150
2	50	75	200	300
3	75	125	300	450
4	100	150	400	600
5	150	225	600	900
6	250	375	1000	Max.
7	350	550	Max.	Max.
8	500	750	Max.	Max.
9	750	1000	Max.	Max.

Max., maximum dose of the ECT device.

The first dosing column (seizure threshold dose) is used incrementally to establish the seizure threshold in the first session. In subsequent sessions the treatment dose is a multiple of the established seizure threshold, for example 1.5 times seizure threshold for bitemporal electroconvulsive therapy (ECT), and, in this example, 4 times seizure threshold or 6 times seizure threshold for unilateral ECT.

lowest level, i.e. 25 mC. However, if she was over 65 years old, taking regular benzodiazepines and was about to start instead with bitemporal ECT, the initial stimulus could be increased by three levels up to 100 mC (see case vignette in Box 4.1).

When stimulated at a subthreshold dose, the patient may grimace due to stimulation of facial muscles (a one-sided grimace often occurs during unilateral ECT) and there may be vagal stimulation causing bradycardia or brief asystole, but there will be no generalised seizure on the EEG or visible motor seizure. However, seizures may develop gradually over 10–15 s, slowly generalising to physical movements. Therefore, it is advisable to wait at least 20 s before re-stimulating to ensure that no seizure is developing. Re-stimulation should then proceed at a moderately higher dose, for example the next threshold dose level in the protocol in Table 4.1.

There should be a maximum of two re-stimulations per titration session in order to adequately safeguard patient oxygenation and ensure that the seizure will be modified. Anaesthetists should be made aware at the start of the treatment that the patient may require re-stimulation and may take appropriate precautions, including extra anaesthesia if they feel it is warranted. If a third stimulation is indicated, then one threshold dose level could be skipped in the protocol (Table 4.1). Each subconvulsive stimulation raises the seizure threshold, so if re-stimulation has been necessary, it may be overestimated. This should be borne in mind when estimating seizure threshold. If this third stimulation results in an adequate

---

Box 4.1 Case vignette

A 72-year-old man is referred for ECT with a 3-month history of treatment-resistant severe depression with suicidal ideation. He is on diazepam (5 mg four times daily), venlafaxine (modified release 225 mg once daily) and mirtazapine (45 mg at night). According to protocol (Table 4.1), his dose titration is started at 100 mC. He fails to have a seizure at this dose, so the dose is increased and he is re-stimulated with 150 mC after 30 s. Again, only diffuse cortical activity similar to baseline is shown on EEG with no unequivocal ictal activity and no physical movement. The anaesthetist is satisfied with oxygenation and muscle tone throughout the procedure. The patient is re-stimulated with 350 mC and he has a successful 43 s generalised motor seizure with classical tonic and clonic phases and unequivocal 3–5 Hz spike–wave activity on EEG. He recovers uneventfully.

The administering physician notes in the treatment record that stimulation should be tried at 250 mC next session as (a) the patient has been re-stimulated and his seizure threshold may thus have been elevated, and (b) the seizure threshold may well lie between 150 and 350 mC. However, at the second session, 250 mC fails to elicit a seizure, so the man is treated with 550 mC (1.5 times the initially established seizure threshold of 350 mC) at re-stimulation with good effect. It is recommended that for the third session, the initial treatment dose should be 550 mC.

---

seizure, the patient should be stimulated with the 'skipped' threshold dose level at the next session to determine whether this might be the real seizure threshold and then treated with suprathreshold ECT thereafter. If after three stimulations a seizure is not elicited, then stimulation should resume at the next daily session with the highest dose used at the last, unsuccessful session.

Why should I measure the seizure threshold?

It is necessary to induce a seizure for ECT to have an antidepressant benefit. Therefore, it is necessary, at a minimum, to ensure that stimulation is suprathreshold so that it reliably induces a seizure. However, the cognitive side-effects of ECT are also proportional to how much the stimulus dose is above threshold (McCall *et al*, 2000). Fixed high dosing has the drawback that many patients will be exposed to significantly more cognitive risk, whether treated with unilateral or bitemporal ECT. The majority of clinicians now favour at least some attempt to estimate seizure threshold and tailor the treatment to the individual patient. Two methods used are direct measurement through titration as described earlier and estimation based on age (i.e. an 'age method').

Differences in age predict differences in seizure threshold between patients, with older patients on average having higher seizure thresholds than younger patients. However, age accounts for only a small proportion of the variability in seizure threshold between individual patients. Repeatedly, studies have found that use of age-based methods for dosing can result in either over- or underdosing (Colenda & McCall, 1996; Heikman *et al*, 1999; Girish *et al*, 2000; Tiller & Ingram, 2006). Moreover, studies that measure the accuracy of age to estimate seizure threshold often do not take into account confounding factors between patients – such as medication, anaesthetic dose and sleep (Gilabert *et al*, 2004) – as well as variations between clinics' anaesthetic practices, ECT machines and prescribing practices. This suggests that age-based dosing may be even more inaccurate in routine practice than estimated in research studies. Direct measurement of the seizure threshold offers the patient the best balance between clinical effectiveness and risk of side-effects and gives us more confidence in the information we give to patients.

For patients in whom a rapid response is required, necessitating a break in treatment routine, the treating team could consider bitemporal treatment thrice weekly or at a higher dose above threshold (e.g. 2.5 times seizure threshold). However, we need to bear in mind that the evidence for a faster response is slim and that bitemporal ECT at 2.5 times seizure threshold is likely to be associated with more cognitive side-effects than at 1.5 times seizure threshold.

What if the seizure threshold is too high?

Most devices in use in the UK and Ireland allow up to 1000 mC stimulation, whereas in the USA the Food and Drug Administration has restricted devices used in routine clinical practice to about 500 mC. Fortunately, the vast majority of patients have seizure thresholds well below this. However, adequately suprathreshold stimulation may be difficult in older patients, for high-dose (e.g. 6 times seizure threshold) unilateral ECT, or those on medications with an anticonvulsive effect (see Chapter 5). The practice of 'holding' such medication doses before each treatment may not be rational if they have a long half-life. For example, diazepam has a half life of 20–50 h, perhaps even longer once active metabolites are considered. So omitting a night-time dose before ECT may result in patient distress and possibly insomnia before their treatment. However, reducing the dose prior to the start of a course of ECT may make a real difference to the threshold and prevent changes in seizure threshold across a treatment course as the need for anxiolytic medication diminishes while the patient improves.

If after modification of the medication regime there is still difficulty giving adequately suprathreshold stimulation, then a number of procedures to lower the seizure threshold may be considered. Hyperventilation to reduce the circulating carbon dioxide/bicarbonate concentration can lower the seizure threshold and is best discussed with the anaesthetist beforehand. Some groups advocate the use of caffeine before treatment (Shapira *et al*, 1987). Methylxanthines such as caffeine antagonise adenosine receptors, reducing the seizure threshold and prolonging seizures. More serious consideration must be given before the use of theophylline or aminophylline, especially in those with heart disease, where they are more likely to cause cardiac complications and both of which have been associated with prolonged seizures in selected patients (Swartz & Lewis, 1991; Rasmussen & Zorumski, 1993; Schak *et al*, 2008).

What if the seizure is too long?

When a prolonged (i.e. >90s) seizure occurs it should be terminated according to a standard protocol, usually involving either extra doses of the initial anaesthetic or intravenous benzodiazepine medication. This occurs in only 1–2% of treatments (Benbow *et al*, 2003; Whittaker *et al*, 2007). Practitioners should be aware that this is more likely in younger, female patients on high doses of medications shown to lower the seizure threshold (e.g. chlorpromazine, venlafaxine or clozapine). If a prolonged seizure occurs during the ECT treatment course which requires medical intervention to terminate it, then a lower dose (Table 4.1) should be used at the next session or the seizure threshold measured again.

What if the seizure threshold is very low?

When a seizure of any duration occurs during the administration of an anaesthetic agent alone, no further stimulus should be given. The seizure should be terminated as quickly as possible. This is an adverse drug reaction and discussion should occur about using alternative anaesthetic agents (see Chapter 3) and investigating possible causes of such a low seizure threshold.

What if the seizure becomes too short during the ECT course?

After seizures demonstrating 15s or longer of typical 3–5Hz spike–wave complexes, patients should not be re-stimulated. If a short seizure of 5–10s is elicited and there has as yet been no clinical response (either because it is early in the treatment course or the patient has failed to respond because of short seizures), then the patient should be re-stimulated at the next higher level in the treatment dosing protocol (Table 4.1) to ensure an adequate treatment. For patients who have shorter seizures later in the treatment course but are having continuing satisfactory clinical improvement, then re-stimulation is not necessary but the treatment dose could be increased by one level at the next treatment session.

Why is the seizure duration falling?

Seizure threshold rises across the ECT treatment course (Chanpattana *et al*, 2000). However, the seizure threshold may only tenuously relate to seizure duration (Fink *et al*, 2008). There is a suggestion by some groups that at low doses above seizure threshold there is a linear relationship between dose and duration, but that this breaks down at higher doses, producing shorter seizures. Indeed, some groups have found a negative relationship between dose and duration of seizure; this is frequently observed at higher doses (Krystal *et al*, 1993). However, in order to give adequate suprathreshold dosages, one must 'stay ahead' of a rising seizure threshold. Therefore, we recommend increasing the initial treatment dose by one level when seizure duration begins to shorten by >20% relative to the second session. If there is an inadequate seizure at the next session, then re-stimulate at the next treatment dose. If successful, use this new dose level as the initial treatment dose at the following session.

How do bitemporal and unilateral ECT compare?

Unilateral ECT induces seizures at lower doses than bitemporal ECT. The precise reason for this is not known but may be due to the increased density of administered charge in cortical areas owing to a shorter traversed path (McCall *et al*, 1993). Therefore, if switching from one version of ECT to the other, it will be necessary to re-establish the seizure threshold for the new electrode placement.

Although bitemporal ECT has been shown to be efficacious at doses minimally above seizure threshold, the efficacy of unilateral ECT depends on using higher doses (Sackeim *et al*, 1987*a*, 1993). Unilateral ECT has been reported to be as efficacious as bitemporal ECT at fixed moderate doses (378 mC) (Abrams *et al*, 1991) and higher doses (McCall *et al*, 2002; Tew *et al*, 2002; Stoppe *et al*, 2006; Kellner *et al*, 2010).

The rationale for using right unilateral ECT is that it causes fewer cognitive side-effects. However, at moderate multiples of the seizure threshold (2–4 times seizure threshold) it appears to be less powerful than bitemporal ECT at 2.5 times seizure threshold (Sackeim *et al*, 1993). At higher doses (6–8 times seizure threshold), this cognitive advantage may be lost, with equivalent antidepressant power coming at the expense of equivalent cognitive side-effects when used thrice weekly (McCall *et al*, 2000; Tew *et al*, 2002; Kellner *et al*, 2010). However, practitioners should be aware that the optimal stimulus dose for unilateral ECT has not yet been established (Semkovska *et al*, 2011).

Unilateral ECT at 4 times seizure threshold given twice weekly may therefore be considered in patients who have suffered severely from cognitive side-effects during previous ECT courses. It may be also considered in those with pre-existing mild cognitive impairment or because of informed patient choice. Patients who are responding to bitemporal ECT at 1.5 times seizure threshold but who have clinically significant cognitive side-effects may be usefully switched to 4 times seizure threshold unilateral treatment at the expense of possibly requiring more treatments during their ECT course. If there is little or no response to 4 times seizure threshold unilateral ECT after six sessions, then the charge could be increased to 6 times seizure threshold, although this may be more likely to be associated with cognitive side-effects.

What about bifrontal ECT?

The majority of studies to date have been small (Bailine *et al*, 2000; Ranjkesh *et al*, 2005; Barekatain *et al*, 2008; Sienaert *et al*, 2009, 2010). However, the most recent and largest study has found no difference in clinical response or cognitive side-effects between thrice weekly 6 times seizure threshold right unilateral treatment, 1.5 times seizure threshold bitemporal treatment and 1.5 times seizure threshold bifrontal treatment (Kellner *et al*, 2010).

What does changing the pulse width do?

One of the main refinements in ECT practice over the past 70 years is the alteration of the stimulus waveform from sine wave to square wave and the shortening of the pulse width (the actual time during which energy is transmitted) as used in contemporary brief pulse ECT (i.e. 0.5–1.0 ms). This is associated with fewer cognitive difficulties after ECT (Sackeim *et al*, 2007).

One preliminary randomised controlled study has reported that 'ultra-brief' pulse ECT, in which the pulse width has been narrowed even more (i.e. <0.5 ms), can further reduce cognitive side-effects (Sackeim *et al*, 2008). However, other studies have found decreased efficacy, possibly interacting with electrode placement (McCormick *et al*, 2009). Remission rates of such studies are generally low, with most reporting response rates instead. Studies are generally limited by their methodology, but unrandomised studies (Loo *et al*, 2008) and restrospective analyses (Niemantsverdriet *et al*, 2011) have all found results in the same direction. Much of the research is confounded by the tendency to change two factors – electrode placement and pulse width – together. There is resultant lack of clarity regarding the possible interaction of electrode placement and stimulus parameters. Roepke *et al* (2011) reported that differences in frequency of the ultra-brief stimulus had no effect. In summary, there is currently not enough evidence of maintained efficacy with ultra-brief pulse width ECT to recommend its routine use. However, it represents a possibility for refined treatment in the future.

Key points

- The majority of ECT research to date has been on depression rather than other disorders such as mania and schizophrenia, but the general principles of ECT practice probably apply.
- Electroconvulsive therapy should be normally administered twice weekly except where continuation or maintenance ECT are considered.
- It is not possible to predetermine the number of ECT treatments that will be required. Therefore, prescribing a set number of treatments is not warranted. The number of treatments will be determined by the patient's response, with the ultimate aim of achieving remission.

- Treating teams should be encouraged to consult with patients and liaise with the ECT team about dosage and laterality, balancing the benefits and risks for the individual patient.
- Bitemporal ECT has been used for 80 years and has a robust evidence base. It is recommended as the first-line electrode placement for severely ill patients (e.g. life-threatening catatonia) or when rapid response is required.
- In cases of informed patient preference, patients with underlying cognitive deficits, patients who have previously suffered severe confusion or memory disturbance, or those with a previous good response to unilateral ECT, it is advisable to treat with at least moderate-dose (4 times seizure threshold), if not high-dose (6 times seizure threshold), right unilateral ECT.
- For patients who have severe cognitive difficulties or memory disturbance during their bitemporal ECT, unilateral ECT should be offered as an alternative.
- For patients who fail to respond to moderate- or high-dose unilateral ECT, bitemporal ECT should be offered. This should be considered as a fresh course of ECT and the seizure threshold will need to be re-established.
- There is currently an insufficient evidence base to recommend bifrontal ECT over bitemporal ECT or recommend ultra-brief pulse over brief-pulse ECT.

Research topics

- What is the relationship between doses above threshold, cognitive side-effects and efficacy for unilateral ECT?
- What is the optimum dose above threshold for unilateral ECT?
- What is the relationship between stimulus dose and seizure duration?
- What is the briefest possible pulse width to maintain efficacy in ECT?
- Does ultra-brief pulse ECT reduce cognitive side-effects?
- What are the long-term outcomes following different forms of ECT, regarding electrode placement and stimulus dose?
- What is the role of bifrontal ECT in clinical practice?

References

Abrams, R. & Taylor, M. A. (1973) Anterior bifrontal ECT. A clinical trial. *British Jornal of Psychiatry*, **122**, 587–590.

Abrams, R., Swartz, C. M. & Vedak, C. (1991) Antidepressant effects of high-dose right unilateral electroconvulsive therapy. *Archives of General Psychiatry*, **48**, 746–748.

Annett, M., Hudson, P. T. W. & Turner, A. (1974) Effects of right and left unilateral ECT on naming and visual discrimination analysed in relation to handedness. *British Journal of Psychiatry*, **124**, 260–264.

Bailine, S. H., Rifkin, A. & Kayne, E. (2000) Comparison of bifrontal and bitemporal ECT for major depression. *American Journal of Psychiatry*, **157**, 121–123.

Barekatain, M., Jahangard, L., Haghighi, M., *et al* (2008) Bifrontal versus bitemporal electroconvulsive therapy in severe manic patients. *Journal of ECT*, **24**, 199–202.

Bauer, J., Hageman, I., Dam, H., *et al* (2009) Comparison of propofol and thiopental as anesthetic agents for electroconvulsive therapy: a randomized, blinded comparison of seizure duration, stimulus charge, clinical effect, and cognitive side effects. *Journal of ECT*, **25**, 85–90.

Benbow, S. M., Benbow, J. & Tomenson, B. (2003) Electroconvulsive therapy clinics in the United Kingdom should routinely monitor electroencephalographic seizures. *Journal of ECT*, **19**, 217–220.

Caliyurt, O., Vardar, E., Tuglu, C., *et al* (2004) Effects of propofol on electroconvulsive therapy seizure duration. *Canadian Journal of Psychiatry*, **49**, 707–708.

Cannicott, S. M. (1962) Unilateral electro-convulsive therapy. *Postgraduate Medical Journal*, **38**, 451–459.

Chanpattana, W., Buppanharun, W., Raksakietisak, S., *et al* (2000) Seizure threshold rise during electroconvulsive therapy in schizophrenic patients. *Psychiatry Research*, **96**, 31–40.

Chung, K. F. (2002) Relationships between seizure duration and seizure threshold and stimulus dosage at electroconvulsive therapy: implications for electroconvulsive therapy practice. *Psychiatry and Clinical Neuroscience*, **56**, 521–526.

Colenda, C. C. & McCall, W. V. (1996) A statistical model predicting the seizure threshold for right unilateral ECT in 106 patients. *Convulsive Therapy*, **12**, 3–12.

d'Elia, G. (1970) Unilateral electroconvulsive therapy. *Acta Psychiatrica Scandinavica Supplement*, **215**, 1–98.

d'Elia, G. & Widepalm, K. (1974) Comparison of frontoparietal and temporoparietal unilateral electroconvulsive therapy. *Acta Psychiatrica Scandinavica*, **50**, 225–232.

Dunne, R. A. & McLoughlin, D. M. (2012) Systematic review and meta-analysis of bifrontal electroconvulsive therapy versus bilateral and unilateral electroconvulsive therapy in depression. *World Journal of Biological Psychiatry*, **13**, 248–258.

Eranti, S., Mogg, A., Pluck, G., *et al* (2007) A randomized, controlled trial with 6-month follow-up of repetitive transcranial magnetic stimulation and electroconvulsive therapy for severe depression. *American Journal of Psychiatry*, **164**, 73–81.

Eranti, S. V., Mogg, A. J., Pluck, G. C., *et al* (2009) Methohexitone, propofol and etomidate in electroconvulsive therapy for depression: a naturalistic comparison study. *Journal of Affective Disorders*, **113**, 165–171.

Eser, D., Nothdurfter, C., Schule, C., *et al* (2009) The influence of anaesthetic medication on safety, tolerability and clinical effectiveness of electroconvulsive therapy. *World Journal of Biological Psychiatry*, **11**, 1–10.

Fear, C. F., Littlejohns, C. S., Rouse, E., *et al* (1994) Propofol anaesthesia in electroconvulsive therapy. Reduced seizure duration may not be relevant. *British Journal of Psychiatry*, **165**, 506–509.

Fink, M., Petrides, G., Kellner, C., *et al* (2008) Change in seizure threshold during electroconvulsive therapy. *Journal of ECT*, **24**, 114–116.

Fleminger, J. J., De Horne, D. J. & Nott, P. N. (1970) Unilateral electroconvulsive therapy and cerebral dominance: effect of right- and left-sided electrode placement on verbal memory. *Journal of Neurology and Neurosurgery Psychiatry*, **33**, 408–411.

Gangadhar, B. N., Janakiramaiah, N., Subbakrishna, D. K., *et al* (1993) Twice versus thrice weekly ECT in melancholia: a double-blind prospective comparison. *Journal of Affective Disorders*, **27**, 273–278.

Geschwind, N. & Levitsky, W. (1968) Human brain: left–right asymmetries in temporal speech region. *Science*, **161**, 186–187.

Gilabert, E., Rojo, E. & Vallejo, J. (2004) Augmentation of electroconvulsive therapy seizures with sleep deprivation. *Journal of ECT*, **20**, 242–247.

Girish, K., Mayur, P. M., Saravanan, E. S., *et al* (2000) Seizure threshold estimation by formula method: a prospective study in unilateral ECT. *Journal of ECT*, **16**, 258–262.

Heikman, P., Tuunainen, A. & Kuoppasalmi, K. (1999) Value of the initial stimulus dose in right unilateral and bifrontal electroconvulsive therapy. *Psychological Medicine*, **29**, 1417–1423.

Hooten, W. M. & Rasmussen, K. G. (2008) Effects of general anesthetic agents in adults receiving electroconvulsive therapy: a systematic review. *Journal of ECT*, **24**, 208–223.

Husain, M. M., Rush, A. J., Fink, M., *et al* (2004) Speed of response and remission in major depressive disorder with acute electroconvulsive therapy (ECT): a Consortium for Research in ECT (CORE) report. *Journal of Clinical Psychiatry*, **65**, 485–491.

Impastato, D. J. & Karliner, W. (1966) Control of memory impairment in EST by unilateral stimulation of the non-dominant hemisphere. *Diseases of the Nervous System*, **27**, 183–188.

Janakiramaiah, N., Motreja, S., Gangadhar, B. N., *et al* (1998) Once vs. three times weekly ECT in melancholia: a randomized controlled trial. *Acta Psychiatrica Scandanavica*, **98**, 316–320.

Kales, H., Raz, J., Tandon, R., *et al* (1997) Relationship of seizure duration to antidepressant efficacy in electroconvulsive therapy. *Psychological Medicine*, **27**, 1373–1380.

Kellner, C. H., Monroe Jr, R. R., Pritchett, J., *et al* (1992) Weekly ECT in geriatric depression. *Convulsive Therapy*, **8**, 245–252.

Kellner, C. H., Knapp, R., Husain, M. M., *et al* (2010) Bifrontal, bitemporal and right unilateral electrode placement in ECT: randomised trial. *British Journal of Psychiatry*, **196**, 226–234.

Kimball, J. N., Rosenquist, P. B., Dunn, A., *et al* (2009) Prediction of antidepressant response in both 2.25 null threshold RUL and fixed high dose RUL ECT. *Journal of Affective Disorders*, **112**, 85–91.

Knecht, S., Drager, B., Deppe, M., *et al* (2000) Handedness and hemispheric language dominance in healthy humans. *Brain*, **123** (Pt 12), 2512–2518.

Krystal, A. D., Weiner, R. D., McCall, W. V., *et al* (1993) The effects of ECT stimulus dose and electrode placement on the ictal electroencephalogram – an intraindividual crossover study. *Biological Psychiatry*, **34**, 759–767.

Lambourn, J. & Gill, D. (1978) A controlled comparison of simulated and real ECT. *British Journal of Psychiatry*, **133**, 514–519.

Lancaster, N. P., Steinert, R. R. & Frost, I. (1958) Unilateral electro-convulsive therapy. *Journal of Mental Science*, **104**, 221–227.

Lerer, B., Shapira, B., Calev, A., *et al* (1995) Antidepressant and cognitive effects of twice- versus three-times-weekly ECT. *American Journal of Psychiatry*, **152**, 564–570.

Letemendia, F. J., Delva, N. J., Rodenburg, M., *et al* (1993) Therapeutic advantage of bifrontal electrode placement in ECT. *Psychological Medicine*, **23**, 349–360.

Loo, C. K., Sainsbury, K., Sheehan, P., *et al* (2008) A comparison of RUL ultrabrief pulse (0.3 ms) ECT and standard RUL ECT. *International Journal of Neuropsychopharmacology*, **11**, 883–890.

Martin, W. L., Ford, H. F., McDanald, E. C., *et al* (1965) Clinical evaluation of unilateral EST. *American Journal of Psychiatry*, **121**, 1087–1090.

McAllister, D. A., Perri, M. G. & Jordan, R. C. (1987) Effects of ECT given two vs. three times weekly. *Psychiatry Research*, **21**, 63–69.

McAndrew, J., Berkey, B. & Matthews, C. (1967) The effects of dominant and nondominant unilateral ECT as compared to bilateral ECT. *American Journal of Psychiatry*, **124**, 483–490.

McCall, W. V., Shelp, F. E., Weiner, R. D., *et al* (1993) Convulsive threshold differences in right unilateral and bilateral ECT. *Biological Psychiatry*, **34**, 606–611.

McCall, W. V., Reboussin, D. M., Weiner, R. D., *et al* (2000) Titrated moderately suprathreshold vs fixed high-dose right unilateral electroconvulsive therapy: acute antidepressant and cognitive effects. *Archives of General Psychiatry*, **57**, 438–444.

McCall, W. V., Dunn, A., Rosenquist, P. B., *et al* (2002) Markedly suprathreshold right unilateral ECT versus minimally suprathreshold bilateral ECT: antidepressant and memory effects. *Journal of ECT*, **18**, 126–129.

McCormick, L. M., Brumm, M. C., Benede, A. K., *et al* (2009) Relative ineffectiveness of ultrabrief right unilateral versus bilateral electroconvulsive therapy in depression. *Journal of ECT*, **25**, 238–242.

Mitchell, P., Torda, T., Hickie, I., *et al* (1991) Propofol as an anaesthetic agent for ECT: effect on outcome and length of course. *Australian and New Zealand Journal of Psychiatry*, **25**, 255–261.

Niemantsverdriet, L., Birkenhager T. K. & van den Broek W. W. (2011) The efficacy of ultrabrief-pulse (0.25 millisecond) versus brief-pulse (0.50 millisecond) bilateral electroconvulsive therapy in major depression. *Journal of ECT*, **27**, 55–58.

Pratt, R. T. C., Warrington, E. K. & Halliday, A. M. (1971) Unilateral ECT as a test for cerebral dominance, with a strategy for treating left-handers. *British Journal of Psychiatry*, **119**, 79–83.

Ranjkesh, F., Barekatain, M. & Akuchakian, S. (2005) Bifrontal versus right unilateral and bitemporal electroconvulsive therapy in major depressive disorder. *Journal of ECT*, **21**, 207–210.

Rasmussen, K. G. & Zorumski, C. F. (1993) Electroconvulsive therapy in patients taking theophylline. *Journal of Clinical Psychiatry*, **54**, 427–431.

Roepke, S., Luborzewski, A., Schindler, F., *et al* (2011) Stimulus pulse-frequency-dependent efficacy and cognitive adverse effects of ultrabrief-pulse electroconvulsive therapy in patients with major depression. *Journal of ECT*, **27**, 109–113.

Sackeim, H. A., Decina, P., Kanzler, M., *et al* (1987*a*) Effects of electrode placement on the efficacy of titrated, low-dose ECT. *American Journal of Psychiatry*, **144**, 1449–1455.

Sackeim, H. A., Decina, P., Portnoy, S., *et al* (1987*b*) Studies of dosage, seizure threshold, and seizure duration in ECT. *Biological Psychiatry*, **22**, 249–268.

Sackeim, H. A., Devanand, D. P. & Prudic, J. (1991) Stimulus intensity, seizure threshold, and seizure duration: impact on the efficacy and safety of electroconvulsive therapy. *Psychiatric Clinics of North America*, **14**, 803–843.

Sackeim, H. A., Prudic, J., Devanand, D. P., *et al* (1993) Effects of stimulus intensity and electrode placement on the efficacy and cognitive effects of electroconvulsive therapy. *New England Journal of Medicine*, **328**, 839–846.

Sackeim, H. A., Prudic, J., Fuller, R., *et al* (2007) The cognitive effects of electroconvulsive therapy in community settings. *Neuropsychopharmacology*, **32**, 244–254.

Sackeim, H. A., Prudic, J., Nobler, M. S., *et al* (2008) Effects of pulse width and electrode placement on the efficacy and cognitive effects of electroconvulsive therapy. *Brain Stimulation*, **1**, 71–83.

Schak, K. M., Mueller, P. S., Barnes, R. D., *et al* (2008) The safety of ECT in patients with chronic obstructive pulmonary disease. *Psychosomatics*, **49**, 208–211.

Semkovska, M., Keane, D., Babalola, O., *et al* (2011) Unilateral brief-pulse electroconvulsive therapy and cognition: effects of electrode placement, stimulus dosage and time. *Journal of Psychiatric Research*, **45**, 770–780.

Shapira, B., Lerer, B., Gilboa, D., *et al* (1987) Facilitation of ECT by caffeine pretreatment. *American Journal of Psychiatry*, **144**, 1199–1202.

Shapira, B., Tubi, N., Drexler, H., *et al* (1998) Cost and benefit in the choice of ECT schedule. Twice versus three times weekly ECT. *British Journal of Psychiatry*, **172**, 44–48.

Sienaert, P., Vansteelandt, K., Demyttenaere, K., *et al* (2009) Randomized comparison of ultra-brief bifrontal and unilateral electroconvulsive therapy for major depression: clinical efficacy. *Journal of Affective Disorders*, **116**, 106–112.

Sienaert, P., Vansteelandt, K., Demyttenaere, K., *et al* (2010) Randomized comparison of ultra-brief bifrontal and unilateral electroconvulsive therapy for major depression: cognitive side-effects. *Journal of Affective Disorders*, **122**, 60–67.

Simpson, K. H., Halsall, P. J., Carr, C. M., *et al* (1988) Propofol reduces seizure duration in patients having anaesthesia for electroconvulsive therapy. *British Journal of Anaesthesia*, **61**, 343–344.

Squire, S. R. & Slater, P. C. (1978) Bilateral and unilateral ECT: effects on verbal and nonverbal memory. *American Journal of Psychiatry*, **135**, 1316–1320.

Stoppe, A., Louza, M., Rosa, M., *et al* (2006) Fixed high-dose electroconvulsive therapy in the elderly with depression: a double-blind, randomized comparison of efficacy and tolerability between unilateral and bilateral electrode placement. *Journal of ECT*, **22**, 92–99.

Stromgren, L. S. (1975) Therapeutic results in brief-interval unilateral ECT. *Acta Psychiatrica Scandinavica*, **52**, 246–255.

Stromgren, L. S., Christensen, A. L. & Fromholt, P. (1976) The effects of unilateral brief-interval ECT on memory. *Acta Psychiatrica Scandinavica*, **54**, 336–346.

Svoboda, E., McKinnon, M. C. & Levine, B. (2006) The functional neuroanatomy of autobiographical memory: a meta-analysis. *Neuropsychologia*, **44**, 2189–2208.

Swartz, C. M. & Lewis, R. K. (1991) Theophylline reversal of electroconvulsive therapy (ECT) seizure inhibition. *Psychosomatics*, **32**, 47–51.

Tew Jr, J. D., Mulsant, B. H., Haskett, R. F., *et al* (2002) A randomized comparison of high-charge right unilateral electroconvulsive therapy and bilateral electroconvulsive therapy in older depressed patients who failed to respond to 5 to 8 moderate-charge right unilateral treatments. *Journal of Clinical Psychiatry*, **63**, 1102–1105.

Tiller, J. W. & Ingram, N. (2006) Seizure threshold determination for electroconvulsive therapy: stimulus dose titration versus age-based estimations. *Australian and New Zealand Journal of Psychiatry*, **40**, 188–192.

UK ECT Review Group (2003) Efficacy and safety of electroconvulsive therapy in depressive disorders: a systematic review and meta-analysis. *Lancet*, **361**, 799–808.

Vieweg, R. S. C. (1998) A trial to determine any difference between two and three times a week ECT in the rate of recovery from depression. *Journal of Mental Health*, **7**, 403–409.

Warrington, E. K. & Pratt, R. T. (1973) Language laterality in left-handers assessed by unilateral ECT. *Neuropsychologia*, **11**, 423–428.

Whittaker, R., Scott, A. & Gardner, M. (2007) The prevalence of prolonged cerebral seizures at the first treatment in a course of electroconvulsive therapy. *Journal of ECT*, **23**, 11–13.

CHAPTER 5

Psychotropic drug treatment during and after ECT

Michael Dixon and Angelica Santiago

This chapter reviews the evidence for the use of psychotropic medicines during and after ECT. There is limited research into the effects of psychotropic medication on ECT. Most patients will be taking medication during a course of ECT which may alter the length of seizure or the seizure threshold. The information in this chapter should be used in conjunction with other sources to make sure the most up-to-date information is followed.

Antipsychotics

The majority of papers in the literature on the use of antipsychotics with ECT involve typical antipsychotics. There have been some studies using atypical antipsychotics including clozapine, olanzapine and risperidone. One systematic review appraised 42 papers including 1371 patients. There were eight double-blind studies involved (Braga & Petrides, 2005). The typical antipsychotics studied were chlorpromazine, haloperidol, trifluoperazine, perphenazine, loxapine, flupentixol, fluphenazine and thiothixene. Most of the reports describe the combination of antipsychotic and ECT as safe or do not mention adverse effects of this combination. Clozapine can cause EEG abnormalities and can reduce the seizure threshold in a dose-dependent manner (Electronic Medicines Compendium, 2010). However, there are reports of clozapine being used successfully in combination with ECT without any serious problems (Braga & Petrides, 2005).

There is a case report of olanzapine being used in combination with duloxetine in a patient receiving ECT without any problems (Hanratta & Malek-Ahmadi, 2006).

There have been case reports of aripiprazole being used in combination with other psychotropic drugs (venlafaxine, levomepromazine, quetiapine, haloperidol and clozapine) in patients receiving ECT with minimal adverse effects (Masdrakis *et al*, 2008*a*; Lopez-Garcia *et al*, 2009).

A review of 11 Indian studies (Painuly & Chakrabarti, 2006) on the use of antipsychotics (chlorpromazine, haloperidol or trifluoperazine) with ECT reported few side-effects, which were minor and/or transient.

Northdurfter *et al* (2006) performed a retrospective study on the effect of antipsychotics on ECT. Of 5482 ECT treatments involving 455 patients, 452 ECT treatments used concomitant antipsychotics. Patients received unilateral or bilateral ECT and a variety of anaesthetic agents (thiopental, propofol, methohexital and etomidate). Suxamethonium, pyridostigmine and atracurium were used as muscle relaxants. Overall, 37% of ECT treatments were carried out with atypical antipsychotics, 17% with high-potency typical antipsychotics, 8% with medium-potency typicals and 37% with low-potency typicals. There were significant differences in seizure duration measured using EEG and electromyography. Use of low-potency antipsychotics was associated with significantly longer EEG seizures compared with no antipsychotic medication. Patients taking atypical antipsychotics experienced shorter electromyography seizures than those receiving high-potency antipsychotics. Taking antipsychotic medication at the time of ECT caused no differences in terms of memory impairment and cardiovascular side-effects. There was a trend towards high-potency typical antipsychotics causing cardiac arrhythmias during ECT.

Clozapine and general anaesthesia

The Clozaril Patient Monitoring Service (2010) recommends caution when people receiving clozapine have general anaesthetic. They recommend that clozapine is withheld for 12 h before surgery and that the patient has their next dose after surgery at the usual time if physically able.

Patients taking clozapine may require bigger doses of noradrenaline and may experience paradoxical hypotension after the administration of adrenaline.

Drug interactions to consider

- Antipsychotics can potentiate the effects of central nervous system (CNS) depressants (Naguib & Koorn, 2002).
- Caffeine can inhibit the metabolism of clozapine causing an increase in clozapine levels. This should be taken into account if caffeine is used during ECT (Bazire, 2009).
- Lower doses of etomidate may be required when using antipsychotics (MedicinesComplete, 2013).
- Chlorpromazine levels are reduced by phenobarbital and barbiturate levels can be reduced by phenothiazines (MedicinesComplete, 2013).

Key points

- Antipsychotics may have an effect on ECT; there is conflicting evidence.
- Clozapine and zotepine can reduce the seizure threshold in a dose-dependent manner (Bazire, 2009).
- Beware of interactions of antipsychotics with agents used during ECT (e.g. caffeine and clozapine).

Mood stabilisers

Electroconvulsive therapy itself may decrease seizure duration and increase seizure threshold as it exerts various anticonvulsant properties. If an anti-epileptic medicine is being used for epilepsy, then the medication should be continued during the course of ECT and the anaesthetist informed about the patient's condition (Sienaert & Peuskens, 2007).

Lithium

Lithium may increase the incidence of adverse effects from ECT, such as memory loss, neurological abnormalities and prolonged seizures (Sartorius *et al*, 2005). It has been reported that time to recovery after ECT is delayed by lithium, with the delay in recovery correlated with the serum lithium level (Thirthalli *et al*, 2011). It has been suggested that lithium should be withheld for 48h prior to ECT to decrease the risk of neurotoxicity. If lithium is used during ECT, the level should be closely monitored; it is prudent to keep the serum level at the lower end of the therapeutic range. There are reports of patients receiving the combination of lithium and ECT without any problems (Dolenc & Rasmussen, 2005; Thirthalli *et al*, 2011). Suddenly stopping lithium may increase the risk of precipitating mood elevation in patients with bipolar disorder.

It has been suggested that lithium prophylaxis needs to be continued for at least 2 years for the benefit of prophylaxis to outweigh the risk of relapse associated with discontinuation (Goodwin, 2003).

Drug interactions to consider (Naguib & Koorn, 2002)

- The pressor effects of noradrenaline are slightly reduced by lithium carbonate.
- Lithium can potentiate the effects of suxamethonium.

Recommendations

There are different recommendations in the literature ranging from lithium should be stopped before ECT and that there should be a suitable washout period before ECT is commenced, to the combination can be used safely. The following guidance is offered for patients taking lithium in whom ECT is being considered.

- If lithium is not having any benefit, stop it before ECT is commenced.
- If lithium is effective then continue during ECT but monitor the patient closely for signs of adverse effects (e.g. delirium, confusion) and maintain the patient on the lowest effective lithium level.
- If there are any concerns about using lithium during ECT, then the patient could be switched to an alternative mood stabiliser such as an antipsychotic if the risks outweigh the benefits of continuing lithium.

Anti-epileptics

Anti-epileptics are commonly used as mood stabilisers but their pharmacological action would be expected to raise the seizure threshold during ECT.

A study looked at seven patients who had received carbamazepine or valproate and ECT. The group receiving anticonvulsants had a shorter duration of seizures and a higher stimulus dose for ECT was required. The authors stated that anticonvulsants did not affect the production of seizures, adverse effects, outcome or number of ECT sessions (Zarate *et al*, 1997). Sienaert & Peuskens (2007) make the following observations:

- Carbamazepine has been shown to either have no effect or to increase seizure threshold in case reports.
- Valproate has been shown to prevent seizures during ECT in case reports. Sometimes the anaesthetic agent was changed or the valproate dose was withheld on the morning of ECT to help elicit a seizure.
- The use of lamotrigine with ECT has been reported in several papers. Lamotrigine has been found to have minimal effect on seizures during ECT.
- There is a case report of gabapentin not having any effect on seizures during ECT.
- There are no data about the use of topiramate and ECT.

Drug interactions to consider

Anti-epileptics have many drug interactions and can either induce (e.g. carbamazepine) or inhibit (e.g. valproate) the metabolism of other drugs.

Carbamazepine can reduce response and recovery times to non-depolarising neuromuscular blocking agents. Conversely, patients may show increased sensitivity to suxamethonium (Naguib & Koorn, 2002).

Recommendations

If anticonvulsants are used for a mood disorder, consider the benefits and risks of continuing them during ECT (see Chapter 4). If it is difficult to produce a seizure when a patient is taking anticonvulsants, try the following:

- change the anaesthetic agent
- withhold the morning dose of the anticonvulsant before ECT
- review the anticonvulsant dose
- if the anticonvulsant is to be discontinued, it should be tapered off to reduce the risk of precipitating seizures/deterioration in mood.

Antidepressants

There are varying reports to the extent to which antidepressants can affect seizure threshold and therefore have an influence on ECT.

Sackeim *et al* (2009) looked at the use of placebo, nortriptyline and venlafaxine in combination with right unilateral or bilateral ECT ($n=340$). The most common adverse event was tachycardia. Nortriptyline and venlafaxine increased the incidence of tachycardia. Patients treated with nortriptyline improved or had no change in cognitive function, whereas patients in the venlafaxine group remained unchanged or worsened.

Selective serotonin reuptake inhibitors

There are several reports of selective serotonin reuptake inhibitors (SSRIs) causing prolonged seizures during ECT, although they probably have little effect on seizure threshold, and overall they are thought to have a low proconvulsive effect (Bazire, 2009; Taylor *et al*, 2009). There is a case report of three patients treated with ECT and escitalopram as well as with other psychotropic drugs. Adverse effects were minimal and transient (Masdrakis *et al*, 2008*b*).

Monoamine oxidase inhibitors

There is little information on the use of ECT and MAOIs (Naguib & Koorn, 2002). They have little effect on seizure threshold. Monoamine oxidase inhibitors have serious interactions with other medicines and foods, which may lead to hypertensive crisis and serotonin syndrome. The anaesthetist must be informed whether the patient is on this type of drug. There is a risk of hypotension. It is recommended that moclobemide is stopped 24 h before ECT as a precaution.

Tricyclic antidepressants

The combination of tricyclic antidepressants and ECT has often been used without problems.

One study (Naguib & Koorn, 2002) showed a shorter seizure time with tricyclic antidepressants than ECT alone and no difference in cardiac adverse effects or confusion.

Although tricyclic antidepressants may lower seizure threshold, they are also associated with arrhythmias following ECT and may cause hypotension and prolonged seizures.

Venlafaxine

This agent can be epileptogenic at high doses. There is an increased risk of asystole at doses greater than 300 mg/day. It may attenuate the beneficial effects of ECT and exacerbate cognitive adverse effects (Sackeim *et al*, 2009).

Duloxetine

There is a case report of a patient on olanzapine and duloxetine having no apparent problems (Hanretta & Malek-Ahmadi, 2006).

49

Animal studies have shown that the seizure threshold increased in mice treated with increasing doses of duloxetine. In placebo-controlled trials, duloxetine had a rate of seizures/convulsions of 0.03% (3/9445) compared with 0.01% (1/6770) with placebo (Hanretta & Malek-Ahmadi, 2006).

Mirtazapine

An open study (n=19) and a case report (n=2) indicate that there were no problems (Bazire, 2009).

Trazodone

A review commented that trazodone significantly potentiated the hypnotic effect of hexobarbital, even more than tricyclic antidepressants. There are reports of it potentially causing cardiac problems (e.g. ventricular arrhythmias) or prolonged seizures in some patients. The authors concluded that it should be used with caution during ECT maintenance therapy (Jarvis *et al*, 1992).

Agomelatine

There are no published reports on the use of agomelatine and ECT but it should not have any pro- or anticonvulsant properties (European Medicines Agency, 2008; Bazire, 2012).

Bupropion

This drug may cause seizures (Pesola & Avasarala, 2002) and has the potential to produce delirium in patients.

Drug interactions to consider

- Monoamine oxidase inhibitors can be continued as long as close monitoring is carried out and the patient is monitored for any rare, unexpected adverse effects. The MAOI may need to be stopped for longer than 20 days to allow the depressed adrenergic receptor function to recover. Hypertensive crisis can occur with indirect-acting sympathomimetic agents (e.g. ephedrine). The pressor effects of direct-acting sympathomimetic agents such as adrenaline and noradrenaline may be increased, especially in patients with hypotension. Moclobemide does not appear to alter the pressor effect of noradrenaline. Great care is needed when using opiates with MAOIs and avoid using opiates with serotonergic properties (e.g. pethidine, tramadol). The anaesthetist needs to know that the patient is taking an MAOI.
- Tricyclic antidepressants can increase the length of barbiturate anaesthesia and can increase the risk of hypotension and arrhythmias during anaesthesia. Tricyclic antidepressants increase the response to noradrenaline and adrenaline, which may lead to hypertension and cardiac arrhythmias.

- Barbiturates can lower the levels of some tricyclic antidepressants.
- Paroxetine and methohexital – case report of a seizure (Folkerts, 1995).
- Selective serotonin reuptake inhibitors and beta blockers – atrioventricular block has occurred with paroxetine/metoprolol, severe bradycardia with fluoxetine and fluvoxamine with beta blockers. All beta blockers metabolised by cytochrome P450 2D6 may interact with fluoxetine or paroxetine.
- Flecainide levels can be increased by paroxetine, fluoxetine and escitalopram.
- Bupropion can cause bradycardia with metoprolol via inhibition of cytochrome P450 2D6.
- Hypotension, CNS and respiratory depression may increase if MAOIs are given with barbiturates, propofol and benzodiazepines.
- Selective serotonin reuptake inhibitors can reduce the clearance of class 1c anti-arrhythmics and beta blockers.

Recommendations

There are limited data available on these drugs with ECT. Selective serotonin reuptake inhibitors probably have a minimal effect on ECT, although you may have to consider drug interactions, especially with fluoxetine, paroxetine and fluvoxamine. If MAOIs are used during a course of ECT, the anaesthetist needs to be aware of this; the patient needs to be carefully monitored for any drug interactions. Tricyclic antidepressants and venlafaxine have been used during ECT but the patient needs to be monitored for cardiac adverse effects. There are very limited data on the newer antidepressants.

Acetylcholinesterase inhibitors

Concerns have been raised (Boman, 2002) about the potential effect that cholinesterase inhibitor drugs might have during ECT treatment, especially when suxamethonium is used as the muscle relaxant. In theory, the duration of neuromuscular blockade could be prolonged as a result of reduced butyrylcholinesterase activity, causing prolonged apnoea. There are no reports if this.

Other side-effects that may occur include bradycardia, cardiac arrhythmias and asystole via an increase in vagal parasympathetic activity. Acetylcholinesterase inhibitors also have the potential to cause generalised convulsions, possibly reducing the threshold for convulsions and increasing the risk of prolonged seizures. There are no reports of this problem from ECT clinics but events have occurred during surgical procedures (Crowe & Collins, 2003; Baruah et al, 2008).

The evidence available suggests that not only is it safe to take an acetylcholinesterase inhibitor while receiving ECT, but that it may have beneficial effects in protecting the individual from cognitive impairment after ECT. Prakash *et al* (2006) conducted a prospective randomised controlled trial (*n*=45) of the potential benefits of donepezil 5 mg/day in reducing cognitive adverse effects after ECT. Patients on donepezil had a significantly faster recovery of cognitive deficits after ECT, especially orientation in time and personal memory.

A non-randomised controlled trial (*n*=17) studied in-patients receiving right unilateral ECT on galantamine 4 mg twice daily compared with controls (Matthews *et al*, 2008). Galantamine was well tolerated, with no significant differences in adverse effects among the groups. The galantamine group had less impairment of delayed memory and abstract reasoning at the completion of ECT, with no differences in word generation. No differences between the groups were found regarding seizure length or energy used to induce seizures. There was no prolongation of muscle paralysis when galantamine was given in combination with suxamethonium and no prolonged period of asystole.

Single case reports have been published on patients receiving donepezil and rivastigmine without problems (Zink *et al*, 2002; Rao *et al*, 2009).

Drug interactions to consider

- Cholinesterase inhibitors could enhance the effects of suxamethonium.
- There is a risk of additional adverse effects if amiodarone is given with cholinesterase inhibitors (e.g. bradycardia).

Recommendations

Cholinesterase inhibitors can be used during a course of ECT and may improve post-ECT confusion. Butyrylcholinesterase inhibitors may enhance the effects of suxamethonium.

Benzodiazepines

Benzodiazepines may decrease the efficacy of unilateral ECT and reduce the effectiveness of ECT (even months after treatment has been stopped) by increasing the seizure threshold. Unilateral ECT can be less effective in patients who are receiving long-term treatment with benzodiazepines (Naguib & Koorn, 2002).

Abruptly withdrawing benzodiazepines can cause confusion, convulsions and toxic psychosis (British Medical Association & Royal Pharmaceutical Society, 2012).

Drug interactions to consider

The majority of interactions with benzodiazepines are predictable and reflect the effects of two (or more) drugs with sedative properties. There is a synergistic interaction during induction of anaesthesia.

Recommendations

All benzodiazepines may raise seizure threshold, so it is desirable to discontinue them prior to ECT. Long-standing prescription of benzodiazepine medication should not be suddenly stopped before a course of ECT, but attempts should be made to reduce the dose of such drugs as far a possible.

Hypnotics

Northdurfter *et al* (2006) report on 787 ECT treatments given without psychiatric medication and 1075 treatments administered with concomitant non-benzodiazepine hypnotics. There were no clinically relevant or statistically significant differences on electrophysiological or clinical parameters between these groups.

Zopiclone can reduce seizure length when used the previous night (Tobiansky, 1991). If it is difficult to produce adequate seizures in patients taking this medication, it should be stopped.

Buspirone

There are no reports of interactions with ECT (Jarvis *et al*, 1992; Naguib & Koorn, 2002).

Central nervous system stimulants

Methylphenidate, dexamfetamine and modafinil can cause increased blood pressure. Central nervous system stimulants pose a potential risk for potentiating seizure activity, leading to prolonged seizures or a risk of status epilepticus (Naguib & Koorn, 2002).

Drug interactions to consider

Benzodiazepines and opiates increase sedation and respiratory depression.

Recommendations

As far as possible, hypnotics should be avoided during a course of ECT. A sedative antipsychotic or antidepressant may be preferable.

Caffeine

Caffeine has been used to prolong seizures during ECT. Caffeine is a non-selective antagonist at adenosine A_1 and A_{2a} receptors and is an inhibitor of a number of phosphodiesterases (Sawynok, 1995). When ECT is used for the treatment of depression there can be a progressive decrease in seizure duration during the course of treatment. Caffeine can prolong the seizure length without altering the seizure threshold. Adenosine analogues produce central anticonvulsant activity via the activation of A_1 receptors. The prolongation of seizures by caffeine is believed to be due to the antagonism of the A_1 receptor.

Caffeine is completely and rapidly absorbed, with peak plasma concentrations reached at 5–90 min and it has a half life of 4.9 h (range 1.9–12.2 h).

Efficacy

An adequate seizure during ECT was traditionally thought to be a generalised seizure lasting 20–30 s and if it lasted less than 15 s it was unlikely to be therapeutic. Current evidence suggests that the relationship between seizures and efficacy is more complex (see Chapter 4).

Caffeine has been shown to increase seizure duration without altering the seizure threshold. It has been reported to increase seizure duration by a mean of 127% (Sawynok, 1995). However, case reports of cardiac dysrhythmia have been reported. Rosenquist et al (1994) found that:

- intravenous caffeine increased seizure duration but did not affect seizure threshold in patients who were not initially resistant to seizure generation – the seizure duration declined as treatment continued, requiring increasing caffeine doses ($n=8$);
- the use of caffeine in six patients with depression led to increased seizure duration – these patients did not develop seizures when on maximal stimulation before the use of caffeine;
- in 20 patients with depression, caffeine was found to increase seizure duration in a dose-dependent manner.

A double-blind, placebo-controlled study compared caffeine augmentation with increasing electrical stimulus intensity plus placebo for 40 in-patients with depression having unilateral ECT (Coffey et al, 1990). The placebo group required a 49% increase in mean electrical stimulus, whereas the caffeine group had a 7.9% decrease in electrical stimulation. The highest dose of caffeine required was 726 mg. There were temporary side-effects, such as anxiety and increased blood pressure post seizure after the use of caffeine.

In an open-controlled study of 21 patients receiving bilateral ECT (Calev et al, 1993), the seizure duration was longer in the caffeine group. The rate of recovery from depression was faster in the caffeine group (5.7 v. 7.9 ECT treatments). In a double-blind, randomised, placebo-controlled study of 12 patients (mean age 62.7 years), methohexital was the anaesthetic agent (Rosenquist et al, 1994) and caffeine was found to have no effect on seizure quality using EEG measures. Oral caffeine was reported to increase seizure duration in 30 elderly patients (Ancil & Carlyle, 1992).

Datto et al (2002) reviewed augmentation strategies and found no evidence of difference in cognitive assessments, minor cognitive effects or delayed orientation time after in-patients were given caffeine prior to

ECT, but cardiac dysrhythmias, prolonged seizures, anxiety, tremors and olfactory sensations were reported.

Drug interactions to consider

- Caffeine can reduce the effects of benzodiazepines.
- Fluvoxamine increases caffeine levels.
- Caffeine increases clozapine levels.
- Large doses of caffeine can cause a reduction in lithium levels.
- There are rare reports of MAOIs increasing the CNS stimulant effects of caffeine.

Recommendations

Caffeine should only be used to prolong the seizure threshold during ECT when other options have failed to work, for example changing the anaesthetic or reviewing the patient's current prescribed medication.

Prophylactic treatment to prevent relapse after ECT

It is well established that there is a high risk of relapse in the first few weeks after a successful course of ECT if a patient is left untreated (Sackeim *et al*, 2001).

In the prophylaxis and prevention of relapse following a depressive illness, NICE (2009) recommends that after successful pharmacological treatment patients should continue to take antidepressant medication at a full treatment dosage for at least 6 months. In high-risk patients, this could extend to 2 or more years. The use of antidepressants reduces the risk of relapse in depressive disorder and continued treatment with antidepressants appears to benefit many patients with recurrent depressive disorder. There are guidelines on continuation treatments for depression, bipolar affective disorder and schizophrenia (e.g. Anderson *et al*, 2008; National Institute for Health and Clinical Excellence, 2009).

If a person's depression has responded to a course of ECT, antidepressant medication should be started or continued to prevent relapse and lithium should also be considered (National Institute for Health and Clinical Excellence, 2009). Most patients treated with ECT have recurrent and refractory illnesses and are likely to require more intensive continuation treatment and longer-term prophylactic treatment to reduce the risk of future episodes of illness. It has been previously recommended (Scott, 2005) that 6 months of continuation treatment must be seen as the bare minimum, and at least 12 months of continuation treatment has been recommended for depressive illness in the elderly (see Chapter 14).

Evidence

The National Institute for Health and Clinical Excellence reported studies looking at continuation treatment after successful treatment with ECT, two of which included maintenance ECT (National Institute for Health and Clinical Excellence, 2009). There was no difference after 6 months between ECT/nortriptyline and nortriptyline alone (relative risk of relapse 0.5, 95% confidence interval (CI) 0.05–4.98), or between ECT alone and a combination of nortriptyline and lithium. At 12 months, ECT/nortriptyline was superior to nortriptyline alone (relative risk of relapse 0.12, 95% CI 0.02–0.89). The relative risk scores for relapse for four trials following successful ECT mentioned by NICE were (National Institute for Health and Clinical Excellence, 2009):

- fluoxetine/placebo v. fluoxetine/melatonin, 1.17 (95% CI 0.4–3.39) (12 weeks)
- nortriptyline/lithium v. placebo, 0.44 (95% CI 0.25–0.8) (6 months)
- nortriptyline v. placebo, 0.77 (95% CI 0.51–1.15) (6 months)
- nortriptyline/lithium v. nortriptyline, 0.6 (95% CI 0.32–1.14) (6 months).

The National Institute for Health and Clinical Excellence (2009) also commented that a trial comparing maintenance ECT v. ECT and an antidepressant showed that the Mini-Mental State Examination (MMSE) scores in both groups improved over 6 months.

In a trial involving maintenance ECT and pharmacotherapy which included a placebo plus ECT arm, the relapse rate for placebo was 84% (95% CI 70–90) (Sackeim et al, 2001). Rates of 18–60% have been quoted for tricyclic antidepressants, 26% for paroxetine and 39% for a combination of nortriptyline and lithium (Anderson et al, 2008). There was no difference in measures of cognitive impairment over the 6 months in the trial of ECT v. lithium/nortriptyline (Kellner et al, 2006).

A retrospective case-note study found that the probability of patients remaining well over 5 years on continuation ECT was 73%, compared with 18% of patients acutely treated with ECT and then maintained on medication (Anderson et al, 2008).

A further small study randomised 74 patients following response to ECT to paroxetine v. placebo or paroxetine v. imipramine for 6 months depending on advice from a cardiologist (Lauritzen et al, 1996). The mean dose of paroxetine in both groups was about 28 mg/day and 138 mg/day for imipramine. Kaplan–Meier survival curves showed a significant benefit for paroxetine over imipramine at 3 and 6 months ($P \leq 0.05$), but paroxetine was found to be statistically different from placebo at 3 months ($P \leq 0.05$) but not 6 months ($P \leq 0.10$).

The NICE technology appraisal on ECT (2003) concluded that compared with placebo, continuation pharmacotherapy with tricyclic antidepressants and/or lithium reduced the rate of relapse in people who had responded to ECT.

Yildiz et al (2010) looked specifically at the combination of pharmacotherapy with ECT in preventing relapse in adults with a diagnosis of major depression. This prospective randomised trial ($n=32$) looked at relapse rates after 18 weeks post randomisation to three treatment arms (ECT with sertraline started after 2 weeks, ECT with sertraline commenced after 4 weeks, and the third group received ECT and placebo). The group that received sertraline during the second week of ECT showed a significant difference compared with the placebo group but not compared with the group that commenced sertraline after ECT application number 8 (fourth week into the trial). These results suggest that SSRIs could be efficacious in the prevention of relapse after successful ECT, and the recommendation would be to start the antidepressant before cessation of the ECT treatment course.

A Cochrane review on the use of ECT in schizophrenia (Tharyan & Adams, 2005) showed that maintenance ECT combined with antipsychotics was more effective than antipsychotics alone ($n=30$, Global Assessment of Functioning weighted mean differences 19.06, 95% CI 9.65 to 28.47 v. –20.30, 95% CI –11.48 to –29.12). The authors commented that a small study showed that the combination of ECT and antipsychotics caused more memory impairment than antipsychotics alone.

Recommendations

- If a patient has responded to an antidepressant it should be continued for at least 6 months after the end of a course of ECT.
- Relapse rates are high after remission is achieved in depression and antidepressants reduce the risk of relapse by about 70%.
- The combination of lithium/antidepressant may reduce the risk of relapse after ECT.
- Maintenance ECT may be considered in patients who have frequent relapses and who have not responded to medication.

Gaps in evidence

There is limited data on the use of medication during ECT, with conflicting data or recommendations available for various medications (e.g. lithium). There is also controversy whether medication should be started with the course of ECT, during or after the course has finished. More data need to be produced for the use of maintenance ECT alone or with pharmacotherapy in preventing relapse of depression.

References

Ancil, R. & Carlyle, W. (1992) Oral caffeine augmentation of ECT. *American Journal of Psychiatry*, **149**, 137.

Anderson, I. M., Ferrier, I. N., Baldwin, R. C., *et al* (2008) Evidence-based guidelines for treating depressive disorders with antidepressants: a revision of the 2000 British Association for Psychopharmacology guidelines. *Journal of Psychopharmacology*, **22**, 343–396.

Baruah, J., Easby, J. & Kessell, G. (2008) Effects of acetylcholinesterase inhibitor therapy for Alzheimer's disease on neuromuscular block. *British Journal of Anaesthesia*, **100**, 420.

Bazire, S. (2009) *Psychotropic Drug Directory 2009. The Professionals' Pocket Handbook and Aide Memoire*. Healthcomm UK.

Bazire, S. (2012) *Psychotropic Drug Directory 2012. The Professionals' Pocket Handbook and Aide Memoire*. Lloyd-Reinhold Communications.

Boman, B. (2002) Concurrent use of ECT and cholinesterase inhibitor medications. *Australian and New Zealand Journal of Psychiatry*, **36**, 816.

Braga, R. J. & Petrides, G. (2005) The combined use of electroconvulsive therapy and antipsychotics in patients with schizophrenia. *Journal of ECT*, **21**, 75–83.

British Medical Association & Royal Pharmaceutical Society (2012) 4.1 Hypnotics and anxiolytics. In *British National Formulary BNF 64*: pp. 213–221. BMJ Group and Pharmaceutical Press.

Calev, A., Fink, M., Petrides, G., *et al* (1993) Caffeine pretreatment enhances clinical efficacy and reduces cognitive effects of electroconvulsive therapy. *Convulsive Therapy*, **9**, 95–100.

Clozaril Patient Monitoring Service (2010) *Clozaril and General Anaesthesia Factsheet*. CPMS.

Coffey, C., Figiel, G., Weiner, R., *et al* (1990) Caffeine augmentation of ECT. *American Journal of Psychiatry*, **147**, 579–585.

Crowe, S. & Collins, L. (2003) Suxamethonium and donepezil: a cause of prolonged paralysis. *Anesthesiology*, **98**, 574–575.

Datto, C., Rai, A., Ilivicky, H., *et al* (2002) Augmentation of seizure induction in electroconvulsive therapy: a clinical reappraisal. *Journal of ECT*, **18**, 118–125.

Dolenc, T. & Rasmussen, K. (2005) The safety of electroconvulsive therapy and lithium in combination: a case series and review of the literature. *Journal of ECT*, **21**, 165–170.

Electronic Medicines Compendium (2010) Summary of Product Characteristics: Clozaril 25mg and 100mg Tablets. Available online at: http://www.medicines.org.uk/EMC/medicine/1277/SPC/Clozaril+25mg+and+100mg+Tablets/.

European Medicines Agency (2008) *CHMP Assessment Report for Valdoxan*. EMEA.

Folkerts, H. (1995) Spontaneous seizure after concurrent use of methohexital anesthesia for electroconvulsive therapy and paroxetine: a case report. *Journal of Nervous and Mental Disorders*, **183**, 115–116.

Goodwin, G. M. (2003) Evidence-based guidelines for treating bipolar disorder. *Journal of Psychopharmacology*, **17**, 149–173.

Hanretta, A. T. & Malek-Ahmadi, P. (2006) Combined use of ECT with duloxetine and olanzapine: a case report. *Journal of ECT*, **22**, 139–141.

Jarvis, M., Goewert, A. & Zorumski, C. (1992) Novel antidepressants and maintenance electroconvulsive therapy: a review. *Annals of Clinical Psychiatry*, **4**, 275–284.

Kellner, C. H., Knapp, R. G., Petrides, G., *et al* (2006) Continuation electroconvulsive therapy vs pharmacotherapy for relapse prevention in major depression: a multisite study from the consortium for research in electroconvulsive therapy (CORE). *Archives of General Psychiatry*, **63**, 1337–1344.

Lauritzen, L., Odgaard, K., Clemmesen, L., *et al* (1996) Relapse prevention by means of paroxetine in ECT-treated patients with major depression: a comparison with imipramine and placebo in medium-term continuation therapy. *Acta Psychiatrica Scandinavica*, **94**, 241–251.

Lopez-Garcia, P. L., Chiclana, C. & Gonzalez R. (2009) Combined use of ECT with aripiprazole. *World Journal of Biological Psychiatry*, **10**, 942–943.

Masdrakis, V., Oulis, P., Zervas, I. M., *et al* (2008*a*) The safety of the electroconvulsive therapy-aripiprazole combination: four case reports. *Journal of ECT*, **24**, 236–238.

Masdrakis, V., Oulis, P., Florakis, A., *et al* (2008*b*) The safety of the electroconvulsive therapy-escitalopram combination. *Journal of ECT*, **24**, 289–291.

Matthews, J., Blais, M., Park, L., *et al* (2008) The impact of galantamine on cognition and mood during electroconvulsive therapy: a pilot study. *Journal of Psychiatric Research*, **42**, 526–531.

MedicincesComplete (2013) *Stockley's Drug Interactions*. Phamaceutical Press (http://www.medicinescomplete.com/mc/stockley/current).

Naguib, M. & Koorn, R. (2002) Interactions between psychotropics, anaesthetics and electroconvulsive therapy. Implications for drug choice and patient management. *CNS Drugs*, **16**, 229–247.

National Institute for Clinical Excellence (2003) *Guidance on the Use of Electroconvulsive Therapy* (Technical Appraisal TA59). NICE.

National Institute for Health and Clinical Excellence (2009) *Depression: The Treatment and Management of Depression in Adults (Update)* (Clinical Guideline CG90). NICE.

Northdurfter, C., Eser, D., Schule, C., *et al* (2006) The influence of concomitant narcoleptic medication on safety, tolerability and clinical effectiveness of electroconvulsive therapy. *World Journal of Biological Psychiatry*, **7**, 162–170.

Painuly, N. & Chakrabarti, S. (2006) Combined use of electroconvulsive therapy and antipsychotics in schizophrenia: the Indian evidence: a review and meta-analysis. *Journal of ECT*, **22**, 59–66.

Pesola, G. R. & Avasarala, J. (2002) Bupropion seizure proportion among new-onset generalized seizures and drug related seizures presenting to an emergency department. *Journal of Emergency Medicine*, **22**, 235–239.

Prakash, J., Kotwal, A. & Prabhu, H. R. A. (2006) Therapeutic and prophylactic utility of the memory-enhancing drug donepezil hydrochloride on cognition of patients undergoing electroconvulsive therapy: a randomized controlled trial. *Journal of ECT*, **22**, 163–168.

Rao, N., Palaniyappan, P., Chandur, J., *et al* (2009) Successful use of donepezil in treatment of cognitive impairment caused by maintenance electroconvulsive therapy: a case report. *Journal of ECT*, **25**, 216–218.

Rosenquist, P., McCall, W., Farah, A., *et al* (1994) Effects of caffeine pretreatment on measures of seizure impact. *Convulsive Therapy*, **10**, 181–185.

Sackeim, H., Haskett, R., Mulsant, B., *et al* (2001) Continuation pharmacotherapy in the prevention of relapse following electroconvulsive therapy: a randomized controlled trial. *JAMA*, **285**, 1299–1307.

Sackeim, H., Dillingham, E., Prudic, J., *et al* (2009) Effect of concomitant pharmacotherapy on electroconvulsive therapy outcomes. Short-term efficacy and adverse effects. *Archives of General Psychiatry*, **66**, 729–773.

Sartorius, A., Wolf, J. & Henn, F. A. (2005) Lithium and ECT-concurrent use still demands attention: three case reports. *World Journal of Biological Psychiatry*, **6**, 121–124.

Sawynok, J. (1995) Pharmacological rationale for the clinical use of caffeine. *Drugs*, **49**, 37–50.

Scott, A. (ed.) (2005) *The ECT Handbook: The Third Report of the Royal College of Psychiatrists' Special Committee on ECT* (2nd edn) (Council Report CR128). Royal College of Psychiatrists.

Sienaert, P. & Peuskens, J. (2007) Anticonvulsants during electroconvulsive therapy: review and recommendations. *Journal of ECT*, **23**, 120–123.

Taylor, D., Paton, C. & Kapur, S. (2009) *The Maudsley Prescribing Guidelines in Psychiatry* (10th edn). Informa Healthcare.

Tharyan, P. & Adams, C. E. (2005) Electroconvulsive therapy for schizophrenia. *Cochrane Database of Systematic Reviews*, **2**, CD000076.

Thirthalli, J., Harish, T. & Gangadhar, B. N. (2011) A prospective comparative study of interaction between lithium and modified electroconvulsive therapy. *World Journal of Biological Psychiatry*, **12**, 149–155.

Tobiansky, R. I. (1991) Effect of the cyclopyrrolone hypnotic zopiclone on ECT seizure duration. *Journal of Psychopharmacology*, **5**, 268–269.

Yildiz, A., Mantar, A., Simsek, S., *et al* (2010) Combination of pharmacotherapy with electroconvulsive therapy in prevention of depressive relapse: a pilot controlled trial. *Journal of ECT*, **26**, 104–110.

Zarate, C., Tohen M. & Baraibar, G. (1997) Combined valproate or carbamazepine and electroconvulsive therapy. *Annals of Clinical Psychiatry*, **9**, 19–25.

Zink, M., Sartorius, A., Lederbogen, F., *et al* (2002) Electroconvulsive therapy in a patient receiving rivastigmine. *Journal of ECT*, **18**, 162–164.

CHAPTER 6

Monitoring a course of ECT

Allan I. F. Scott and Jonathan Waite

It is important to evaluate any patient's response to any treatment. This is especially the case for an emotive and serious intervention such as ECT. This chapter will offer advice on evaluating response, in terms of the relief of the patient's psychiatric symptoms, monitoring seizures in the ECT clinic and assessing the cognitive effects of ECT.

Establishing a baseline

It is necessary to quantify the severity of the patient's symptoms before starting treatment. Assessments should be undertaken by the referring team before, during and after the course of treatment.

Disease symptoms

Depression is the most common indication for ECT. The Montgomery–Åsberg Depression Rating Scale (MADRS) (Montgomery & Åsberg, 1979) has been widely used for assessing auditing response to ECT. It has been found to be acceptable to both patients and practitioners and is recommended for routine use. The Hamilton Rating Scale for Depression (Hamilton, 1960), which has often been used in research, would be an alternative. For patients receiving ECT for other indications such as mania or catatonia, the Brief Psychiatric Rating Scale (BPRS) (Lukoff et al, 1986) or Global Assessment of Functioning (GAF) (Piersma & Boes, 1997) could be considered. Whatever the indication for treatment is, a baseline level of severity on the Clinical Global Impression of Severity (CGI-S) (Guy & Bonato, 1976) should be documented before the course starts (Box 6.1).

Cognition

Before starting a course of ECT, the patient's level of functioning in memory, verbal and non-verbal cognitive domains should be established. Most patients starting a course of ECT will be severely ill. They may be reluctant or unable to participate in detailed neuropsychological

---

Box 6.1 Clinical Global Impression of Severity (CGI-S): score at baseline

1 = Normal, not at all ill

2 = Borderline mentally ill

3 = Mildly ill

4 = Moderately ill

5 = Severely ill

6 = Among the most severely ill

Guy & Bonato (1976)

---

assessment. Most UK clinics use the MMSE (Folstein *et al*, 1975). This is not an entirely satisfactory instrument, but it has the advantage that most clinical staff are familiar with its use. It is suggested that clinics continue to use the MMSE until it is demonstrated that a better alternative exists. Practitioners should be aware that the MMSE is copyright and that there may be clinically relevant cognitive impairment which the MMSE cannot detect (see Chapter 8).

A clinical assessment of recent memory, autobiographical memory and subjective memory difficulties should be undertaken and clearly documented. This will help the clinical team to decide whether any cognitive impairment has been caused by the treatment. Interviewing the patient, preferably with an informant, should be sufficient. Suggestions for formal memory tests can be found in Chapter 8. Routine use of the Autobiographical Memory Interview (McIlhiney *et al*, 2001) is not recommended.

Physical symptoms

Electroconvulsive therapy frequently causes physical adverse effects such as headache, nausea, dental problems and muscle aches (see Chapter 7). The presence of physical symptoms prior to treatment should be documented. The patient's dental health should also be recorded (see Chapter 9).

Monitoring during ECT and recovery

Any patient receiving a general anaesthetic needs to be monitored with pulse oximetry, ECG, capnography and non-invasive blood pressure monitoring (see Chapter 3). At the end of the procedure the time to re-orientation should be documented and a check made as to whether physical side-effects (headache, muscle pains, nausea/vomiting or confusion) have occurred, before the patient leaves the ECT clinic. If such symptoms have not resolved before the patient leaves the clinic, the ward team should record how long they persist.

The seizure must be monitored visually and on a (at least) two-channel EEG. Manufacturers of ECT machines can supply self-adhesive, pre-gelled, disposable EEG electrodes. Most ECT practitioners prefer to position these away from the hairy scalp and far apart, to maximise the amplitude of the EEG tracing – that is, over the manubrium, just above the middle of the eyebrow on the forehead and on the skin over the ipsilateral mastoid process, the so-called prefrontal–mastoid positioning (Fig. 6.1).

The hallmark of generalised cerebral seizure activity is the tonic–clonic (or grand mal) convulsion; after an initial tonic contraction of the muscles, there is a longer, clonic phase of rhythmic alternating contraction and relaxation of the muscles on both sides of the body. There may be a delay of a few seconds after the end of electrical stimulation before any convulsion is seen – this is known as the latent phase.

The clinical efficacy of ECT depends on the induction of generalised cerebral seizure activity. This is by the appearance on the EEG of widespread high-frequency spike waves (polyspike activity) followed by slower spike and wave complexes, typically around 3 Hz. Typically, generalised cerebral seizure activity is followed by a phase of relative or complete suppression of electrical activity (post-ictal suppression).

Methods of monitoring

It is recommended that the convulsion is timed from the end of electrical stimulation to the end of generalised (bilateral) clonic activity. If there is a significant discrepancy between the end of generalised clonic activity and the end of clonic activity in one limb, it would be prudent to record

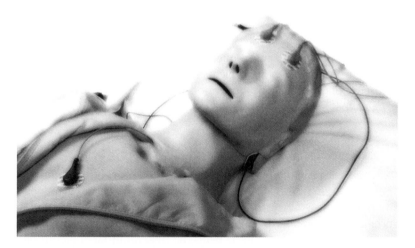

Fig. 6.1 Prefrontal–mastoid positioning of electrodes for EEG tracing.

both times. Convulsive activity of the muscles of the face can be seen with focal cerebral seizure activity and cannot be relied on as an indicator of generalised seizure activity.

The purpose of asking the clinic team to record visible seizure duration is to ensure that the patient is observed closely during the seizure. A brief convulsion should prompt the ECT team to ensure that the necessary quality of seizure activity has been induced. It is not wise to rely on EEG monitoring alone to time seizures. This method is vulnerable to technical problems: the EEG tracing may be unreadable because of artefact, connecting cables may become disconnected, or the machine may run out of paper. On some occasions clinically evident generalised convulsions are not associated with detectable EEG evidence of cerebral seizure activity (Whittaker *et al*, 2007). The brain is well protected by the skull and scalp, which may prevent seizure activity being picked up by skin electrodes.

Electroencephalogram monitoring is the simplest means of assessing cerebral seizure activity (Scott, 2007). The routine use of EEG monitoring has revealed that patients may demonstrate prolonged seizure activity, even where the observed clonic movements cease after about 30 s (Benbow *et al*, 2003). These EEG features are illustrated in Fig. 6.2 and discussed in more detail by Weiner *et al* (1991). The duration of the cerebral seizure activity or the tonic–clonic convulsion is not related to clinical efficacy (Sackeim *et al*, 1991; Weiner *et al*, 1991). However, it is difficult to be certain whether a seizure has occurred unless either tonic–clonic muscle activity or an EEG showing polyspike followed by 3 Hz spike-and-wave activity is observed. Three possible problems may arise:

1   The cerebral seizure activity may end not abruptly, but gradually.
2   The cerebral seizure may be followed by only limited, that is, relative post-ictal suppression.
3   The analysis of the EEG recording may be difficult or impossible because of the presence of artefact.

These difficulties mean that it is impossible for ECT machines to accurately determine seizure duration in many instances, despite the manufacturer's claims. The figures produced by the machine's computers cannot be relied on to give a correct value for seizure duration.

Figure 6.3 shows an example of a recording of the termination phase in which the end-point of the cerebral seizure is almost totally obscured by artefact. Nevertheless, there are about 2 s (between 39 and 41 s) when the EEG recording is less affected by artefact, and it is possible to see that no clear-cut cerebral seizure activity is visible.

Figure 6.4(a) is an example of an EEG recording of a termination phase in which the determination of the end-point is difficult, not because of artefact, but because the degree of post-ictal suppression is insufficient to lead to a flat tracing after the cerebral seizure. A large-amplitude slow wave, just before 34 s, is followed by only relative post-ictal suppression.

63

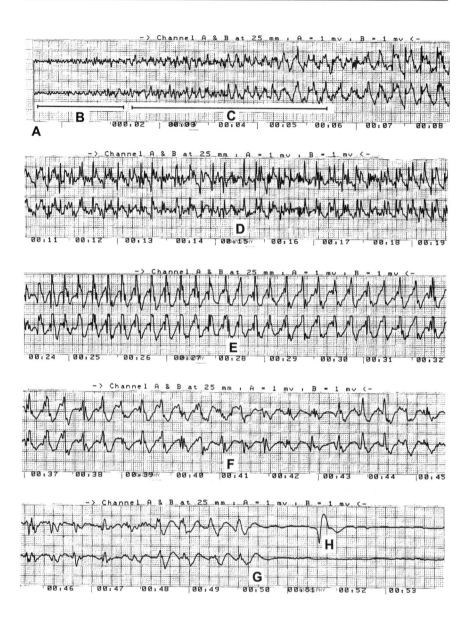

Fig. 6.2 Electroencephalogram (EEG) features of the necessary generalised cerebral seizure activity. Compare left (top) and right (bottom) hemisphere tracings to confirm generalisation. A: End of electrical stimulation. B: Latent phase – no visible convulsion, only low-amplitude, high-frequency polyspike activity EEG pattern. C: Increasing amplitude of EEG polyspike and gradual slowing of frequency. D: Start of clonic phase of convulsion. E: Classic 3 Hz spike-and-wave activity. F: Gradual loss of spike-and-wave pattern. G: End-point, after which EEG tracing has lower amplitude and frequency than at baseline (post-ictal suppression). H: Movement artefact from anaesthetist reapplying face mask.

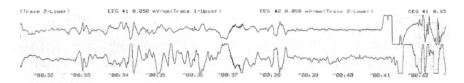

Fig. 6.3 Electroencephalogram recording where the termination phase is obscured by aretefact. Reproduced from Scott (2007).

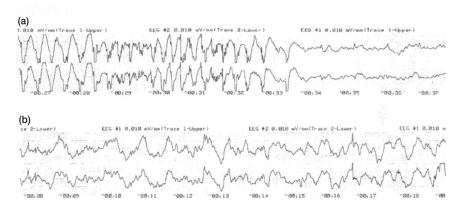

Fig. 6.4 Recording of (a) the resultant cerebral seizure followed by only relative post-ictal suppression and (b) the tracing recorded just before electrical stimulation. Reproduced from Scott (2007).

The tracing in Fig. 6.4(b) was recorded just before electrical stimulation and is included for comparison.

If seizures are not terminated within 3–5 min, then there is a risk of increased confusion and memory impairment. It is recommended that seizures should be terminated after 2 min with either a short-acting intravenous benzodiazepine or a bolus of the anaesthetic induction agent (see Chapter 3).

Assessment of seizure adequacy by EEG

Seizure threshold may, but will not inevitably, rise over a course of treatment, and if this happens, then the electrical dose should rise *pari passu* to maintain the dosing strategy. In the absence of obvious evidence such as a missed seizure, any change in the length of the convulsions is only modestly correlated with any rise in the seizure threshold. Clinical monitoring remains the best guide to what change in electrical dose is required. There has been much research interest in the potential of EEG monitoring to contribute to the assessment of seizure adequacy; unfortunately, there are no clear answers. Contemporary ECT machines provide computer-derived measurements of aspects of an individual tracing, but there is no evidence in the public domain to suggest that these increase predictive accuracy. Once the necessary cerebral seizure activity has been induced and recorded by EEG, it is not possible for the ECT team to examine an individual EEG tracing and make accurate predictions about the clinical outcome after a course of treatment (Nobler *et al*, 2000; Scott, 2007). Nevertheless, the availability of EEG monitoring will assist decisions on the need to increase the electrical dose over a course of treatment.

If high-amplitude synchronous typical cerebral seizure activity and typical post-ictal suppression appear on the EEG early in the course of treatment, but progressively the EEG tracings show less clear-cut or fewer typical features, then this suggests that the seizure threshold may be rising. Progressive EEG changes must, however, be assessed in the context of the necessary clinical monitoring; the ECT team are treating the patient, not the EEG tracing.

Electroencephalogram findings are also helpful in making a decision to discontinue ECT in a patient who is not showing clinical response. If high-amplitude synchronous typical cerebral seizure activity of adequate duration and typical post-ictal suppression appear consistently on the EEG, the lack of response cannot be attributed to poor technique from the ECT team. If it is not possible to obtain a therapeutic seizure with the first choice of anaesthetic regime, it is worthwhile trying an alternative induction agent (e.g. etomidate rather than propofol) or an anaesthetic sparing agent such as remifentanil.

Cuff technique

This is a simple technique that minimises the influence of the muscle relaxant on the assessment of convulsive activity (Hamilton, 1987). It involves isolating one limb by inflating a blood pressure cuff to above systolic pressure as the patient is becoming unconscious but before the muscle relaxant is administered. If the pressure in the cuff remains above systolic blood pressure, then the distal part of the limb is isolated from circulating muscle relaxant, allowing unmodified convulsions to be observed. It is important to maintain the pressure in the cuff well above systolic pressure during seizure activity, because if circulating muscle relaxant leaks into the distal part of the limb, it might be concentrated there, as venous return is occluded. The length of time the cuff is kept inflated is kept to a minimum by deflating it as soon as the convulsion has ended. When unilateral ECT is given, it is suggested that the cuff be applied to one of the ipsilateral limbs to ensure that a bilateral convulsion occurs.

This technique is not widely used. This is partly the result of a study that found no difference between the length of the convulsion in cuffed and uncuffed limbs in one English ECT clinic (Wise *et al*, 2000). Although use of the cuff technique cannot be recommended for routine use, it may still be helpful if only brief convulsive activity has been seen at the outset of the course of treatment. There may be typical generalised cerebral seizure activity in a substantial proportion of patients who display brief convulsive activity (Scott *et al*, 1989). The cuff technique may also be used where an unusually large dose of muscle relaxant is administered with the aim of total muscle paralysis, for example in a patient who has recently sustained a fracture of a long bone.

Monitoring during the course of ECT

After each treatment, clinical status should be assessed using a formal validated outcome measure (National Institute for Health and Clinical Excellence, 2009). The Clinical Global Impression of Improvement (Guy & Bonato, 1976) fulfils this requirement (Box 6.2). The patient's subjective assessment of their response to treatment should also be recorded. Assessment of mood needs to take into account diurnal variations. Guidance on when to stop a course of ECT is given in Chapter 4.

Cognitive function should be kept under review during treatment. The NICE (2009) guidance only requires formal testing (e.g. MMSE) to be undertaken every three or four treatments and at the end of treatment, but it is especially important to ensure that there is no worsening of cognition after the first treatment. If delirium or prolonged confusion occurs after an initial bilateral application of current, the need for ECT should be re-examined and the possibility of unilateral treatment considered. The psychiatric team should discuss with the anaesthetist whether using an alternative induction agent would reduce the risk of delirium recurring.

Box 6.2 Clinical Global Impression of Improvement (CGI-I): score after treatment

1 = Very much improved

2 = Much improved

3 = Improved

4 = No change

5 = Minimally worse

6 = Much worse

7 = Very much worse

Guy & Bonato (1976)

Every patient receiving ECT should have a clinical interview 24–48 h after treatment to explore whether any problems with new learning, retrograde amnesia and subjective memory impairment have arisen. It will not usually be feasible for this assessment to be carried out by a member of the ECT team, but the results need to be shared with clinic staff to give an opportunity for changes in how ECT is given to be considered.

Post-ECT nausea and muscle pains (Dinwiddie *et al*, 2010) are most common after the first treatment – these often become less troublesome as the course progresses, but if they are upsetting to the patient, pre-treatment with ondansetron for gastrointestinal symptoms or mivacurium for muscle aches (Scottish ECT Accreditation Network, 2011) is worthwhile. Pre-treatment with paracetamol can be used for recurrent headache. Sumatriptan may be of value if headache is severe (Markowitz *et al*, 2001).

Monitoring after a course of ECT

At the end of the course the assessment procedures undertaken prior to starting ECT should be repeated. If there is any impairment in cognitive functioning at the end of treatment, further neuropsychological evaluation should take place. Recommendations on appropriate assessment are given in Chapter 8. Most studies of cognitive adverse effects have shown that performance on neuropsychological tests 15 days after ECT have improved beyond baseline levels (Semkovska & McLoughlin, 2010), although there may be subtle impairment of visuospatial memory for at least 1 month after ECT (Falconer *et al*, 2010).

Assessment of mood will be helpful in determining what treatment for relapse prevention will be needed, whether continuation or maintenance ECT (Chapter 17) is indicated or whether changes should be made in pharmacotherapy, such as the introduction of lithium (Chapter 5). Psychological therapy, such as individual cognitive–behavioural therapy or mindfulness-based cognitive therapy could also be considered (National Institute for Health and Clinical Excellence, 2009).

Recommendations

- Monitoring of patients' clinical symptoms, cognitive functioning and physical health before, during and after the course of ECT is an essential requirement for the safe and effective practice of ECT.
- Clinical inspection alone is inadequate to assess seizures produced in ECT; the EEG is an essential tool to ensure that potentially therapeutic seizures have been generated, although there are no specific features on the EEG which can establish whether a seizure actually has produced benefit for the patient.
- Members of the ECT clinic team need to maintain close liaison with the team providing care for the patient throughout the course of ECT.

Acknowledgement

Dr Andrew Whitehouse contributed to the original draft of this chapter, but has not been involved in its revision for this edition of *The ECT Handbook*.

References

Benbow, S., Benbow, J. & Tomenson, B. (2003) Electroconvulsive therapy clinics in the UK should routinely monitor electroencephalographic seizures. *Journal of ECT*, **19**, 217–220.

Dinwiddie, S. H., Huo, D. & Gottlieb, O. (2010) The course of myalgia and headache after electroconvulsive therapy. *Journal of ECT*, **26**, 116–120.

Falconer, D. W., Cleland, J. & Reid, I. C. (2010) Using the Cambridge Neuropsychological Test Automated Battery (CANTAB) to assess the cognitive impact of electroconvulsive therapy on visual and visuo spatial memory. *Psychological Medicine*, **40**, 1017–1025.

Folstein, M., Folstein, S. & McHugh, P. R. (1975) 'Mini-mental state'. A practical method for grading the cognitive state of patients for the clinician. *Journal of Psychiatric Research*, **12**, 189–198.

Guy, W. & Bonato R. R. (1976) *CGI: Clinical Global Impressions in ECDEU Assessment Manual for Psychopharmacology* (revised edn). National Institute for Mental Health.

Hamilton, M. (1960) A rating scale for depression. *Journal of Neurology, Neurosurgery and Psychiatry*, **23**, 56–62.

Hamilton, M. (1987) Electrodermal response as a monitor in ECT. *British Journal of Psychiatry*, **151**, 559.

Lukoff, D., Nuechterlein, K. H. & Ventura, J. (1986) Manual for expanded Brief Psychiatric Rating Scale (BPRS). *Schizophrenia Bulletin*, **12**, 594–602.

Markowitz, J. S., Kellner, C. H., de Vane, C. L., *et al* (2001) Intranasal sumatriptan in post-ECT headache: results of an open-label trial. *Journal of ECT*, **17**, 280–283.

McIlhiney, M. C., Moody, B. J. & Sackeim H. A. (2001) *Autobiograhpical Memory Interview – Short Form: Manual for Administration and Scoring*. Department of Biological Psychiatry, Columbia University.

Montgomery, S. A. & Åsberg, M. (1979) A new depression scale designed to be sensitive to change. *British Journal of Psychiatry*, **134**, 382–389.

National Institute for Health and Clinical Excellence (2009) *Depression: The Treatment and Management of Depression in Adults (Update)* (Clinical Guideline CG90). NICE.

Nobler, M. S., Luber, B., Moeller, J. R., *et al* (2000) Quantitative EEG during seizures induced by electroconvulsive therapy: relations to treatment modality and clinical features. I. Global analyses. *Journal of ECT*, **16**, 211–228.

Piersma, H. L. & Boes, J. L. (1997) The GAF and psychiatric outcome: a descriptive report. *Community Mental Health Journal*, **33**, 35–41.

Sackeim, H. A., Devanand, D. P. & Prudic, J. (1991) Stimulus intensity, seizure threshold, and seizure duration: impact on the efficacy and safety of electroconvulsive therapy. *Psychiatric Clinics of North America*, **14**, 843–844.

Scott A. I. F. (2007) Monitoring electroconvulsive therapy by electroencephalogram: an update for ECT practitioners. *Advances in Psychiatric Treatment*, **13**, 298–304.

Scott, A. I., Shering, P. A. & Dykes, S. (1989) Would monitoring by electroencephalogram improve the practice of electroconvulsive therapy? *British Journal of Psychiatry*, **154**, 853–857.

Scottish ECT Accreditation Network (2011) *Scottish ECT Accreditation Network: Annual Report 2011. A Summary of ECT in Scotland for 2010*. NHS National Services Scotland.

Semkovska, M. & McLoughlin, D. M. (2010) Objective cognitive performance associated with electroconvulsive therapy for depression: a systematic review and meta-analysis. *Biological Psychiatry*, **68**, 568–577.

Weiner, R. D., Coffey, C. E. & Krystal, A. D. (1991) The monitoring and management of electrically induced seizures. *Psychiatric Clinics of North America*, **14**, 845–870.

Whittaker, R., Scott, A. I. & Gardner, M. (2007) The prevalence of prolonged cerebral seizures at the first treatment in a course of electroconvulsive therapy. *Journal of ECT*, **23**, 11–13.

Wise, M. E. J., Mackie, F., Zamar, A. C., *et al* (2000) Investigation of the 'cuff' method for assessing seizure duration in electroconvulsive therapy. *Psychiatric Bulletin*, **24**, 301.

CHAPTER 7

Non-cognitive adverse effects of ECT

Susan M. Benbow and Jonathan Waite

Assessment before ECT

The adverse effects of ECT are a major concern for people treated with ECT, their families and the public. During the assessment process, before the person consents to treatment, the risk–benefit balance for a particular person will be considered and discussed. If there are reasons why this person might be at greater risk of particular adverse effects, ways in which the risk might be minimised should be considered. For example, people with concurrent dementia may be at increased risk of developing cognitive adverse effects during ECT (Griesemer *et al*, 1997; Krystal & Coffey, 1997) and for this reason unilateral ECT may be preferred to bilateral ECT (see Chapter 4). Similarly, people with existing cardiac disease may be at risk of adverse cardiac events during treatment and therefore may be treated more safely in a cardiac care unit with specialist staff to hand (see Chapter 19).

Informed consent

As far as possible, patients and their families should be involved in discussions about the treatment, its likely adverse effects, its possible benefits, any alternative treatments and the risks (if any) of not having the treatment. The use of written as well as verbal information is good practice.

Mortality rate

Electroconvulsive therapy is a low-risk procedure with a mortality rate similar to that of anaesthesia for minor surgical procedures, despite its frequent use in elderly people and those with major medical problems (Sackeim, 1998; Weiner *et al*, 2000). An audit in the USA found that there were no deaths directly related to ECT reported in any Veterans Affairs hospital between 1999 and 2010 (Watts *et al*, 2011). This suggests – based on the number of treatments given – that ECT mortality is less than 1 death per 73 440 treatments.

In earlier studies, Shiwach *et al* (2001) reported on 8148 patients receiving 49 048 ECT treatments in Texas between 1993 and 1998. No patient died during ECT. Thirty patients died within 2 weeks of receiving ECT; the authors felt that one death, which occurred on the day of treatment, could specifically be linked to ECT and four others could plausibly be linked to the treatment. They estimated mortality associated with ECT to be <2/100 000 treatments. A Danish case-register study found a lower mortality rate from natural causes for in-patients treated with ECT compared with other psychiatric patients (Munk-Olsen *et al*, 2007). Rates of death for stroke and cancer were the same for both groups but ECT patients had lower rates of death from cardiac and respiratory disease. The American Psychiatric Association (2001) stated that a reasonable current estimate of the ECT-related adverse effects of ECT mortality rate was 1 per 10 000 patients or 1 per 80 000 treatments; recent studies suggest a lower figure of 1 per 73 440 treatments (Watts *et al*, 2011). This small mortality as a result of treatment must be set in the context of any risks involved in not having ECT. For some people, morbidity and mortality rates with ECT are believed to be lower than with antidepressant drug treatments (Sackeim, 1998).

Cardiovascular and pulmonary complications are the most frequent physical causes of death and serious morbidity (Shiwach *et al*, 2001; Nuttall *et al*, 2004; Munk-Olsen *et al*, 2007). Electroconvulsive therapy clinic protocols and processes should identify individuals who present a high risk and ensure that they are carefully assessed and treated to minimise the risks of ECT (Tess & Smetana, 2009). Such patients require close monitoring during and after the procedure in an environment that will allow rapid intervention should complications occur (see Chapter 19).

Suicide

In the published outcome data from Texas (Shiwach *et al*, 2001) and Denmark (Munk-Olsen *et al*, 2007), several patients died by suicide within a few days of receiving ECT. Neither study included a control group of patients with psychiatric disorder of a severity to warrant ECT: in the Danish study the rate of suicide following ECT was only marginally higher than the rate in all psychiatric in-patients with a relative risk of 1.2. The authors concluded that the most likely explanation for the increased rate of suicide in ECT-treated patients was that patients with suicidal ideation are especially likely to be administered ECT. The US Veterans survey (Watts *et al*, 2011) reports two deaths by suicide, both of which occurred more than a week after the last ECT treatment: poor communication between the ECT team and the out-patient providers was cited as a contributory factor in both cases.

Prolonged seizures

Prolonged seizures and status epilepticus are more likely in people on medication that lowers their seizure threshold, such as theophylline

(Abrams, 2002), or with pre-existing medical conditions that lower their seizure threshold, such as electrolyte imbalance (Finlayson *et al*, 1989). Non-convulsive status epilepticus following ECT may be difficult to diagnose; EEG monitoring will indicate whether or not seizure activity has ceased (Weiner & Krystal, 1993).

Mania

In follow-up studies, about 20% of patients with unipolar depression develop elevated mood (Bailine *et al*, 2010). The natural risk of a switch from depression to mania during recovery in a patient with bipolar disorder is from 4 to 8% (Grunze *et al*, 2010). Similar rates of treatment-emergent affective switches (Tohen *et al*, 2009) are reported among patients treated for depression with ECT (Medda *et al*, 2009; Bailine *et al*, 2010) and antidepressant medication (Grunze *et al*, 2010).

Other non-cognitive adverse effects

After treatment, patients may have headaches (reported after 22% of episodes), muscular aches (9%) or nausea (6%) (Scottish ECT Accreditation Network, 2011). Anorexia, weakness and drowsiness are other frequent adverse effects. Although common, these are usually mild (Dinwiddie *et al*, 2010) and respond to symptomatic treatments (e.g. ondansetron for nausea). People who commonly experience post-ECT headaches may benefit from prophylactic treatment immediately after ECT (e.g. aspirin or a non-steroidal anti-inflammatory drug). Sumatriptan may also be helpful (Markowitz *et al*, 2001). Watts *et al* (2011) found that the most commonly reported more significant adverse effects were injuries to the mouth (see Chapter 9) and problems related to muscle relaxants (see Chapter 3).

Adverse psychological reactions to ECT are rare, but may involve the person developing an intense fear of treatment (Fox, 1993). Support and information are critical in preventing and managing this side-effect.

Regular review during the course of treatment

Regular review is necessary during the course of treatment to detect the possible adverse effects listed above (see also Chapter 6). If any are detected, this should prompt consideration of whether they could be avoided, minimised or treated. Staff in the ECT clinic, in conjunction with other ward or community staff caring for people being treated with ECT, may wish to develop and use standardised assessments of possible treatment-emergent adverse effects.

Recommendations

- During pre-ECT assessment, ways of minimising potential adverse effects should be considered, particularly for individuals who are deemed at high risk of adverse effects during treatment.

- During the consent process, patients should be informed of the likely adverse effects related to treatment within the context of considering the risks and benefits of treatment.
- Doctors prescribing or administering ECT should be aware of particular possible adverse effects of treatment.
- All ECT clinics should have a protocol for the management of prolonged seizures (see Chapter 6).
- People receiving ECT should be regularly monitored during the course of treatment for treatment-emergent objective and subjective adverse effects.
- Ways of preventing, minimising and treating adverse effects should be considered.

References

Abrams, R. (2002) *Electroconvulsive Therapy* (4th edn). Oxford University Press.

American Psychiatric Association (2001) Adverse effects. In *The Practice of Electroconvulsive Therapy: Recommendations for Treatment, Training and Privileging* (2nd edn), pp. 59–76. APA.

Bailine, S., Fink, M., Knapp, R., *et al* (2010) Electroconvulsive therapy is equally effective in unipolar and bipolar depression. *Acta Psychiatrica Scandinavica*, **121**, 431–436.

Dinwiddie, S. H., Huo, D. & Gottlieb, O. (2010) The course of myalgia and headache after electroconvulsive therapy. *Journal of ECT*, **26**, 116–120.

Finlayson, A. J., Vieweg, W. V., Wiley, W. D., *et al* (1989) Hyponatraemic seizure following ECT. *Canadian Journal of Psychiatry*, **34**, 463–464.

Fox, H. A. (1993) Patients' fear of and objection to electroconvulsive therapy. *Hospital and Community Psychiatry*, **44**, 357–360.

Griesemer, D. A., Kellner, C. H., Beale, M. D., *et al* (1997) Electroconvulsive therapy for treatment of intractable seizures: initial findings in two children. *Neurology*, **49**, 1389–1392.

Grunze, H., Vieta, E., Goodwin, G. M., *et al* (2010) The World Federation of Societies of Biological Psychiatry (WFSBP) Guidelines for the Biological Treatment of Bipolar Disorders: Update 2010 on the Treatment of Acute Bipolar Depression. *World Journal of Biological Psychiatry*, **11**, 81–109.

Krystal, A. D. & Coffey, C. E. (1997) Neuropsychiatric considerations in the use of electroconvulsive therapy. *Journal of Neuropsychiatry and Clinical Neurosciences*, **9**, 283–292.

Markowitz, J. S., Kellner, C. H., de Vane, C. L., *et al* (2001) Intranasal sumatriptan in post-ECT headache: results of an open-label trial. *Journal of ECT*, **17**, 280–283.

Medda, P., Perugi, G., Zanello, S., *et al* (2009) Response to ECT in bipolar I, bipolar II and unipolar depression. *Journal of Affective Disorders*, **118**, 55–59.

Munk-Olsen, T., Munk Laursen, T., Videbech, P., *et al* (2007) All-cause mortality among recipients of electroconvulsive therapy. Register-based cohort study. *British Journal of Psychiatry*, **190**, 435–439.

Nuttall, G. A., Bowersox, M. R., Douglass, S. B., *et al* (2004) Morbidity and mortality in the use of electroconvulsive therapy. *Journal of ECT*, **20**, 237–241.

Sackeim, H. A. (1998) The use of electroconvulsive therapy in late-life depression. In *Geriatric Psychopharmacology* (3rd edn) (ed. C. Salzman), pp. 262–309. Williams & Wilkins.

Scottish ECT Accreditation Network (2011) *Annual Report 2011: A Summary of ECT in Scotland for 2010*. NHS National Services Scotland.

Shiwach, R. S., Reid, W. H. & Carmody, T. J. (2001) An analysis of reported deaths following electroconvulsive therapy in Texas, 1993–1998. *Psychiatric Services*, **52**, 1095–1097.

Tess, A. V. & Smetana, G. W. (2009) Medical evaluation of patients undergoing electroconvulsive therapy. *New England Journal of Medicine*, **360**, 1437–1444.

Tohen, M., Frank, E., Bowden, C. L., *et al* (2009) The International Society for Bipolar Disorders (ISBD) Task Force report on the nomenclature of course and outcome in bipolar disorders. *Bipolar Disorders*, **11**, 453–473.

Watts, B. V., Groft, A., Bagian, J. P., *et al* (2011) An examination of mortality and other adverse events related to electroconvulsive therapy using a national adverse event report system. *Journal of ECT*, **27**, 105–108.

Weiner, R. D. & Krystal, A. D. (1993) EEG monitoring of ECT seizures. In *The Clinical Science of Electroconvulsive Therapy* (ed. C. E. Coffey), pp. 93–109. American Psychiatric Press.

Weiner, R. D., Coffey, C. E. & Krystal, A. D. (2000) Electroconvulsive therapy in the medical and neurologic patient. In *Psychiatric Care of the Medical Patient* (2nd edn) (eds A. Stoudemire, B. S. Fogel & D. Greenberg), pp. 419–428. Oxford University Press.

CHAPTER 8

Cognitive adverse effects of ECT

Chris P. Freeman

The study of the impact of ECT on memory begins with Janis's studies (1950), when most ECT was given unmodified and with a sine wave stimulus. Sine wave ECT has not been used in the UK for the past 25 years, although it is still used around the world and, surprisingly, still used in the USA (Sackeim *et al*, 2007). Previous reviews have combined studies undertaken using different electrode placements (see Chapter 4) and different pulse widths, which has made the interpretation of the nature and severity of memory impairment difficult to assess. The recommendations in this chapter are based on studies that have used brief pulse and ultra-brief pulse stimuli carried out mainly from the mid-1980s onwards.

A couple of studies that do not quite fit into the mould are worthy of comment. Ottoson's (1960) landmark research compared three groups with case-matched controls. The groups were high-dose bilateral ECT, a suprathreshold group and a group where the seizure was triggered with a suprathreshold stimulus and then aborted by intravenous lidocaine. The results led to the influential conclusion that it was the electricity rather than the seizure that caused memory impairment, because the high-dose stimulus caused more memory impairment than the suprathreshold and shortening the seizure length with lidocaine did not protect memory. These results have not entirely been borne out by more modern research and are difficult to interpret because Ottoson used a partial (quarter-wave) sine wave stimulus which lies somewhere between traditional sine wave and brief-pulse stimulus. Further research in this area has not clarified the situation. For example:

- Weiner *et al* (1986) found no relationship between stimulus dose and autobiographical memory using brief pulse unilateral and bilateral ECT
- Coffey *et al* (1990) found no relationship between electrical dose and Wechsler Memory Scale scores or time to orientation using brief pulse right unilateral ECT
- Miller *et al* (1985) found a significant relationship between memory impairment and seizure duration with brief pulse right unilateral ECT

- Sackeim *et al* (1986) found a significant correlation between seizure duration and post-ictal disorientation brief pulse right unilateral ECT
- Calev *et al* (1991) found a significant correlation between seizure duration and post-ictal disorientation using brief pulse bitemporal ECT.

Given the above studies, there is probably just sufficient evidence to continue measuring time to re-orientation after each treatment.

Definitions of memory loss

Some definitions of memory loss are given in Box 8.1. None of the types of memory described in Box 8.1 are discrete functions. Memory overlaps with and subsumes other cognitive functions such as learning, attention and overall intelligence.

Does ECT cause cognitive impairment?

The clear answer to this is yes, although the severity, permanence and spectrum of such deficits remain contentious. The most detailed, up-to-date and accurate evidence we have is from two meta-analyses (Semkovska & McLoughlin, 2010; Semkovska *et al*, 2011). The conclusions in this section rely heavily on these papers.

One area that is more difficult to address is the clear difference that has emerged between studies that have involved objective testing of memory and those that have recorded subjective findings, with the latter often reporting much more severe and persistent memory deficits. It is also the case that a small number of patients complain of extremely severe, ubiquitous memory impairment, cognitive changes and sometimes even personality change. There have been no such findings in carefully controlled follow-up studies.

Box 8.1 Types of memory loss

Anterograde amnesia: amnesia for the period after ECT.

Autobiographical memory: store of knowledge of past experiences and learning, sometimes rather confusingly referred to as personal remote memories.

Retrograde amnesia: amnesia for the period prior to ECT.

Working memory: the ability to store and access information in everyday life; often involves accessing both autobiographical memory and new memories that have been laid down after ECT.

What do other bodies say?

The current ECT guidelines from the American Psychiatric Association (2001) do not contain warnings about adverse effects on cognition but advise that most patients report that memory is actually improved by ECT. The American Psychiatric Association practice guidelines on major depressive disorder (2010) acknowledge that ECT may be associated with cognitive adverse effects, including anterograde amnesia.

In all types of information gathered for the review by Philpot *et al* (2004), it was evident that memory loss was a persistent side-effect for at least a third of recipients of ECT. For some, this memory loss profoundly affected their lives and sense of self. The NICE guidelines on ECT (2003) do conclude that cognitive impairment occurs and comment that evidence from users is that cognitive impairment after ECT often outweighed the perception of any benefit from it (p. 16, para. 4.3.8).

Does depression cause cognitive impairment?

Clearly it can and pseudodementia is the most dramatic illustration of this. Many patients show overall improvement after a course of ECT. This is because the balance between ECT caused deficits and relief of depression improving cognitive function is in favour of the latter. These are all pre-post ECT assessments, so markedly improved patients may still have significant cognitive impairment as their pre-ECT functioning may have been very poor.

Squire *et al* (1979) designed the Subjective Memory Questionnaire specifically to distinguish between cognitive impairments caused by depression and those caused by ECT. This is an 18-item self-report questionnaire where patients are asked to compare their memory pre- and post-ECT, rating each item on a 9-point scale (−4, much worse; through to 0, no change; to +4, much improved). The Subjective Memory Questionnaire has stood the test of time and has been shown to have adequate reliability and good construct validity. Van Bergen *et al* (2010) have shown that depression does have marked effects on attention and concentration and new learning, whereas ECT has more marked effect on retrograde amnesia and perhaps visuospacial tasks.

Unfortunately, patients with the most severe depression are usually unable to complete any cognitive tests and assessing their pre-ECT performance is almost impossible. It is worth remembering that most studies on memory and ECT and memory and depression have not included these patients. To state that to confuse the 'temporary effects of depression on cognition (especially attention) and the long-lasting effects of ECT on a range of cognitive functions [...] is unnecessary and could be avoided' somewhat over simplifies a complex clinical area (Robertson & Pryor, 2006: p. 230).

Recent systematic reviews

Semkovsa & McLoughlin (2010) reviewed objective cognitive performance associated with ECT in patients with depression. They included 84 studies (2981 patients) in their meta-analysis and analysed 24 different cognitive variables. One clear problem they had was that they could not identify any standardised retrograde amnesia tests (tests that would measure autobiographical memory). What they found was:

- over 70% of tests showed significant decreases in cognitive performance at 0–3 days after the last ECT
- improvement in test results occurred between 4 and 15 days post-ECT
- by 15 days after the last treatment, no negative effects on cognitive function were measurable
- nearly 60% of tests at 15 days showed improvement with the testing carried out before ECT.

They concluded: 'After 15 days, processing speed, working memory, anterograde memory and some aspects of executive function improved beyond baseline levels'. This study combined patients who had received unilateral and bilateral ECT.

In a second study, Semkovsa *et al* (2011) tried to clarify the differential effects, if any, of unilateral *v.* bilateral ECT. They identified 39 studies, comprising 1415 patients and some 24 cognitive variables. The overall results were similar to the analysis described above but in addition they found:

- bitemporal ECT was associated with more deficits in verbal and visual episodic memory
- brief pulse ECT caused less impairment on visual episodic memory than sine wave ECT
- no relation was found between cognitive change and age
- no relation was found between total number of ECT treatments and cognitive change
- no relation was found between mean electrical dosage and cognitive change.

The authors caution against the premature conclusion that these latter factors may not be associated with increased cognitive impairment, pointing out that many of these factors interact with each other. The authors again come to the conclusion that it is not possible to make any clear statement about retrograde amnesia and comment that this is remarkable given the amount of research that has been done, that this is the area of cognitive function that patients complain about most and that it may be the memory impairment that persists the longest.

Fraser *et al* (2008) conducted a systematic review of autobiographical memory studies, covering papers from 1980 to 2007, yielding 15 studies of ECT and autobiographical memory. Their conclusions were as follows:

- Autobiographical memory impairment does occur as a result of ECT.
- Objective measures found memory loss to be relatively short term (less than 6 months post-treatment).
- Subjective accounts reported amnesia to be more persistent (longer than 6 months post-ECT).
- Electroconvulsive therapy predominantly affects memory of prior personal events that are near the treatment (the 6 months before).
- Autobiographical memory loss is reduced by using brief pulse ECT compared with sine wave ECT.
- Unilateral ECT causes less autobiographical memory loss than bilateral ECT.
- There is less autobiographical memory loss if the electrical current is titrated relative to the patient's own seizure threshold.

There are clearly individual studies which contradict the findings of the three meta-analyses described but picking out individual studies can only be done on an ad hoc (and therefore potentially biased) basis.

Visuospatial memory

It is possible that the earlier-mentioned, very large studies underestimate the cognitive impact of ECT because they concentrate on verbal rather than visuospatial memory. Falconer *et al* (2010) showed more enduring effects, particularly on spatial recognition, using the Cambridge Neuropsychological Test Automated Battery (CANTAB). Although most deficits resolved between testing 1 week and 1 month after ECT, deficits in spatial recognition persisted at 1 month. They concluded that aspects of cognitive function dependant on the use of the right medial temporal lobe and perhaps frontal lobe were most affected. This fits with what patients say about getting lost in the supermarket and not recognising faces (prosopagnosia) after ECT. It clearly has implications for the use of non-dominant unilateral ECT and may mean we should alter our advice about driving after ECT.

What do patients complain of?

Typical complaints are of:

- not being able to hold on to information that has recently been acquired
- memory not being as good as it was before, or not as good as others of their age
- forgetting simple things, such as where they have left their keys
- having to make lists all the time
- not being able to recognise or remember faces or put names to them
- losing the thread of what they are saying as they are saying it
- getting lost in hospital corridors or supermarkets that they could previously easily navigate

- losing important or significant autobiographical memories of holidays, birthdays or important interpersonal events.

What to tell patients and relatives

Patients and their families should be informed in line with the earlier conclusions. They should be told that:

- ECT does cause memory problems
- difficulties with their everyday memory, learning and retaining new information will be relatively short-lived
- because these abilities are affected by both ECT and depression, their everyday memory may function better a few weeks after the end of a course of ECT.

They should be told separately about autobiographical memory, that the effects on this can be longer lasting and may continue for up to 6 months and that, even after that period, some patients complain of gaps or holes in their memory which last much longer.

In addition, they should be told that depression has very marked effects on a wide range of cognitive abilities and that the longer this goes on, the more persistent and enduring those memory problems will become, and therefore relieving depression is important.

How and when to test

Having reviewed all the literature, we have concluded that there are currently no valid, reliable and repeatable tests that can be easily used in routine clinical practice. We are aware that the MMSE (Folstein et al, 1975) is now very widely used in the UK and that some clinics are using the Autobiographical Memory Interview (McIliney et al, 2001). The MMSE was produced as a dementia screening scale. It is almost certainly the wrong test used in the wrong place at the wrong time but has retained its place because it is well known, and clinicians are familiar with using it in other settings. Surprisingly, it has picked up deficits, has shown change and has shown differences between unilateral and bilateral ECT in some studies (Prudic, 2008).

Robertson & Pryor (2006) have recommended a battery of tests which they say are suitable for use after ECT (Box 8.2). Interestingly, they too have no recommendation for autobiographical memory. Their battery is comprehensive and covers non-verbal and visuospatial memory and reasoning, working memory, executive function and reasoning. To carry out even a subset of these tests would take 30–40 min per patient. Although such test batteries might be applicable to research settings or to particular individual cases, they cannot be recommended for routine clinical practice.

Box 8.2 Neuropsychological batteries suitable for use after ECT

Non-verbal and visuospatial memory and reasoning
Benton Visual Retention Test (Sivan, 1992)

Bender Gestalt (Bender, 1938)

Test of Non-verbal Intelligence (Brown *et al*, 1982)

Working memory
Digits Backwards (Wechsler, 1997)

Speaking Span Test (Daneman & Green, 1986)

Executive function
Wisconsin Card Sort (Heaton, 1981)

Halstead Category (Reitan & Wolfson, 1993)

Booklet Category (de Filippis *et al*, 1979)

Reasoning and working memory
Subtests of the Wechsler (1997) such as Arithmetic and Picture arrangement

Reproduced from Robertson & Pryor (2006)

The ethics of cognitive testing

The patient should not be exposed to detailed and repeated cognitive testing, unless part of an ethically approved research study, if that testing is not going to lead to any change of treatment or benefit for the patient. Clearly, testing after a course of ECT is not then going to alter what treatment has already been given. To test during a course of ECT leads to results that are difficult to interpret. Patients should also not be subjected to tests that are lengthy and/or that are not valid or standardised.

The problems of assessing autobiographical memory

This is exemplified by the Autobiographical Memory Test (Williams & Broadbent, 1986). This test has been widely used in research studies, particularly in the USA, and does detect retrograde amnesia at 2 and 6 months post-ECT. There are some problems with it, for example it has not been standardised on a general population and it is only possible to score negatively on it; in other words, it can only measure memories that have been lost. It concentrates on a great deal of overlearned and old information (e.g. grandparents' names, telephone numbers of close relatives) and Robertson & Pryor (2006) have estimated that some 60%

of the 200–300 test items are of this type. Trying to capture unique and idiosyncratic memories that have been lost is clearly a difficult task – putting it simply, the patient does not know what they have forgotten until they are asked to retrieve it, and their assessment that previously they did know something which now they do not remember is a complex and possibly flawed judgement. Janis (1950) came closest to capturing this experience, but he interviewed patients for 1–2 h before treatment, which has no routine clinical utility. Attempts have been made to construct tests of impersonal remote memories (world events) such as the Amsterdam Short-Term Memory Test (Schagen *et al*, 1997) which are constantly kept up to date. Although these are fun to do, they are hugely influenced by culture, intelligence, employment status, etc., and need to be done before and after treatment. They are far too complex for pre-ECT patients with depression. The Kopelman Autobiographical Memory Test (Kopelman *et al*, 1989) is the best we have at present: it has been validated on normal samples and does allow for improvement; however, currently it remains a research rather than a clinical tool.

We currently have no valid, reliable test of remote memory, be it autobiographical or impersonal, that we can use clinically in routine ECT practice.

Key points

- Electroconvulsive therapy causes dysfunction in a wide variety of cognitive skills that is over and above that caused by the patient's pre-existing depression.
- This is clearly and significantly present in the first few days after ECT but then begins to improve and usually remits within 2–3 weeks of the end of a course of ECT.
- After this time, patients function as well on all tests (and better on some) than they could before ECT was started, although patients may still have significant impairment.
- There is a difference in the amount and quality of evidence for deficits and improvement in anterograde amnesia and working memory as compared to retrograde amnesia/autobiographical memory.
- Given several caveats about the quality of the evidence, autobiographical memory is affected by ECT for up to 6 months after the end of an ECT course and then returns to pre-ECT levels.
- For autobiographical memory there are consistent reports of more severe and more persistent dysfunction when subjective and objective reports are compared.

Recommendations

- Measure time to re-orientation using a structured protocol so that this can be estimated to within a few minutes (Box 8.3).

- Reassess the stimulus dose and electrode position if this is markedly prolonged (see Chapter 4).
- Continue to use the MMSE until a more appropriate, reliable, valid and repeatable test is available but recognise that this is the least unacceptable of current tests which can be used in routine clinical practice.
- Make a careful and systematic enquiry of subjective memory complaints at the end of a course of treatment and at 3 and 6 months post-ECT.
- Take subjective complaints of memory impairments seriously and help patients with simple strategies to cope with and overcome these (Box 8.4).

Box 8.3 Protocol for time to re-orientation

1 Develop local protocol depending on clinical population
2 Measure time from stimulus to fully oriented time, place and person
3 Recovery nurse should be responsible for timing and recording
4 Ensure questioning is not too intrusive and not repeated too frequently (e.g. not every 5 mins; usually 15 + mins); timing will depend on how quickly your patients typically recover
5 Ensure information is readily available before next treatment session and available to ward team

---

Box 8.4 Ten points to help patients who complain of persistent memory impairment

1 Take the complaints seriously and enquire in detail
2 Explain again the nature of the memory impairment to the patient and family if appropriate
3 Explain things in everyday terms
4 Encourage the patient to practice specific memory tasks that they find difficult
5 Explain how to use compensation strategies such as lists and labelling, e.g. keeping keys, diary/notebook/wallet or purse in the same labelled drawer
6 Explain the relationship between low mood and memory and check level of depression
7 Consider appropriate accounts from patients; the paper by Donahue (2000) may be a good basis to adapt from
8 Help the patient rehearse strategies if caught out by memory failures, e.g. not recognising a neighbour
9 Consider referral for formal neuropsychological testing if the patient's complaints are marked and very persistent
10 Consider forming links with other clinical services that may routinely be dealing with similar problems, e.g. epilepsy services

References

American Psychiatric Association (2001) *The Practice of Electroconvulsive Therapy: Recommendations for Treatment, Training, and Privileging* (2nd edn). APA.

American Psychiatric Association (2010) *Practice Guideline: Treatment of Patients with Major Depressive Disorder* (3rd edn). APA.

Bender, L. (1938) *A Visual Motor Gestalt Test and Its Clinical Use. Research Monographs 3.* American Orthopsychiatric Association.

Brown, L., Sherbenou, L. J. & Johnsen, S. K. (1982) *Test of Non-Verbal Intelligence.* Pro-Ed.

Calev, A., Nigal, D., Shapira, B., *et al* (1991) Early and long-term effects of electroconvulsive therapy and depression on memory and other cognitive functions. *Journal of Nervous and Mental Diseases*, **179**, 526–533.

Coffey, C. E., Figiel, G. S., Weiner, R .D., *et al* (1990) Caffeine augmentation of ECT. *American Journal of Psychiatry*, **147**, 579–585.

Daneman, M. & Green, I. (1986) Individual differences in comprehending and producing words in context. *Journal of Memory and Language*, **25**, 1–18.

de Filippis, N. A., McCampbell, E. & Rogers, P. (1979) Development of a booklet form of the Category Test: normative and validatory data. *Journal of Clinical Neuropsychology*, **1**, 339–342.

Donahue, A. (2000) Electroconvulsive therapy and memory loss: a personal journey. *Journal of ECT*, **16**, 133–143.

Falconer, D. W., Cleland, J., Fielding, S., *et al* (2010) Using the Cambridge Neuropsychological Test Automated Battery (CANTAB) to assess the cognitive impact of electroconvulsive therapy on visual and visuospatial memory. *Psychological Medicine*, **40**, 1017–1025.

Folstein, M. F., Folstein, S. E. & McHugh P. R. (1975) 'Mini-mental state'. A practical method for gading the cognitive state of patients for the clinician. *Journal of Psychiatric Research*, **12**, 189–198.

Fraser, L. M., O'Carroll R. E. & Ebmeier, K. P. (2008) The effect of electroconvulsive therapy on autobiographical memory: a systematic review. *Journal of ECT*, **24**, 10–17.

Heaton, R. K. (1981) *Wisconsin Card Sorting Test (WCST).* Psychological Assessment Resources.

Janis, I. L. (1950) Psychologic effects of electric convulsive treatments. *Journal of Nervous and Mental Diseases*, **111**, 383–397.

Kopelman, M. D., Wilson, B. A. & Baddeley, A. D. (1989) The autobiographical memory interview: A new assessment of autobiographical and personal semantic memory in amnesic patients. *Journal of Clinical and Experimental Neuropsychology*, **11**, 724–744.

McIliney, M. C., Moody, B. T. & Sackeim, H. A. (2001) *Autobiographical Memory Interview – Short Form: Manual for Administration and Scoring.* Department of Biological Psychiatry, Columbia University.

Miller, A. L., Faber, R. A., Hatch, J. P., *et al* (1985) Factors affecting amnesia, seizure duration, and efficacy in ECT. *American Journal of Psychiatry*, **142**, 692–696.

National Institute for Clinical Excellence (2003) *Guidance on the Use of Electroconvulsive Therapy (Update)* (Technology Appraisal TA59). NICE.

Ottoson, J. O. (1960) Experimental studies of the mode of action of electroconvulsive therapy. *Acta Psychiatrica et Neurologica Scandinavica*, **145**, 1141.

Philpot, M., Collins, C., Trivedi, P., *et al* (2004) Eliciting users views of ECT in two mental health trusts with a user-designed questionnaire. *Journal of Mental Health*, **13**, 403–413.

Prudic, J. (2008) Strategies to minimize cognitive side effects with ECT: aspects of ECT technique. *Journal of ECT*, **24**, 46–51.

Reitan, R. M. & Wolfson, D. (1993) *The Halstead–Reitan Neuropsychological Test Battery: Theory and Clinical Application* (2nd edn). Neuropsychology Press.

Robertson, H. & Pryor, R. (2006) Memory and cognitive effects of ECT: informing and assessing patients. *Advances in Psychiatric Treatment*, **12**, 228–238.

Sackeim, H. A., Portnoy, S., Neeley, P., *et al* (1986) Cognitive consequences of low-dosage electroconvulsive therapy. *Annals of the New York Academy of Sciences*, **462**, 326–340.

Sackeim, H. A., Prudic, J., Fuller, R., *et al* (2007) The cognitive effects of ECT in community settings. *Neuropsychologia*, **32**, 244–254.

Schagen, S., Schmand, B., de Sterke, S., *et al* (1997) Amsterdam Short-Term Memory Test: a new procedure for the detection of feigned memory deficits. *Journal of Clinical and Experimental Neuropsychology*, **19**, 43–51.

Semkovska, M. & McLoughlin, D. M. (2010) Objective cognitive performance associated with electroconvulsive therapy for depression: a systematic review and meta-analysis. *Biological Psychiatry*, **68**, 568–577.

Semkovska, M., Keane, D., Babalola, O., *et al* (2011) Unilateral brief-pulse electroconvulsive therapy and cognition: effects of electrode placement, stimulus dosage and time. *Journal of Psychiatric Research*, **45**, 770–780.

Sivan, A. B. (1992) *Benton Visual Retention Test* (5th edn). Psychological Corporation.

Squire, L. R., Wetzel, C. D. & Slater, P. C. (1979) Memory complaint after electroconvulsive therapy: assessment with a new self-rating instrument. *Biological Psychiatry*, **14**, 791–801.

van Bergen, S., Brands, I., Jelicic, M., *et al* (2010) Assessing trait memory distrust: psychometric properties of the Squire Subjective Memory Questionnaire. *Legal and Criminological Psychology*, **15**, 373–384.

Wechsler, D. (1997) *Wechsler Adult Intelligence Scale III*. Psychological Corporation.

Weiner, R. D., Rogers, H. J., Davidson, J. R. T., *et al* (1986) Effect of stimulus parameters on cognitive side effects. *Annals of the New York Academy of Sciences*, **462**, 315–325.

Williams, J. M. & Broadbent, K. (1986) Autobiographical memory in suicide attempters. *Journal of Abnormal Psychology*, **95**, 144–149.

CHAPTER 9

Dental issues related to ECT

Denis Martin

This chapter is designed to raise awareness of the risks of damage to dental tissue during ECT, with the possible consequences to the patient, ECT team, psychiatrists and anaesthetists, and to place dental risk into context. Although the first section of the chapter is more applicable to psychiatrists and the second section to anaesthetists, the issue of dental risk bridges both specialties. The entire chapter should be read by all staff involved with the delivery of ECT.

Dental issues for psychiatrists

There is a general view among psychiatrists that any dental or jaw problems associated with ECT should be managed by the anaesthetist at the time of the treatment. It is expected that the anaesthetist, during their pre-anaesthetic assessment, will identify any dental risks and work towards their safe management.

Recent research from the USA (Watts *et al*, 2011) indicates that oral (dental and tongue) injuries are the most common complication of ECT. Patients seem to accept this risk identification and management process as being part of the anaesthetist's domain and do not see it as being related to the ECT itself. A literature search found that the risk of dental injury (excluding soft tissue injury) is about 1–2% (Beli & Bentham, 1998) and suggests that this process has worked well. Information from the Medical Defence Union indicates that litigation following dental injury or damage is rare and this is mirrored in American psychiatry (Slawson, 1989). However, recent developments including legal issues of risk management and consent, patient attitude to dental health, the role of private dentistry and technological advances in dentistry make a reappraisal of dental risk management within ECT appropriate.

Although the management of dental risks during the ECT session is likely to remain with the anaesthetist, the overall management of risks from ECT are the psychiatrist's responsibility. Injury to the teeth during ECT is a well-established risk (Beli & Bentham,1998) and therefore needs to be considered in the process of obtaining consent. See Chapter 22 for details on consenting and risk factors in ECT.

Risks to jaws and teeth during ECT are the direct result of the ECT and not the anaesthetic. Electroconvulsive therapy can cause dental damage by two means. First, bitemporal electrode placement leads directly to stimulation of the muscles of mastication during treatment (Fig. 9.1). Temporalis, being beneath the electrode, is totally stimulated. The lateral spread of the stimulus current causes depolarisation of the muscles of expression, which accounts for the observed grimacing of the patient and also the masseter muscle. The medial pterygoids are too deep to be affected.

This direct stimulation bypasses neuromuscular blockade (see Chapter 3) – as a result, the jaw muscles are stimulated to 60–75% of their maximal contractive force during the stimulus current phase.

Second, as the patient is unconscious during ECT, pressures on the teeth, usually limited by conscious control, can be exceeded and result in damage.

The potential for damage to the teeth and jaw is greatest during the passage of the stimulus current. Once the stimulus current has finished, during the stage of the modified convulsion, all impulses to the jaw muscles from the brain via the motor branch of the trigeminal nerve are blocked by the muscle relaxant.

The primary function of the anaesthetist is to manage the anaesthetic and safeguard the patient's airway. Minimising the risks due to forceful striated muscle contraction throughout the body and protecting the teeth is a secondary role.

Psychiatrists need to be aware of potential dental injuries occurring during electrical stimulation. Recent technological advances, especially dental implants and modern ceramics, have allowed the development of complex restorations with excellent aesthetics. This has replaced the need for dentures and unacceptable aesthetic restorations. It is now possible to implant teeth in the upper posterior jaw region by the ablation of the maxillary sinus, and in both jaws it is possible to support artificial teeth on intraosseous implants.

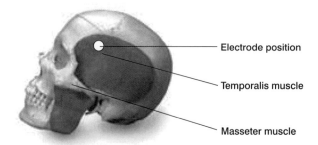

Electrode position

Temporalis muscle

Masseter muscle

Fig. 9.1 Position of electrode in bilateral ECT and the relation to the muscles of mastication.

There may now be candidates for ECT who have a high dental awareness and possess complex dental restoration work. Any damage to these dental structures occurring during ECT will therefore, almost certainly, constitute a 'serious injury' for that individual patient, with the potential for a claim for compensation or other legal redress. As a result of the ongoing trends in dentistry, this group of patients will increase in number and could become a significant potential risk area for ECT. It is therefore necessary to identify patients with cosmetic dentistry in advance, in order to establish valid consent and manage the identified dental risks appropriately.

There is considerable overlap in the management of these patients and those in the 'at risk group' identified by Beli & Bentham (1998). Here, the risks were as a direct result of dental negligence, where decayed teeth and periodontal disease dominated the clinical picture. The expectation is therefore that all patients presenting for ECT with identified dental risks should be managed prospectively. The following is a risk management strategy adapted and evolved from the suggestions of Beli & Bentham (1998) and Morris (2002). The proposed strategy is in four stages: the risks, risk awareness, risk identification and risk management.

The risks

Electroconvulsive therapy exposes the dental tissue to the risk of damage. This includes the soft tissue as well as the teeth and dental restorations. Tongue and lip trauma occur in about 20% of cases, damage to hard tissues in 1% to 2% (Beli & Bentham, 1998). Consideration must also be given to the risk of claims for negligence and compensation. If the consent process did not address the possibility of dental damage, then that consent may be invalid.

Risk awareness

This section provides specialist information to professionals involved with the consent process and pre-ECT assessment, to raise awareness of the existence of dental risk from ECT. Dental risk can be seen as the product of the ECT process and the dental status of the individual patient. Psychiatric patients commonly have poor dental health (Stevens et al, 2010). The presence of the following is related to an increase in the risk of dental damage for an individual patient:

- crowns, bridges, implants or veneers
- periodontal disease and gum recession
- heavily filled or root-filled teeth
- gaps where teeth have been lost, the presence of dentures
- loose teeth
- teeth that are painful or on which the patient is afraid to bite for fear of damage
- jaw or temporomandibular joint disease or previous jaw surgery.

Risk identification

The assessment process should consist of a dental history taken to identify the risk factors mentioned earlier. This may need to be supplemented by information from the patient's dental surgeon or relatives. An examination of the mouth and teeth must be performed to verify the presence of any risk factors. Dentures should be checked for evidence of intraosseous fixation devices, and jaw opening and closing assessed.

The examination should be carried out by dentally experienced personnel (Morris, 2002), preferably a dentist with experience of ECT. The possibility of this role being carried out by suitably trained ECT staff should be considered, although access to dental services is a requirement for the accreditation of acute in-patient mental health services by the Royal College of Psychiatrists' AIMS scheme (Lelliott *et al*, 2006).

Risk management

For consent to be valid, all risks that may produce a significant event to the patient must be considered. It is necessary to balance the risk of dental damage against the need for ECT. The following points should be taken into account:

- The identified risks should be discussed with the patient by the consenting psychiatrist.
- Renegotiation of consent to include the identified dental risks may be necessary in order to establish 'valid consent'.
- Liaison with the anaesthetist is essential; if risk factors are identified the use of appropriate techniques by the anaesthetist at the time of treatment can minimise these.
- Specialist dental referral may be needed for advice or the provision of specially constructed bite guards. It may be appropriate to postpone ECT until this stage is completed.
- Prescribing unilateral ECT will reduce jaw pressures by 50%, as only one side of the jaw muscles are stimulated.
- Patients who will not comply with or consent to an oral examination because they lack capacity should be managed within the framework of mental health and mental capacity legislation; legal advice may be needed. Appropriate documentation and records are essential.
- A post-treatment review of the patient's dental status, with appropriate documentation, should be performed.

Dental issues for anaesthetists

During the stimulus current phase of ECT, teeth with large restorations or crowns are at risk of fracture, and teeth with bridges and implants are vulnerable to being dislodged or displaced. This is due to considerable axial or non-axial forces acting on the teeth. The force is transmitted to the jaws by direct stimulation of the muscles of mastication. Practical management is directed at reducing these axial or non-axial forces to safe levels. As all patients are different dentally, it is difficult to be specific in offering advice on management. The following points are general points to consider:

- Has a dental examination been completed?
- Have any risks been identified?
- Has the consent process of the psychiatrist drawn attention to dental risks?
- Are you able to minimise the identified risks by use of a bite guard and its judicious placement in the mouth?
- Consider obtaining specialist advice (patient's dental surgeon or oral surgery department) and the provision of individually made bite guards.
- Consider suggesting withholding treatment if further assessment or advice is needed.
- Consider requesting unilateral ECT – this will reduce the possible jaw pressures by 50%.
- Initiate a post-treatment dental review.

Brief review of specific dental restorations and associated risks

Veneers

Avoid 'point loading' on the incisal edges or contact with metal objects to minimise the risk of fracture.

Crowns

Unless a tooth has been crowned for purely cosmetic reasons, consider that beneath the crown is likely to be a heavily restored tooth, which may have been root-filled. Such non-vital teeth may be brittle and more liable to fracture. There may be apical pathology, so the root may be relatively unsupported. Anterior teeth restored by the 'post crown' procedure are at increased risk of damage.

Bridges

These are designed to replace a lost tooth with a non-removable prosthesis. If both supporting teeth are sound, there should be no increased risk with ECT. A problem exists when one of the supporting teeth becomes weakened, perhaps due to periodontal disease. When the patient is conscious, the pressure applied to the bridge can be consciously limited to safe levels. When the patient is unconscious during ECT, excessive pressure on the bridge may move the weakened tooth and apply damaging torsional forces to the other support tooth. It would be prudent to test all bridge 'support teeth' independently prior to ECT and off-load the bridge if concern exists.

Anterior bridges are at considerable risk if loaded during ECT, especially if the bite guard becomes pushed up behind the front teeth. The risk increases if the teeth on the bridge follow the curve of the dental arch.

Implants

Implants fill gaps in the dental arches with non-removable teeth and like bridges obviate the need for dentures. The artificial teeth are supported on pegs that are inserted into alveolar bone and in time become integral with it. These teeth have no periodontal membrane and therefore lack the ability to move slightly under pressure. This, together with the fact that the peg is usually much smaller than the natural root, means that they are more likely to be dislodged during ECT. They should not be loaded if at all possible.

Intraosseous denture supports

It is now possible to fix screws, bars or bolts into the alveolar bone or facial skeleton on which dentures can be located. The decision to be made is whether to remove the denture or give ECT with it kept in the mouth. Specialist advice should be sought on this point.

Clinical situations that require different management strategies

The fully dentate patient

Choose the thinnest bite guard possible to avoid excessive pressure on the back teeth. If the overbite or overjet is large, do not allow the bite guard to be forced up behind the upper anterior teeth by the lower anterior teeth. This could displace the upper teeth forwards, especially in the elderly patient or in the presence of gum disease.

The mouth with complex restorations

The presence of crowns, bridges and implants can cause management problems, as they may not be capable of withstanding the forces applied to the teeth during the stimulus current phase. Implants are supported by about 50% or less of the root size of the natural tooth that it replaces and must be considered to be at risk during ECT. In general, it is best to 'off-load' any of the above by the judicious placement of the bite guard.

If it is not possible to avoid such teeth, then their ability to withstand pressure could be assessed by a 'dry-run', with the teeth being loaded by jaw pressure in the patient during the pre-ECT assessment stage.

Implants that are most vulnerable to axial overloading forces are posterior teeth implants, especially those in the upper jaw where they may be sited over an ablated maxillary antrum. Anterior teeth implants are vulnerable to lateral (anterior) forces and could be dislodged by the bite guard during the stimulus current phase. Consider requesting unilateral ECT and off-loading such teeth.

The edentulous patient

Do not allow the jaw to overclose beyond centric during treatment to avoid gum, muscle or joint damage. The articulating disc can be damaged if the joint is put under pressure in the overclosed position. Use packs or consider using the dentures to maintain the jaw in the correct position during treatment. Upper acrylic dentures may be vulnerable to midline fractures if pressure is applied to both sides of the jaws. Consider limiting the pressure to one side by using a small prop on one side only. Consider requesting the use of unilateral ECT to reduce jaw pressure.

The partially dentate patient

This is the situation where one or both jaws have had teeth extracted. The resultant gaps may or may not be filled by dentures. The main issue is that solitary standing teeth are at risk of being exposed to excessive forces. It may be appropriate to consider using the dentures to support the teeth and spread the load. However, acrylic dentures may fracture, but metal-based dentures should not. The other option is to request that a specially designed bite guard is constructed to spread the load on to the alveolar ridges as well as support these solitary teeth. Solitary teeth that cannot be supported should not be loaded at all.

Key points

- Dental injuries are a common complication of ECT.
- Dental injuries are a direct result of contraction of the muscles during ECT.
- Psychiatric patients often have poor dental health.
- Modern techniques of dental restoration are costly and the resulting structures are vulnerable to damage.
- The consent process must address issues of dental risk.

References

Beli, N. & Bentham, B. (1998) Nature and extent of dental pathology and complications arising in patients receiving ECT. *Psychiatric Bulletin*, **22**, 562–565.

Lelliott, P., Bennett, H., McGeorge, M., *et al* (2006) Accreditation of acute in-patient mental health services. *Psychiatric Bulletin*, **30**, 361–363.

Morris, A. (2002) A dental risk management protocol for electroconvulsive therapy. *Journal of ECT*, **18**, 84–89.

Slawson, P. (1989) Psychiatric malpractice and ECT: a review of national loss experience. *Convulsive Therapy*, **5**, 126–130.

Stevens, T., Spoors, J., Hale, R., *et al* (2010) Perceived oral health needs in psychiatric in-patients: impact of a dedicated dental clinic. *The Psychiatrist*, **34**, 518–521.

Watts, B. V., Groft, A., Bagian, J. P., *et al* (2011) An examination of mortality and other adverse events related to electroconvulsive therapy using a national adverse event report system. *Journal of ECT*, **27**, 105–108.

CHAPTER 10

Training, supervision and professional development: achieving competency

Grace M. Fergusson, Daniel M. Bennett and Susan M. Benbow

The Royal College of Psychiatrists (2009) recommend that a senior psychiatrist, preferably a consultant, is responsible for the ECT clinic. For a standard clinical service, a minimum of one contracted session per week is recommended for the duties of an ECT consultant. The ECT consultant is responsible for making sure that the clinic keeps up to date with developments in ECT practice, achieves the necessary quality standards, and that all medical staff giving ECT are properly trained and supervised.

The duties of the psychiatrist responsible for ECT can be divided into four main areas:

1   organisation of the clinic
2   treatment policy
3   training and supervision; achieving competency
4   achieving and maintaining appropriate service standards.

This chapter outlines the role of the psychiatrist responsible for ECT and describes how medical staff achieve and demonstrate their competencies.

Organisation of the clinic

The location and fabric of the ECT clinic, including the ECT machine, should meet the standards set out in Chapter 2.

The clinic should be served by a small core team of senior anaesthetists, supported by appropriately trained personnel with a special interest in ECT and with whom discussion can take place regarding treatment protocols and responsibilities.

Nurse staffing should be as described in Chapter 11 and there should be good liaison with nurse management to ensure that these guidelines are being adhered to.

The ECT rota should be organised in such a way to ensure that continuity of patient care is maximised and that trainees have the opportunity to treat patients over several consecutive treatments. It is important that doctors training in psychiatry receive training in the practice of ECT, and the core curriculum states that 'all Core training programmes must ensure that there is training and supervision in the use of ECT so that trainees become proficient in the prescribing, administration and monitoring of this treatment' (Royal College of Psychiatrists, 2009). Electroconvulsive therapy consultants who have difficulty in maintaining the attendance of trainees are advised to consider whether this should be treated as an issue of professional practice/probity. These issues should be raised using the standard routes as set out in the *Gold Guide* (Modernising Medical Careers, 2010). This is likely to include discussion with the educational supervisor and training programme director in the first instance.

Although it is considered mandatory that core trainees have access to training in the practice of ECT, other trainees should not be excluded from such training. This will depend on local arrangements, but trainees in general practice, foundation programmes and in higher specialist training should all be able to access ECT training.

Treatment policy

The administration of ECT must take account of many factors to ensure that each treatment is tailored to each individual patient: the aim is to maximise efficacy while minimising side-effects. Knowledge regarding the mechanism of ECT, technical aspects of treatment and factors affecting outcome is continually advancing and this informs the development of optimum treatment protocols.

The relationship between the clinical team and ECT team needs to be defined with clarity and understanding about shared responsibility. In general, the patient's psychiatrist (i.e. from their clinical team) will prescribe ECT and the ECT consultant will determine the dose of electricity to be delivered. The precise details of the relationship between the two will depend on local circumstances, but in all situations there is a need for a clear two-way communication between prescribing and treating teams if the treatment is to be as effective as possible.

Treatment protocols should cover:

- consent to treatment
- prescription of ECT
- pre-ECT work up, including liaison with the anaesthetist if necessary
- ECT for special populations, including day patients, patients going home on leave between treatments, and patients deemed to be at higher risk
- administration of ECT to include:
  - bilateral *v.* unilateral electrode placement
  - determination of the initial treatment dose
  - a stimulus dosing policy, i.e. how to adjust the stimulus dose according to response, in terms of both seizure length and/or clinical response

- termination of prolonged seizures
- procedure for dealing with missed seizures
- treatment records, including details of the machine settings and the observed seizure, stating the method of timing, whether by stopwatch, machine or EEG
- observations in the recovery period to include the recording of any immediate post-ECT confusion or other side-effects
- assessments by staff and patients of outcome, including side-effects, between treatments and at the end of the course.

Training and supervision: achieving competency

Electroconvulsive therapy consultants need to be able to demonstrate that they are competent to undertake the responsibilities of the role. The College has developed a competency framework which sets out the competencies they are expected to achieve and maintain (Appendix II). These cover:

- theory and background
- practical aspects of treatment
- other aspects including: involvement in audit; undertaking 1 day of continuing professional development in ECT practice per year; advising consultant colleagues regarding ECT practice; regular review of policies and procedures; and training and supervision of doctors in training.

Thus responsible consultants will need to include ECT in their continuing professional development programme, to attend formal update training, and to keep up to date with research developments. A module on the prescription of ECT can be found on the College website (www.rcpsych.ac.uk/publications/cpdonline.aspx), and consultants of services that use ECT infrequently should arrange to attend a neighbouring clinic for practical updates.

The competency framework (Appendix II) also sets out the competencies which consultants who prescribe ECT should demonstrate, and updating their colleagues is another role which ECT consultants may undertake.

The training and supervision of staff is probably the most time-consuming duty of the ECT consultant. It is no longer possible to include all the variables of treatment in one simple schedule, therefore trainees administering ECT should not be left unsupervised until they have achieved a range of competencies (Appendix II). The training programme should include:

- the theoretical background of ECT
- awareness of current guidelines and standards
- an introduction to treatment protocols and demonstration of technique

- initial supervision – a minimum of six treatments in total to three different patients is recommended
- continued supervision until competence is achieved; the time taken for this will vary from trainee to trainee and will also depend on how busy the clinic is.

Trainees' competencies for ECT

Electroconvulsive therapy consultants should be aware of the specific competencies for trainees with regard to ECT. These can be found within the MRCPsych curriculum for specialist core training in psychiatry (Royal College of Psychiatrists, 2010).

One method of demonstrating that such competencies have been achieved would be for the trainee to ask the ECT consultant to provide feedback and complete a workplace-based assessment – this would be in addition to trainees being expected to achieve the appropriate ECT competencies. The most common type of workplace-based assessment used is a direct observation of procedural skills (DOPS). The standardised form and guidance on workplace-based assessments can also be found on the College's website (www.rcpsych.ac.uk/traininpsychiatry/corespecialtytraining.aspx).

Where other trainees, such as foundation or general practice, are accessing ECT training, this should be broadly similar to that provided to core trainees. It is also important to remember that these trainees also have workplace-based assessments to complete and the systems are slightly different from those described above.

Achieving and maintaining appropriate service standards

Two systems of audit and accreditation operate in the UK:

1 the ECT Accreditation Service (ECTAS) for England and Wales (www.rcpsych.ac.uk/cru/ECTAS.htm)
2 the Scottish ECT Accreditation Network (SEAN) for Scotland (www.sean.org.uk).

The ECT consultant will be expected to take a lead in discussion with management to make sure that all aspects of the service reach the standards expected for safe and effective delivery of treatment.

Key points

- Doctors prescribing ECT should be competent to do so.
- Supervision should continue until treating doctors are competent.
- All ECT staff should undertake continued professional development.

References

Modernising Medical Careers (2010) *A Reference Guide for Postgraduate Specialty Training in the UK* (4th edn). National Health Service.

Royal College of Psychiatrists (2009) ECT training. In *Specialist Training in Psychiatry: A Comprehensive Guide to Training and Assessment in the UK for Trainees and Local Educational Providers* (Occasional Paper OP69), p. 78. Royal College of Psychiatrists.

Royal College of Psychiatrists (2010) *A Competency Based Curriculum for Specialist Core Training in Psychiatry: Core Training in Psychiatry CT1–CT3*. Royal College of Psychiatrists.

CHAPTER 11

Nursing guidelines for ECT

Linda Cullen, Stephen Finch and Eamonn Heaney

The responsibilities of the ECT nurse specialist have continued to expand and develop over recent years. It is now widely recognised that this is an expert role which is pivotal within the ECT core team. This chapter outlines the guidelines for best practice and describes the main responsibilities of the nurses involved in the ECT process (see also Appendices III and IV).

The role and responsibilities of the ward nurse

The ward nurse should be able to provide care and support for both the patient and their relatives before and after treatment on the ward. They should be familiar with the requirements for the treatment in order for them to accurately and sensitively inform both the patient and their relatives of what to expect during the course of treatment. The ward nurse requires the following knowledge and skills:

- A good knowledge of current national guidelines and standards, including ECTAS (Cresswell *et al*, 2012), SEAN (2010), Royal College of Nursing (Finch, 2005), Royal College of Psychiatrists (Waite & Easton, 2013), Association of Anaesthetists of Great Britain and Ireland (2010), NICE (2003) and Nursing and Midwifery Council (2008).
- A good working knowledge of local ECT guidelines, protocols and policies.
- A good working knowledge of the requirements of legal status and consent to treatment, including prescription.
- A good basic knowledge of the following:
  - referral process
  - indications for ECT
  - risks and benefits of ECT
  - contraindications to ECT
  - pre-ECT investigations and significance of results
  - potential drug interactions with ECT
  - preparation of the patient for ECT

- requirements for day-case/out-patient ECT
- possible side-effects of ECT
- the anaesthetic procedure for ECT including risks and potential side-effects
- the ECT procedure
- unilateral and bilateral ECT differences, risks and benefits
- continuation or maintenance ECT
- drugs used in ECT and their potential side-effects
- post-ECT observations on return to the ward
- the review process between treatments
- protocol for patients going out on pass following ECT.

Role and responsibilities of the escort nurse

Each patient should be individually escorted from the ward through ECT and recovery and back to the ward. The escorting nurse should always be a registered nurse. If the escort role is delegated to an unqualified member of staff/care assistant, then it is the delegating nurse who will be held accountable for the consequences of that delegation. To this end, adequate staffing levels should be agreed with management and provision made to meet the staffing needs on ECT treatment days. This may require treatments to be staggered to ensure adequate staffing levels from wards and this should be arranged at local level between ward staff and the ECT team.

Escorting nurses should know the patients they are escorting and be aware of their legal status, consent and any possible medical complications. They should ensure the safekeeping of patients' valuables or any prosthesis (although any prosthesis should not be removed until immediately before treatment at the ECT clinic). The escorting nurse should know the location of the toilets in the ECT clinic and the arrangements for further appointments for the patient.

The escort nurse should be able to provide care and support for the patient throughout the process of ECT. They should be familiar with the requirements for the treatment in order for them to accurately and sensitively inform and support the patient throughout the treatment.

The escort nurse requires the following knowledge and skills in addition to those required for ward nurses:

- up-to-date training in basic life support
- a good knowledge of the transport requirements for individual patients in accordance with their manual handling risk assessment
- a good knowledge of the ECT process
- to act as an advocate for the patient, assessing concerns and feeding these back to the members of the ECT team
- a good knowledge of what their role is during the treatment and in recovery (in accordance with local protocols)

- a good working knowledge of local ECT guidelines, protocols and policies
- a good basic knowledge of:
  - the layout of the ECT clinic and location of routine and emergency equipment
  - the emergency protocol for the treating hospital (which may be different to that of the prescribing hospital)
  - the fasciculation process
  - the significance of missed seizures
  - the significance of prolonged seizures
  - timing of seizure protocol
  - moving and handling protocol at ECT
  - post-anaesthetic complications
  - completing required documentation
  - discharge from recovery protocol
  - the support required for the individual patient during transfer back to ward or hospital
  - passing on relevant information to the prescribing team.

Role and responsibilities of the ECT nurse specialist

The nurse responsible for the running of the ECT clinic should be a registered nurse who is a minimum of a Band 6, or Band 7 if they are a budget holder (equivalent to CNM2 in Ireland). They should be a designated person who is primarily employed as an ECT nurse specialist or seconded to this role (it should not be left to a nurse or group of nurses drafted in from a ward that are available on the day of treatment). There should be a fully trained deputy who regularly attends ECT and is available to provide cover for the clinic during absence of the nurse in charge. The nurse should have protected time to carry out all the duties required and should not be expected to be covering a ward or have other responsibilities on the days of treatment.

The ECT nurse specialist is best placed to meet with patients and/or relatives to discuss the procedure and any concerns, as they should be in possession of the most up-to-date information. Both written and verbal information on ECT should be given to all patients and specific day-case/out-patient information should be given to those attending for day-case/out-patient ECT. This opportunity can be used to show the patient around the ECT clinic if appropriate. Meeting the ECT nurse specialist before the first treatment session can help to reduce the patient's anxieties as the patient may recognise a familiar face when attending the clinic and this also provides better continuity of care.

The protected time allocated should be adequate to allow the ECT nurse specialist to carry out the following areas of responsibility and should also reflect the level of activity at the clinic:

- spending time with patients and relatives in order to provide support, information and review
- ensuring a safe environment for patients and staff
- liaising with the prescribing teams and ECT team
- organising, coordinating and managing treatment sessions
- updating of protocols, policies and documentation in line with current national standards and guidelines
- audit and risk assessment
- training (staff and personal)
- administration
- maintenance of equipment and environment
- ordering and stocking of treatment suite.

The ECT nurse specialist requires the following knowledge and skills:

- specialist knowledge of ECT related to theory, efficacy, practices and procedures
- in-depth understanding of the legal issues relating to consent to ECT and the relevant mental health and capacity acts (including amendments and codes of practice)
- ability to implement policy and service development in a manner consistent with the principles and standards at national and local level, and to observe recommendations from ECTAS (Cresswell *et al*, 2012), SEAN (2010), Royal College of Nursing (Finch, 2005), Royal College of Psychiatrists (Waite & Easton, 2013), Association of Anaesthetists of Great Britain and Ireland (2010), NICE (2003) and the Nursing and Midwifery Council (2008)
- ability to work without direct supervision in clinical practice.
- management and clinical supervision of all junior staff in the department
- attendance and contributions to regional and national ECT special interest groups
- management of the departmental financial budget to accommodate physical and environmental maintenance, repair and replacement cost (where applicable)
- ability to provide the most up-to-date information and specialist education for service users, relatives and carers in an appropriate manner
- ability to assist the lead ECT consultant in providing specialist training to junior medical staff
- ability to provide specialist training as part of the local induction programme for all new staff (qualified and unqualified)
- ability to manage and provide specialist training in ECT for qualified nursing staff both on the wards and at ECT
- ability to supervise, guide and advise other nursing staff and disciplines as required, to encompass all aspects of managing care, including infection control

- ability to coordinate education of multidisciplinary team and students within their locality
- efficient use of staffing resources in the treatment areas, ensuring that staffing levels are safe, appropriate and contain the necessary skill mix at each treatment session
- ability to provide evidence-based practice
- ability to maintain statistical records
- ability to conduct ongoing audits and provide reports to the senior management team and lead ECT consultant to ensure high standards are achieved and maintained.

Before a treatment session

The ECT nurse specialist should carry out the following:

- ensure all equipment involved with the delivery of ECT has been checked and a record kept of the individual carrying out the check
- ensure there are sufficient supplies of drugs required for the treatment session
- ensure there an adequate number of appropriately trained staff to carry out the treatment session
- liaise with referring wards and the prescribing team to ensure that the information on the patient is up to date and all relevant investigations have been carried out before treatment (then pass on any significant results to the other members of the ECT team)
- organise and schedule appointments for treatments for both in-patients and day-case/out-patients to ensure smooth running of the treatment session and minimise waiting time for individuals
- provide information and support for patients and their relatives (where possible).
- ensure ward-based staff are aware of how to prepare patients (routine investigations required, accompanying documentation, ECT care pathway, etc. – a protocol containing all of this information should be available to all the wards that are likely to refer patients for ECT)
- coordinate the ECT team and keep them informed of times, patient numbers, patient details and any other significant information
- discuss the treatment of the next patient with the team before that patient enters, which may include checking and setting the treatment dose with the psychiatrist (this must be checked again verbally before the treatment button is pressed, as per local protocol).

During a treatment session

The ECT nurse specialist should carry out the following:

- record routine pre-ECT nursing checks on patients when they attend for treatment, or delegate this task to a suitably trained assistant or deputy

- check the patient's legal status, consent and capacity and that all relevant documentation is present (e.g. case notes, nursing notes, consent form, legal documents, record of medication)
- ensure that any concerns or issues arising from nursing checks on patients are passed on to the relevant members of the ECT team (e.g. changes to consent, legal status, capacity, medication or physical condition)
- provide support and reassurance for patients while they are in the clinic
- ensure the safety and comfort of the patient throughout the treatment.
- introduce the ECT team to the patient
- carry out any required preparation of the patient (e.g. applying the ECG and EEG electrodes)
- assist the psychiatrist with the timing of the duration of the seizure by use of the chosen method (e.g. stopwatch, Hamilton cuff technique, EEG monitoring, in accordance with local protocols)
- observe the patient throughout treatment and record observations such as oxygen saturation, blood pressure, heart rate, seizure duration and quality, EEG monitoring, time to spontaneous breathing and any other significant events (unless done by the anaesthetist, anaesthetic assistant or psychiatrist, as agreed by local protocols)
- assist with placing the patient in the recovery position prior to transfer to the recovery area as per local protocol
- escort the patient through to the recovery area and ensure relevant information is passed on to the nurse in charge of recovery (the anaesthetist should pass on any specific instructions to the nurse in charge of recovery); any drugs, intravenous fluids or oxygen to be administered should have a written prescription
- prepare the treatment room for the next patient (change single-use equipment, clean or change electrodes, etc.).
- discuss the treatment of the next patient with the team before the patient enters, including checking and setting the treatment dose with the psychiatrist (this must be checked again verbally before the treatment button is pressed, as per local protocol).

The nurse should be fully conversant with the use of the particular ECT machine in the clinic and should carry out the self-test procedure in accordance with the manufacturer's instructions and local protocol.

The ECT nurse specialist should not administer the treatment but, if suitably trained, could assist the psychiatrist by operating the controls on the fascia of the ECT machine while the psychiatrist applies the electrodes. The nurse should check the dose (which should be set by the psychiatrist) and static impedance, and confirm verbally with the psychiatrist before pressing the treat button. This should be done in accordance with a locally agreed protocol. There should be a minimum of two suitably trained nurses in the treatment room during the administration of the treatment (e.g. ECT nurse specialist and escort nurse). A suitably trained anaesthetic assistant (operating department practitioner, theatre practitioner or anaesthetic assistant) should always be present during the treatment, in accordance with guidelines laid down by the Royal College of Anaesthetists (2011) and the Association of Anaesthetists of Great Britain and Ireland (2010) (this must not be the ECT nurse specialist, who should not be performing a dual role).

After a treatment session

It is advantageous for the ECT nurse specialist (where possible) to be able to visit patients on the afternoon of their treatment as this allows the nurse to follow-up patients and the opportunity to observe any side-effects and address any concerns or anxieties that the patient may have. It also provides better continuity of care, and helps to build a more therapeutic relationship between the patient and the ECT nurse specialist, helping to reduce patients' anxieties for consequent treatments. The ECT nurse specialist should provide feedback to both the prescribing team and ECT team, and ensure that all relevant documentation has been completed. After treatment, the ECT nurse specialist should ensure that day-case/ out-patients are not discharged until fully recovered. (It is good practice for the ECT nurse specialist to have them seen by a doctor before agreeing their discharge home.) Day-case patients must be collected by a responsible adult and should not be allowed to leave alone or drive a vehicle. (Patients and the person collecting them should be reminded of this before they leave and advised to consult the specific day-case/out-patient information they were given at the outset of treatment.)

Administrative duties

The ECT nurse specialist should:

- be familiar with local and national guidelines and should regularly assist in updating protocols and policies accordingly
- complete ECT records on each patient's visit to the ECT clinic in accordance with the local protocol
- carry out regular audits of practice and patient care.

Maintenance of equipment and environment

The ECT nurse specialist should:

- ensure the ECT clinic is a safe environment for patients, staff and visitors
- organise regular maintenance of equipment and the environment and keep detailed records on this
- ensure medical equipment that requires a maintenance contract has one in place (check with medical physics)

- carry out and keep updated risk assessments within the unit and take action to address any issues of concern
- be familiar with the use of all the equipment in the ECT clinic
- check expiry dates on all disposable equipment and order required stock
- check expiry dates on all routine and emergency drugs and order as appropriate.

Staff training and personal development

The ECT nurse specialist should:

- undertake annual training in immediate life support (or equivalent), to meet the requirements of local protocols and national standards from ECTAS, SEAN, the Royal College of Nursing, the Royal College of Psychiatrists, the Royal College of Anaesthetists, NICE and the Nursing and Midwifery Council
- provide training and support to escort and ward nurses
- organise teaching sessions for students and new staff
- attend appropriate ECT nurse specialist training to update their knowledge (adequate time and financial support to attend this type of training should be provided by the employer, as it is important that practice and standards are regularly updated)
- be an active member of a regional and national ECT nurse specialist special interest group.

Role of the nurse in charge of recovery

The guidelines below are in accordance with recommendations of the Royal College of Anaesthetists (2011), ECTAS (Cresswell et al, 2012) and SEAN (2010).

The nurse in charge of the recovery room must hold an up-to-date certificate in immediate life support (or equivalent) and have experience and competencies in recovery procedures and techniques. There should be a minimum of two appropriately trained nurses at all times during the recovery process. Patients must be cared for on a one-to-one basis until they can maintain their airway, breathing and circulation. Responsibilities of the nurse in charge of the recovery room include the following:

- have a good knowledge of the ECT process, especially the possible side-effects (both common and rare) and the nursing actions required in the event of their occurrence
- be familiar with the ECT clinic and location of emergency equipment and be trained and competent in its use
- be competent in all aspects of basic and immediate life support or equivalent

- have received specific training in recovery procedures, airway management and all aspects of recovery care, and be up to date and competent in their practice
- ensure they receive a hand-over from the anaesthetist with regard to each patient and any specific instructions given – any intravenous fluids, drugs or oxygen therapy must be properly prescribed and this information should in turn be passed on to the nurse escort with the patient
- provide a safe environment for patients and staff
- monitor the care of the patient at all stages of recovery
- monitor the patient in recovery in accordance with local protocols, which must include determining heart rate, oxygen saturation, blood pressure, level of responsiveness and level of orientation; they should ensure the patient's safety within the recovery room, and remain with the patient and provide support and orientation throughout the whole process until such time as the patient is suitably recovered as well as ensure that the patient is appropriately escorted back to the ward by a registered nurse (see 'Role and responsibilities of the escort nurse')
- alert the anaesthetist or ECT psychiatrist to any concerns or adverse events during recovery
- orientate patients to their situation and environment
- complete any relevant documentation
- ensure that patients are not discharged back to their area until fully recovered, with their observations stable (the anaesthetist should either discharge patients from recovery or provide the nurse in charge of recovery with strict criteria for discharge)
- remind all day-case/out-patients of the specific instructions for day-case treatment and advise them to refer to the day-case/out-patient information sheet they were given at outset of treatment
- ensure that day-case/out-patients are fully recovered before they leave the main recovery area to further recover either in a secondary recovery area or in a ward.

Acknowledgements

With thanks for advice and support from the Committee of Nurses at ECT in Scotland (CONECTS) and the National Association of Lead Nurses in ECT (NALNECT). This chapter is endorsed by the Royal College of Nursing.

References

Association of Anaesthetists of Great Britain and Ireland (2010) *The Anaesthesia Team 3.* AAGBI.

Cresswell, J., Murphy, G. & Hodge, S. (2012) *The ECT Accreditation Service (ECTAS): Standards for the Administration of ECT* (10th edn). Royal College of Psychiatrists' Centre for Quality Improvement.

Finch, S. (2005) *Nurse Guidance for ECT*. Royal College of Nursing.

National Institute for Clinical Excellence (2003) *Guidance on the Use of Electroconvulsive Therapy* (Technical Appraisal TA59). NICE.

Nursing and Midwifery Council (2008) *The Code: Standards of Conduct, Performance and Ethics for Nurses and Midwives*. NMC.

Royal College of Anaesthetists (2011) *Guidance on the Provision of Anaesthetic Care in the Non-Theatre Environment*. Royal College of Anaesthetists.

Scottish ECT Accreditation Network (2010) *SEAN Standards. Version v1.0*. National Services Scotland.

Waite, J. & Easton, A. (eds) (2013) *The ECT Handbook* (3rd edn). RCPsych Publications.

CHAPTER 12

Inspection of ECT clinics

Chris P. Freeman, Joanne Cresswell, Grace M. Fergusson and Linda Cullen

---

The ECT Accreditation Service (ECTAS)

In the early 1980s there was an editorial in *The Lancet* entitled 'ECT in Britain: a shameful state of affairs' (*Lancet*, 1981). This was at a time when ECT was the main target of the anti-psychiatry movement and there were regular protests outside Royal College of Psychiatrists' meetings about the use of ECT. Paradoxically, several of the UK randomised controlled trials of ECT had been published and others were under way, so the evidence base for the efficacy was stronger than it had ever been. The College had just completed its first survey of the use and practice of ECT, concluding that standards of practice were low, equipment was outdated and regional variations were enormous. The author of *The Lancet* editorial concluded that it was not ECT that was bringing psychiatry in disrepute, it was psychiatrists and the way they practised.

The College conducted further surveys of practice in the late 1980s and early 1990s, sadly showing that standards were improving little. The Special Committee on ECT (now Special Committee on ECT and Related Treatments) began running regular training courses which several thousand psychiatrists have now attended. More recently there have been increasing numbers of anaesthetic and nursing delegates.

Thirty years on, we now have a third edition of *The ECT Handbook*, guidelines from NICE endorsing the use of ECT (National Institute for Clinical Excellence, 2003; National Collaborating Centre for Mental Health, 2010) and we have ECTAS.

Over the first 20 years the rate of ECT steadily fell and if the slope had not levelled out it would have crossed zero in 2012. This did not happen, and the past 10 years have shown a levelling of the rates of giving ECT, with some areas showing a rise. National figures are no longer collected. This contrasts with the situation in North America, where the rates of ECT use have been rising, and raises the view that ECT may be underused, causing patients with severe and chronic depression to suffer for much longer, as antidepressant after antidepressant is changed.

Whatever the future of ECT, it is vitally important that when it is given, it is given appropriately, safely and with due concern to a patient's consent and dignity. The ECT Accreditation Service aims to assure and improve the quality of the administration of ECT. It was launched in May 2003 and is managed by the Royal College of Psychiatrists' Centre for Quality Improvement. As of February 2013, 94 ECT clinics in England and Wales participate in the ECTAS programme. There are also ECTAS members in Northern Ireland.

Participating clinics complete a self-review to measure themselves against a set of evidence-based standards. A 1-day peer review visit from a multidisciplinary team serves to validate this self-review data, and allows for action points and areas of achievement to be highlighted. The accreditation visits are detailed, involving the rating of nearly 200 carefully worded standards. No other country, save for Scotland, has a system like ECTAS. Accreditation is not a toothless exercise – some clinics have not achieved accreditation and often accreditation has been deferred for a short time to allow clinics to appoint extra staff or obtain appropriate equipment.

Accreditation lasts for a 3-year period, subject to satisfactory interim review at 18 months. The Royal College of Nursing and the Royal College of Anaesthetists support the work of ECTAS and are represented on the Accreditation Committee, whose role it is to suggest an accreditation rating for participating clinics. Members receive initial feedback at the end of the peer review visit, and shortly afterwards receive a more detailed report of compliance with the standards, action points and areas of achievement.

Another benefit of participating in ECTAS includes access to the email discussion group, which provides members with a forum to discuss issues relating to ECT. The email discussion group is very active, with regular posting of clinical queries and opinion.

In addition, members are encouraged to train as peer reviewers and visit other ECTAS member clinics, providing invaluable opportunities for networking and the sharing of good practice. The ECT Accreditation Service also provides a 3-day training course for ECT lead nurses (in conjunction with the College's Education and Training Centre and NALNECT).

By October 2011, 18 ECTAS member clinics had completed their third cycle of self-review and peer-review, and all clinics continued to improve in their third review cycle, as indicated by the number of standards met. Overall, the average percentage of standards met between cycle 2 and cycle 3 rose from 92% to 97%. Also during this period, 41 ECTAS member clinics had completed their second cycle of self-review and peer-review. All clinics performed better in their second review cycle than they had in their first, as indicated by the number of standards met and, overall, the average percentage of met standards rose from 90% to 96%. Five clinics met 100% of standards in their second cycle; a feat that none had achieved in their first.

Further information on ECTAS, including a list of accredited clinics, current standards (Cresswell et al, 2012) and reports, can be downloaded from www.rcpsych.ac.uk/workinpsychiatry/qualityimprovement/qualityandaccreditation/ectclinics/ectas.aspx.

The Scottish ECT Accreditation Network (SEAN)

The aims of SEAN are:

- to improve the quality of clinical care and outcomes via the collection and use of process and outcomes data
- the accreditation of all ECT clinics in Scotland
- the development of a clinical network to provide peer support and drive up standards of care using a 'bottom up' approach.

To achieve this, an electronic integrated care pathway is installed in all ECT units in Scotland and data are submitted centrally for validation and analysis.

Coupled to this is a programme of biennial inspection visits to all ECT suites to assess performance against predetermined standards, set in accordance with advice from representatives of the Royal College of Psychiatrists, the Royal College of Anaesthetists and the Royal College of Nursing, and with input from a user reference group. Visits are undertaken by a team comprising a consultant psychiatrist, consultant anaesthetist, ECT nurse and SEAN's clinical coordinator and are timed to link with an actual treatment session. The unit is given immediate feedback during the visit and this is followed up by a formal report along with an accreditation level award, agreed on by members of the SEAN Steering Group. Notification is sent to the chief executive, clinical and medical directors, clinical governance lead, line manager and all members of the ECT team. During the accreditation process, if an issue is identified that puts patients or staff at risk, an escalation policy is followed, immediately alerting the ECT team and senior management to the situation.

Data are fed back to clinical teams, and are also presented at SEAN's annual meeting. The Steering Group identifies factors that improve efficacy and disseminates this information to clinical teams; information on ways to reduce possible side-effects is also disseminated. The clinicians involved aim to improve the confidence of the general public that this form of treatment is effective and fit for the 21st century. The Scottish ECT Accreditation Network has an informative website (www.sean.org.uk), including information for professionals and the general public. The website also has all the SEAN annual reports available, the most recent being 2012 (Scottish ECT Accreditation Network, 2012).

References

Cresswell, J., Murphy, G. & Hodge, S. (2012) *The ECT Accreditation Service (ECTAS): Standards for the Administration of ECT* (10th edn). Royal College of Psychiatrists' Centre for Quality Improvement.

Lancet (1981) ECT in Britain: a shameful state of affairs. *Lancet*, **2**, 1207–1208.

National Collaborating Centre for Mental Health (2010) *Depression: The NICE Guideline on the Treatment and Management of Depression in Adults* (updated edn). British Psychological Society & Royal College of Psychiatrists.

National Institute for Clinical Excellence (2003) *Guidance on the Use of Electroconvulsive Therapy* (Technology Appraisal TA59). NICE.

Scottish ECT Accreditation Network (2012) *Scottish ECT Accreditation Network Annual Report 2011: A Summary of ECT in Scotland for 2011*. NHS National Services.

CHAPTER 13

Other brain stimulation treatments

Sarah Browne, David Christmas, Douglas Steele, M. Sam Eljamel and Keith Matthews

Electroconvulsive therapy prescribers, practitioners and many patients will be aware of an emerging clinical evidence base for non-ECT brain stimulation treatments. Although the previous edition of *The ECT Handbook* made no mention of brain stimulation treatments, a review of the status of the three most studied therapies is now relevant. These therapies are:

- repetitive transcranial magnetic stimulation
- vagus nerve stimulation
- deep brain stimulation.

In this chapter, we consider the use of these therapies in the management of depression and how they might relate to the ECT treatment pathway.

Repetitive transcranial magnetic stimulation (rTMS)

Repetitive transcranial magnetic stimulation is a non-invasive technique causing modification of brain activity by focal stimulation of the superficial layers of the cerebral cortex using a train of magnetic pulses via an external wire coil. The impetus for studies of rTMS in psychiatry has arisen from the need for a viable alternative to ECT with a lower burden of adverse effects and greater patient acceptability. A substantial literature, including several systematic reviews and meta-analyses, now exists on the use of rTMS in the management of depression. In 2008 the US Food and Drug Administration approved a TMS system 'for the treatment of Major Depressive Disorder in adult patients who have failed to achieve satisfactory improvement from one prior antidepressant medication at or above the minimal effective dose and duration in the current episode'.

However, NICE published a technology appraisal in 2007, restating the core recommendations in the 2010 depression guideline update, which is consistent with the absence of convincing evidence of superior efficacy for rTMS over sham treatment and with the paucity of efficacy data extending beyond 4–6 weeks of treatment. The status of the technique is summarised as follows:

'Current evidence suggests that there are no major safety concerns associated with transcranial magnetic stimulation (TMS) for severe depression. There is uncertainty about the procedure's clinical efficacy, which may depend on higher intensity, greater frequency, bilateral application and/or longer treatment durations than have appeared in the evidence to date. TMS should therefore be performed only in research studies designed to investigate these factors.' (National Institute for Health and Clinical Excellence, 2007)

In our opinion, on the basis of current evidence, rTMS remains an interesting but experimental therapy which should not be considered a viable alternative to treatment with ECT. Indeed, scrutiny of the characteristics of individuals in trials of rTMS and those receiving ECT in clinical practice frequently show different refractoriness to previous treatments. Also, only a small number of comparative trials report greater effectiveness of ECT compared with rTMS in the short-term management of depression (Eranti *et al*, 2007).

Vagus nerve stimulation (VNS)

Vagus nerve stimulation is an 'indirect' brain stimulation technique involving the application of small electrical stimuli to the cervical portion of the left vagus nerve. Importantly, VNS does not require intracranial surgery; instead, it uses an implanted programmable neurostimulator which delivers electric pulses through a surgically placed bipolar lead, wrapped around the vagus nerve. The battery-powered pulse-generating device is usually implanted subcutaneously within the soft tissues of the upper left chest. A connecting wire is tunnelled under the skin and connects the device with the cervical portion of the left vagus nerve in the neck. Vagus nerve stimulation implantation requires a general anaesthetic and is usually performed by a neurosurgeon. Stimulation parameters (e.g. pulse width, frequency, current intensity, on/off cycles) are set via a hand-held 'programming wand' and linked computer (typically a hand-held device). A common treatment regimen involves intermittent stimulation for 30 s every 5 min through the day and night. Vagus nerve stimulation has been investigated as a treatment for depression for over a decade, after it was noted to improve mood in patients receiving VNS for refractory epilepsy – its primary clinical indication.

Putative mechanisms of action for VNS remain highly speculative. Approximately 80% of the fibres within the left cervical vagus nerve are afferent fibres terminating in the nucleus tractus solitarius of the brain stem. From there, they project to noradrenergic systems via the locus coeruleus and to serotonergic systems via the raphe nuclei. Additionally, vagal afferents project to the amygdala, thalamus and hypothalamus via the nucleus tractus solitarius. It is therefore hypothesised that by modulating neuronal activity in the vagus nerve, 'upstream' neural systems are affected. Many of these are implicated in controlling the emotions and autonomic–sensory integration. However, the evidence for this remains limited.

Outcomes for VNS as a treatment for major depression

Vagus nerve stimulation was approved by the US Food and Drug Administration in July 2005 as an adjunctive long-term treatment of chronic (symptoms lasting ≥2 years) or treatment-resistant depression, which had not adequately responded to a minimum of four antidepressant treatments.

Table 13.1 summarises the response and remission rates in studies of VNS for major depression to date. Some important caveats are required when interpreting the data in Table 13.1.

- The D-01 study (USA) initially involved 30 patients. A further 30 patients were recruited. So far, data have been reported up to 2 years.
- The D-02 group of studies (USA) comprised a number of different design phases with the same cohort of patients. Patients participating in a 10-week controlled trial continued within an open follow-up study where comparisons were made between outcomes for this group and a separate cohort receiving treatment as usual.
- The D-03 study was a European multicentre replication of the D-02 study and used a similar protocol. Outcomes have been reported for 24 months.
- Each study (D-01 to D-03) generated multiple reports, including longer follow-up studies of previously reported cohorts which do not represent additional numbers of patients treated. The National Institute for Health and Clinical Excellence, in their recent technology appraisal of VNS for depression (2009), did not account for this.
- Within the constraints of interpreting studies with an open-label design, response to VNS appears cumulative. Over time, more patients appear to respond. Although, on average, studies suggest that 15% of people will have responded by 3 months, 18–20%, 25–30% and 30–40% will have responded by 6, 9 and 12 months respectively. It is therefore important to ensure that patients (and clinicians) have realistic expectations. Several months may pass before any improvement is seen.

Contraindications to VNS

The most common contraindications to VNS include:

- significant cardiac disease and/or a predisposition to bradycardia
- a pre-existing cardiac pacemaker
- clinically significant chronic obstructive pulmonary disease
- previous neck surgery
- a history of left or bilateral cervical vagotomy.

Post-implantation, magnetic resonance image scanning of any part of the body as well as shortwave diathermy is contraindicated due to the possibility of current induction in the electrodes.

Table 13.1 Outcomes from published studies of vagus nerve stimulation for major depression

	n	Design	Study	Duration	Response rate, %	Remission rate, %
Rush et al (2000)	30	Open study	D-01	10 weeks	40	17
Sackeim et al (2001)	60	Open study	D-01	10 weeks	30.5	15.3
Marangell et al (2002)	30	Open study	D-01	12 months	46	29
George et al (2005)	329	VNS + TAU (n = 205) v. TAU (n = 124)	D-02	12 months	27 (VNS) 13 (TAU)	15 (VNS) 3.6 (TAU)
Nahas et al (2005)	59	Open study	D-01	2 years	42	22
Rush et al (2005a)	235	RCT	D-02	10 weeks	15.2 (active) 10 (sham)	N/A
Rush et al (2005b)	202	Open study	D-02	12 months	27.2	15.8
Corcoran et al (2006)	11	Open study	D-03	12 months	55	27
Schlaepfer et al (2008)	60	Open study	D-03	12 months	53	33
Bajbouj et al (2010)	49	Open study	D-03	24 months	53	39
Cristancho et al (2011)	15	Open study	Independent	12 months	28.6	7.1
Total[1]	384	At 12 months At 24 months			31 (n = 118/384) 38 (n = 51/134)	18 (n = 69/384) 24 (n = 32/134)

RCT, randomised controlled trial; TAU, treatment as usual; VNS, vagus nerve stimulation.

1. Summary data calculated by expressing total number of responders and remitters at 12 and 24 months as a percentage of the total number of reports available for each time period.

Surgical procedure

The procedure is usually performed under general anaesthetic. A small, helical stimulating electrode is wrapped around the cervical portion of the left vagus nerve by dissecting the nerve out of the carotid sheath. The electrode is then tunnelled under the skin to the programmable pulse generator implanted subcutaneously in the left anterior chest wall. The left vagus nerve is stimulated to avoid the cardiac effects found with right vagus nerve stimulation and because over 80% of fibres in the left vagus are afferents.

The VNS stimulator is usually activated 2 weeks after surgery. The patient is asked to hold the wand over the stimulator while settings are checked and reprogrammed. In the weeks after implantation, the stimulating current is gradually increased within tolerable levels. Shortening the pulse width of the stimulation is often helpful in reducing adverse effects. Most people will receive 30 s of active stimulation every 5 min; a duty cycle of 10% (30 s on out of 300 s). For some, it is possible to increase the duty cycle to 25% or higher.

Adverse effects

So far, no deaths have been reported with VNS surgery. There have been five reports from all implanted patients (approximately 0.02%) of transient bradycardia/asystole when the pulse generator was tested intra-operatively. In each instance, there were no further adverse sequelae.

- One in three patients experiences pain around the surgical wounds in the acute post-operative period. This is usually managed with simple analgesia.
- Post-operative infections occur in 3–6% of patients. Most are successfully treated with oral antibiotics.
- Fewer than 1% of people develop a temporary paralysis of their vocal cords leading to hoarseness and difficulty speaking. This can usually be reversed if the device is removed.
- There have been some reports of altered sensation in the lower face or weakness of the face muscles. This became rare as surgical techniques improved.
- If the patient receives no therapeutic benefit, or for example intractable infection occurs, device removal may be necessary. Typically though, it is difficult to remove the helical wire tip completely as it becomes fibrosed round the vagus nerve. This may potentially cause problems if future magnetic resonance imaging scans are required, as current induction with stimulation and heating can occur.

Adverse effects related to stimulation

Adverse effects are generally similar across all reported studies and are summarised in Table 13.2.

Table 13.2 Adverse effect rates for vagus nerve stimulation

Adverse effect	3 months, %	6 months, %	9 months, %	12 months, %
Headache	5	4	4	4
Neck pain	16	11	14	13
Dysphagia	13	8	7	4
Nausea	6	2	2	2
Increased cough	24	9	7	6
Dyspnoea	14	16	15	16
Voice alteration	58	60	57	54
Worsening depression	5.2	6.7	4.6	5.7
Mania	1	<1	0	0
Suicide	1	1	<1	<1

Most stimulation-related adverse effects are reduced by altering stimulation parameters, although some (e.g. voice alteration) may persist for as long as active stimulation is delivered. Others (e.g. dysphagia, cough) reduce over time.

Vagus nerve stimulation in contemporary psychiatric practice

In their procedure guidance, NICE concluded:

> 'Current evidence on the safety and efficacy of vagus nerve stimulation (VNS) for treatment-resistant depression is inadequate in quantity and quality.' (National Institute for Health and Clinical Excellence, 2009)

In our opinion, on the basis of the current evidence, VNS is a promising but unproven adjunctive therapy for patients with treatment-refractory major depression. Vagus nerve stimulation should not be considered as an alternative to treatment with ECT. It should, however, be considered for patients for whom ECT is not possible and for those whose response is not sustained despite appropriate medication.

We concur with NICE (2009) that:

> 'this procedure should be used only with special arrangements for clinical governance, consent and audit or research. It should be used only in patients with treatment-resistant depression.'

Practical considerations for ECT practitioners

- It is possible to give ECT to patients with an implanted VNS system. There are numerous reports of it being delivered safely. The authors also have experience of giving ECT with VNS stimulators *in situ*.
- The anaesthetist should be alerted to the theoretical possibility of bradycardia. This can be mitigated by switching off the VNS (setting

the output current to zero) while ECT is being given. Following ECT, standard diagnostics are performed and the device is reprogrammed. However, there is some evidence that patients are less likely to respond to VNS where their previous response to ECT is poor (Sackeim *et al*, 2001).

Deep brain stimulation (DBS)

Like VNS, DBS is a surgical approach which has been used to treat a variety of disabling neurological symptoms, including the motor symptoms associated with Parkinson's disease. Although interest in DBS appears relatively recent, it has been an established treatment for movement disorders for several decades and experimentation as a treatment for psychiatric illness dates back at least as far. Implanted intracranial electrodes were tested as a treatment for anxiety in 1975 and obsessive–compulsive disorder (OCD) in 1988. In 1999, Nuttin *et al* in Leuven, Belgium, were first to report improvements in OCD symptoms with stimulation electrodes sited bilaterally in the anterior limbs of the internal capsule, a target similar to that of ablative anterior capsulotomy. Since 2001, further reports have described positive outcomes for small cohorts of patients with OCD and, more recently, for patients with refractory major depression.

Deep brain stimulation is achieved through the use of surgically implanted programmable neurostimulator devices which deliver electrical stimuli to deep brain structures via bilaterally implanted electrodes. A number of different stimulation targets have been investigated with respect to the treatment of major depression with the subgenual anterior cingulate white matter tracts (Lozano *et al*, 2008) and the internal capsule/ventral striatum/ nucleus accumbens region (Malone *et al*, 2009) showing the strongest accruing evidence for efficacy. The battery-powered pulse-generating device is usually implanted under the skin of the upper chest. Either a single device powers two electrodes, or two devices independently stimulate each side. Connecting wires are tunnelled under the skin to connect the device with the implanted electrode. Electrodes have several contacts which can be stimulated independently, offering increased precision of targeting or increasing the total area that can be stimulated. Deep brain stimulation electrodes are implanted by a neurosurgeon under either general or local anaesthesia using stereotactic, image-guidance techniques. Stimulation parameters are programmed into the pulse generator via a programming wand.

Frequently cited advantages for DBS over ablative neurosurgery include the reversibility of the technique and the adjustability of the stimulation parameters, allowing optimal clinical response and accommodating adverse effects of stimulation. There are, however, no published studies comparing the effectiveness, acceptability, tolerability or utility of the two techniques. Also, masked studies have been promised, but are still awaited. In addition, high rates of hardware problems are reported from DBS studies for neurological indications. This should be noted and borne in mind when evaluating the short-term reports of DBS, as short battery life has been a major issue for some DBS-treated patients with OCD and depression.

Mechanisms of action

The mechanisms of action of DBS remain unknown. Several different theories exist. It should be noted that the effects described are not mutually exclusive and may coexist.

- Deep brain stimulation is inhibitory. To some extent, this follows on from research in movement disorders where DBS and ablation reduce tremor by blocking normal neuronal firing.
- Deep brain stimulation is excitatory. Studies have demonstrated increased neurotransmitter release in structures downstream from DBS targets, and neuroimaging studies have shown activation of outflow pathways with thalamic stimulation.
- Deep brain stimulation is modulatory. The principle of stochastic resonance suggests changes can be seen in a system when noise is added. It is hypothesised that DBS may regulate neuronal activity by improving signal transduction in pathways that are abnormally noisy due to disease processes.

Outcomes for DBS as a treatment for major depression

The reported outcomes for DBS in patients with major depression are summarised in Table 13.3. To date, most reports are of small case series with relatively short follow-up (<12 months) and no masking.

Adverse effects with DBS for major depression

Given the small numbers reported, rates of adverse effects require cautious interpretation. Adverse effects from the four largest case series are summarised in Table 13.4. Note that adverse effects are typically not screened for systematically, nor described using the same categorisations.

Deep brain stimulation in contemporary psychiatric practice

There is no NICE guidance on the use of DBS as a treatment for major depression or OCD. However, to paraphrase NICE on VNS, it seems reasonable to conclude that current evidence on the safety and efficacy of DBS for treatment-resistant major depression is inadequate in quantity and quality.

In our opinion, on the basis of the current evidence, DBS is a promising but unproven therapy for patients with treatment-refractory major depression. Compared with VNS, there are substantially greater risks for the patient. Consequently, DBS should not be considered as an alternative to ECT, but

Table 13.3 Summary of outcomes for deep brain stimulation for depression

	n	Target	Follow-up, months	Response,[1] %	Comments
Jiménez et al (2005)	1	Inferior thalamic peduncle	24	N/A	Patient also had borderline personality disorder and bulimia nervosa. Symptoms improved during a period when stimulator was off
Mayberg et al (2005)	6	SGC25	6	66 (n = 4/66)	
Kosel et al (2007)	1	Globus pallidus interna	18	N/A	Patient with tardive dyskinesia and comorbid depression
Lozano et al (2008)[2]	20	SCG	12	60	At month 12, 35% achieved or were within one point of achieving remission
Neimat et al (2008)	1	SGC25	30 months	Yes	Patient underwent deep brain stimulation 6 months after bilateral anterior cingulotomy
Schlaepfer et al (2008)	3	Nucleus accumbens	5–22 weeks	66 (n = 2/3)	Variable follow-up. Two were monozygotic twins
Malone et al (2009)	15	VC/VS	12	53.3	Multiple comorbid diagnoses
Bewernick et al (2010)[2]	10	Nucleus accumbens	12	50	Unclear whether includes patients from Schlaepfer et al (2008)
Lozano et al (2012)	21	SCG	12	62	Initial response rate of 57% at 1 month declined by month 6 to 48%
Total	69				

SCG, subcallosal cingulate gyrus; SGC25, subgenual cingulate gyrus, Brodmann area 25; VC/VS, ventral (internal) capsule/ventral striatum.

1. Response is defined as >50% reduction in baseline score on the Hamilton Rating Scale for Depression (Hamilton, 1960).

2. The Lozano et al (2008) study includes the patients reported in Mayberg et al (2005), and Bewernick et al (2010) may include patients from the Schlaepfer et al (2008) cohort. Therefore, both are omitted from the total.

Table 13.4 Adverse effects and deep brain stimulation for major depression

Adverse effect	Lozano et al (2008) (n = 20)	Malone et al (2009) (n = 15)	Bewernick et al (2010) (n = 10)	Lozano et al (2012) (n = 21)
Target location	SCG	VC/VS	NAcc	SCG
Indication	MDD	MDD	MDD	MDD
Peri-operative headache	4	1	Not reported	6, 1 month post-operatively
Intracranial haemorrhage	Not reported	Not reported	Not reported	Not reported
Wound infection and hardware removal	3	None reported	Not reported	Not reported
Lead fracture/hardware failure	None reported	1	1	2
Wound infection (managed with antibiotics)	1	None reported	None reported	1
Worsening mood/irritability	2	1	None reported	Not reported
Suicidality	None reported	4	2, with 1 suicide	2, with 1 suicide
Peri-operative seizures	1	None reported	None reported	Not reported
Hypomania	0	2	2	Not reported
Other psychopathological states (e.g. anxiety)	None reported	None reported	6	4, including agitation/increasing amplitude
Neurological effects	None reported	None reported	6	14
Neuropsychological impairment	None reported	None reported	'No worsening'	Not reported
Weight gain	None reported	None reported	Not reported	1

MDD, major depressive disorder; NAcc, nucleus accumbens; SCG, subcallosal cingulate gyrus; VC/VS, ventral (internal) capsule/ventral striatum.

as an alternative to ablative neurosurgery. Deep brain stimulation should only be offered to patients with chronic, disabling and demonstrably treatment-refractory major depression within the context of a clinical research study which has been subject to ethics committee approval. Further, DBS should only be offered by multidisciplinary teams with a high level of expertise in the pharmacological and psychological management of refractory major depression and who have experience of providing such care over extended periods. Standardised assessment protocols should be used to audit the intervention pre- and post-surgery and at medium- and long-term follow-up. These protocols should include measures of symptoms, quality of life, social and personality function, as well as comprehensive neuropsychological tests. We further believe that clinical services offering DBS should have access to independent advice on issues such as adequacy of previous treatment and consent. They should be familiar with relevant mental health legislation relating to DBS for psychiatric disorder. Such treatments should also be subject to appropriate external oversight and governance. Services offering DBS should be committed to sharing and publishing audit information.

Practical considerations for ECT practitioners

The safety of ECT in patients who have an implanted DBS system has not been established. Induced electrical currents may damage DBS system components. This may result in a loss of therapeutic effect and/or clinically significant undesirable stimulation effects. It is possible that the DBS system may require to be explanted. Electroconvulsive therapy with a DBS system implanted could, in theory, lead to neurological injury.

Other treatment options – ablative neurosurgery

In addition to the stimulation techniques which represent the focus of this chapter, patients with the most chronic, disabling and refractory forms of major depression should be considered as potential candidates for established ablative neurosurgical treatments. These treatment pathways should certainly be considered for those with major depression who require regular or maintenance ECT, or where ECT fails to elicit a response. Details of the procedures, clinical guidelines and other relevant information can be accessed and downloaded from www.advancedinterventions.org.uk.

Key points

- Despite extensive study, there is limited evidence that rTMS elicits a useful and sustained clinical response as a therapy for major depression. It does not presently represent a viable alternative to ECT. Repetitive transcranial magnetic stimulation should only be offered as part of a research protocol with ethics committee approval.

- There is some evidence from open studies that VNS exerts a useful therapeutic effect as an adjunctive therapy for some patients with chronic major depression. The risks and adverse effects associated with VNS are modest. It does not presently represent a viable alternative to ECT. It should, however, be considered in cases of refractory major depression where ECT is not possible and where responders to ECT fail to sustain that response despite appropriate medication. Vagus nerve stimulation should only be used with special arrangements for clinical governance, consent and audit or research. Electroconvulsive therapy may be administered safely to a patient with an implanted VNS system.

- A limited number of small case series provide evidence that DBS can be an effective therapy for some patients with chronic and treatment-refractory major depression. However, the associated surgical risks, the potential adverse effects of stimulation and potential hardware vulnerabilities should not be underestimated. Deep brain stimulation should only be offered to patients as part of a research protocol with ethics committee approval.

- Other treatment options for patients with highly treatment-refractory major depression include ablative neurosurgery. Modern stereotactic neurosurgical techniques are associated with favourable clinical outcomes for many.

References

Bajbouj, M., Merkl, A., Schlaepfer, T. E., et al (2010) Two-year outcome of vagus nerve stimulation (VNS) in treatment-resistant depression. Journal of Clinical Psychopharmacology, 30, 273–281.

Bewernick, B. H., Hurlemann, R., Matusch, A., et al (2010) Nucleus accumbens deep brain stimulation decreases rating of depression and anxiety in treatment-resistant depression. Biological Psychiatry, 67, 110–116.

Corcoran, C. D, Thomas, P., Phillips, J., et al (2006) Vagus nerve stimulation in chronic treatment-resistant depression. Preliminary findings of an open-label study. British Journal of Psychiatry, 189, 282–283.

Cristancho, P., Cristancho, M. A., Baltuch, G. H., et al (2011) Effectiveness and safety of vagus nerve stimulation for severe treatment-resistant major depression in clinical practice after FDA approval: outcomes at 1 year. Journal of Clinical Psychiatry, 72, 1376–1382.

Eranti, S., Mogg, A., Pluck, G., et al (2007) A randomized, controlled trial with 6-month follow-up of repetitive transcranial magnetic stimulation and electroconvulsive therapy for severe depression. American Journal of Psychiatry, 164, 73–81.

George, M. S., Rush, A. J., Marangell, L. B., et al (2005) A one year comparison of vagus nerve stimulation with treatment as usual for treatment-resistant depression. Biological Psychiatry, 58, 364–373.

Hamilton, M. (1960) A rating scale for depression. Journal of Neurology, Neurosurgery and Psychiatry, 23, 56–62.

Jiménez, F., Velasco, F., Salin-Pascual, R., et al (2005) A patient with a resistant major depression disorder treated with deep brain stimulation in the inferior thalamic peduncle. Neurosurgery, 57, 585–593.

Kosel, M., Sturm, V., Frick C., *et al* (2007) Mood improvement after deep brain stimulation of the internal globus pallidus for tardive dyskinesia in a patient suffering from major depression. *Journal of Psychiatric Research*, **41**, 801–803.

Lozano, A. M., Mayberg, H. S., Giacobbe, P., *et al* (2008) Subcallosal cingulate gyrus deep brain stimulation for treatment-resistant depression. *Biological Psychiatry*, **64**, 461–467.

Lozano, A. M, Giacobbe, P., Hamani, C., *et al* (2012) A multicenter pilot study of subcallosal cingulate area deep brain stimulation for treatment-resistant depression. *Journal of Neurosurgery*, **116**, 315–322.

Malone, D. A, Dougherty, D. D., Rezai, A. R., *et al* (2009) Deep brain stimulation of the ventral capsule/ventral striatum for treatment-resistant depression. *Biological Psychiatry*, **65**, 267–275.

Marangell, L. B., Rush, A. J., George, M. S., *et al* (2002) Vagus nerve stimulation for major depressive episodes: one year outcomes. *Biological Psychiatry*, **51**, 280–287.

Mayberg, H. S., Lozano, A. M., Voon, V., *et al* (2005) Deep brain stimulation for treatment-resistant depression. *Neuron*, **45**, 651–660.

Nahas, Z., Marangell, L. B., Husain, M. M., *et al* (2005) Two year outcome of vagus nerve stimulation for treatment of major depressive episodes. *Journal of Clinical Psychiatry*, **66**, 1097–1104.

National Collaborating Centre for Mental Health (2010) *Depression: The Treatment and Management of Depression in Adults* (update edn) (National Clinical Practice Guideline 90). British Psychological Society & Royal College of Psychiatrists.

National Institute for Health and Clinical Excellence (2007) *Transcranial Magnetic Stimulation for Severe Depression* (Interventional Procedure Guidance IPG242). NICE.

National Institute for Health and Clinical Excellence (2009) *Vagus Nerve Stimulation for Treatment-Resistant Depression* (Interventional Procedure Guidance IPG330). NICE.

Neimat, J. S., Hamani, C. & Giacobbe, P. (2008) Neural stimulation successfullly treats depression in patients with prior ablative cingulotomy. *American Journal of Psychiatry*, **165**, 687–693.

Nuttin, B., Cosyns, B., Demeulemeester, H., *et al* (1999) Electrical stimulation in anterior limbs of internal capsules in patients with obsessive-compulsive disorder. *Lancet*, **354**, 1526.

Rush, A. J., George, M. S., Sackeim, H. A., *et al* (2000) Vagus nerve stimulation for treatment-resistant depressions: a multicenter study. *Biological Psychiatry*, **47**, 276–286.

Rush, A. J., Marangell, L. B., Sackeim, H. A., *et al* (2005a) Vagus nerve stimulation for treatment-resistant depression: a randomized, controlled acute phase trial. *Biological Psychiatry*, **58**, 347–354.

Rush, A. J., Sackeim, H. A., Marangell, L. B., *et al* (2005b) Effects of 12 months of vagus nerve stimulation in treatment-resistant depression: a naturalistic study. *Biological Psychiatry*, **58**, 355–363.

Sackeim, H. A., Rush, A. J., George, M. S., *et al* (2001) Vagus nerve stimulation for treatment-resistant depression: efficacy, side effects and predictors of outcome. *Neuropsychopharamacology*, **25**, 713–728.

Schlaepfer, T. E., Frick, C., Zobel, A., *et al* (2008) Vagus nerve stimulation for depression: efficacy and safety in a European study. *Psychological Medicine*, **38**, 651–661.

US Food and Drug Administration (2008) Repetitive transcranial magnetic stimulator for treatment of major depressive disorder. FDA. Available online at: http://www.accessdata.fda.gov/cdrh_docs/pdf8/K083538.pdf.

CHAPTER 14

The use of ECT in the treatment of depression

Heinrich C. Lamprecht, I. Nicol Ferrier, Alan G. Swann and Jonathan Waite

Depression remains the most frequent disorder for which ECT is required. This chapter summarises the evidence for the efficacy of ECT in depression and practical guidelines for its use. The Department of Health commissioned a systematic review of the safety and efficacy of ECT in depression (UK ECT Review Group, 2003), and for the NICE guidance on depression in adults, a further systematic review was undertaken (National Collaborating Centre for Mental Health, 2010: pp. 509–528.)

Efficacy of ECT in depression

The UK ECT Review Group (2003) examined data from randomised controlled trials identified in an extensive search. The results were independently checked by two reviewers. Data from studies which met inclusion criteria were extracted by paired members of the review team. Identified trials were assessed for methodology, where appropriate and data from individual trials were summarised by meta-analyses.

ECT v. 'sham' ECT

Six randomised controlled trials comparing ECT with 'sham' ECT in the short-term treatment of depression were examined by the UK ECT Review Group (2003). They included data on a total of 256 patients (Wilson *et al*, 1963; Lambourn & Gill, 1978; Freeman *et al*, 1978; Johnstone *et al*, 1980; West, 1981; Gregory *et al*, 1985). Most participants were in-patients under the age of 70 with some form of depressive disorder. The depression ratings at the end of treatment showed the standardised effect size (SES) between real and simulated ECT to be –0.91 (95% CI –1.27 to –0.54), indicating a mean difference in the Hamilton Rating Scale for Depression (HRSD) of 9.67 (95% CI 5.72 to 13.53) in favour of ECT. There have been no trials comparing ECT with sham ECT since the last edition of the *Handbook*.

ECT v. pharmacotherapy

In 18 randomised controlled trials with a total of 1144 patients, ECT was compared with antidepressant medication in the short-term treatment of depression. Of these, 13 trials contained sufficient data to contribute to a pooled analysis. The SES of these trials was –0.80 (95% CI –1.29 to –0.29). This equates to a mean difference of 5.2 (95% CI 1.37 to 8.87) on the HRSD in favour of ECT. None of these trials compared ECT with newer antidepressant medications such as SSRIs, mirtazepine or venlafaxine.

ECT v. rTMS

There have been several well-controlled studies of ECT v. rTMS. These have been reviewed by the Cochrane Collaboration (Martín et al, 2002) and by NICE (2006). Both reviews concluded that there was less evidence for the efficacy of rTMS than ECT and that rTMS should only be used in research studies. Research published since these reviews were undertaken confirms this conclusion (Hansen, et al 2011). Further information on rTMS is given in Chapter 13.

Bilateral v. unilateral ECT

Data from 21 studies were used to calculate an SES of bilateral v. unilateral application of ECT (UK ECT Review Group, 2003). Various electrode placements were used in both bilateral and unilateral ECT. In only eight studies was a duration of treatment described. There was an SES of –0.32 (95% CI –0.46 to –0.20) in favour of bilateral ECT.

Since 2003, six new studies have been published (Table 14.1). The studies published between 2002 and 2009 were analysed by NICE (National Collaborating Centre for Mental Health, 2010). This review concluded that there were few differences in efficacy or cognitive adverse effects between high-dose right unilateral ECT (i.e. treatment given at four (or more) times seizure threshold) and bitemporal ECT.

Kellner et al (2010), in the largest study published so far, demonstrated that bitemporal ECT at given at 1.5 times seizure threshold was more rapidly effective than right unilateral ECT at 6 times seizure threshold. Remission rates were higher (64% v. 55%) for bitemporal electrode placement. The remission rate for bifrontal ECT delivered at 1.5 times seizure threshold was 61%; this form of treatment had no advantages in terms of either efficacy or side-effect profile and was associated with more impairment of executive function.

The cognitive effects of bilateral and unilateral ECT have been reviewed by Semkovska et al (2011), who concluded that significant benefits for unilateral electrode placements are limited to the first 3 days after the end of treatment. The cognitive adverse effects of ECT are considered in more detail in Chapter 8.

Table 14.1 Summary of studies of bilateral v. unilateral ECT in depression

Study	n	Study design	Outcome
Heikman et al (2002)	24	High-dose right unilateral (400% above ST) v. moderate-dose right unilateral (just above ST) v. low-dose bifrontal (150% above ST)	Higher response rate with high-dose right unilateral compared with either moderate dose right unilateral or bifrontal ECT
McCall et al (2002)	77	Right unilateral (8 times ST) v. (1.5 times ST)	The antidepressant response rate was not significantly different for the right unilateral and bilateral groups (60% v. 73%)
Tew et al (2002)	24	Bilateral v. high-charge right unilateral (450% above ST)	No statistically significant differences in clinical response to bilateral or high-charge right unilateral ECT (63.6% and 61.5% respectively) or in depressive symptom remission (18.1% and 46.2% respectively)
Ranjkesh et al (2005)	45	Moderate-dose bifrontal (50% above ST) v. low-dose bitemporal (just above ST) v. high-dose right unilateral (400% ST)	Hamilton Rating Scale for Depression scores were not significantly different across the three groups
Stoppe et al (2006)	39	Unilateral v. bilateral	Remission rates for right unilateral ECT (88.2%) and bilateral ECT (68.2%) were similar ($P = 0.25$). Reduction rates of depressive symptoms were also similar
Eschweiler et al (2007)	92	Right unilateral (250% of ST) v. bifrontal (150% of ST)	Mean Hamilton Rating Scale for Depression score decreased from 27 to 17 points in both groups. No reduction in the modified Mini Mental State Examination score
Sackeim et al (2008)	90	Right unilateral (6 times seizure threshold) v. bilateral (2.5 times seizure threshold)	Remission rate for ultra-brief bilateral was 35% v. 73% for ultra-brief unilateral, 65% for standard pulse width bilateral, and 59% for standard pulse width unilateral
Sienaert et al (2009)	64	Bifrontal (1.5 times ST) v. right unilateral (6 times ST)	No deterioration in any of the neuropsychological measures. Patients rated their memory as clearly improved after treatment
Kellner et al (2010)	230	Bifrontal (1.5 times ST) v. bitemporal (1.5 times ST) v. unilateral (6 times ST)	Remission rates were 55% with right unilateral, 61% with bifrontal and 64% with bitemporal. More rapid decrease in symptom ratings over the early course of treatment with bitemporal

ST, seizure threshold.

Frequency of ECT

In the USA, ECT is generally administered three times a week; in the UK, twice-weekly treatment is the norm. Gangadhar & Thirthalli (2010) reviewed the evidence on ECT frequency and concluded that twice-weekly ECT offers the best balance between therapeutic outcome and adverse effects.

Six trials, involving a total of 210 patients, were assessed by the UK ECT review group (2003). Four trials compared twice-weekly with thrice-weekly ECT (Kellner et al, 1992; Lerer et al, 1995; Janakiramaiah et al, 1998; Vieweg & Shawcross, 1998) and two compared once-weekly with thrice-weekly ECT (Gangadhar et al, 1993; Shapira et al, 1998). There was no difference in favour of ECT given three times a week.

Dose of electrical stimulus

This remains an area of some contention. On the basis of available evidence from 12 studies, the NICE review group was not able to draw any firm conclusions (National Collaborating Centre for Mental Health, 2010: p. 515). They defined low-dose unilateral ECT as treatment up to 1.5 times seizure threshold; doses above this were reported as high dose. High-dose treatment was superior at achieving remission but this was not felt to be clinically important and no differential benefit was suggested with the other outcome measures.

High-dose, ultra-brief unilateral ECT has been reported to produce less cognitive impairment (Sackeim et al, 2008), but may be less effective (McCormick et al, 2009). The use of ultra-brief pulse width ECT is discussed in Chapter 4.

Number of ECT sessions

Guidance on the length of a course of ECT is given in Chapter 4. There is no evidence to indicate what number of sessions of ECT gains the best response. Neither is there any evidence to support the practice of giving two extra ECT sessions after the patient is considered to be well enough to discontinue ECT.

The place of ECT in the treatment of depression

General principles on the use of ECT in depression are given in Chapters 1 and 4; its use in older adults is considered in Chapter 20.

ECT as an emergency treatment in depression

Electroconvulsive therapy is still the treatment of choice for patients with a severe depressive episode, psychomotor retardation and associated problems of poor oral intake or physical deterioration. It is also used in patients with depression who are actively suicidal. The use of ECT in these circumstances is based on its efficacy and speed of action. Early improvement has been reported in all subtypes of depression (Sobin *et al*, 1996) and it can be considered as a possible first-line treatment in all emergencies (Porter & Ferrier, 1999). In urgent situations, bilateral ECT should be administered, as it is more effective than unilateral ECT and it also works faster (Kellner *et al*, 2010). Electroconvulsive therapy administered three times a week may produce a more rapid response (Shapira *et al*, 1998).

The use of ECT in treatment-resistant depression

There is no agreed definition of treatment-resistant depression. The previous edition of the Handbook (Scott, 2005) suggested that, in the absence of severe symptoms or an urgent need for treatment, treatment resistance should be considered as the failure to respond adequately to two successive courses of monotherapy with pharmacologically different antidepressants given in an adequate dose for sufficient time (Souery *et al*, 1999). Open label studies suggest that the proportion of patients who do not respond to either of two antidepressants (whether or not they belong to the same class) is estimated to be 50% (Thase & Rush, 1997).

Treatment resistance does not rule out a favourable response to ECT. Patients who failed one or more adequate medication trials had a diminished but substantial rate of response to ECT (Prudic *et al*, 1990, 1996) compared with non-treatment-resistant patients with depression. When ECT is used to treat unipolar major depression that has not responded despite vigorous antidepressant treatment, the remission rate is still about 50% (Dombrovski *et al*, 2005).

The use of ECT as treatment for depression in perinatal psychiatric disorders

Henshaw *et al* (2009) have produced comprehensive guidance on the management of mental disorders in the perinatal period.

Pregnancy

Anderson & Reti (2009) have reviewed the use of ECT in pregnancy in 339 published cases. There was a partial response of depressive symptoms in 84% of cases (compared with 61% pregnant women treated for schizophrenia). The most common adverse effect on the fetus was bradycardia, and in 3.5% of cases, uterine contractions and/or premature labour were reported. Positioning the patient with the right hip elevated to minimise aortocaval compression should improve placental perfusion and reduce the risk of fetal hypoxia.

Postnatal depression

There is evidence that depression may respond better to ECT in the postnatal period than in other circumstances, with more rapid and complete remission of mood and psychotic symptoms (Reed *et al*, 1999).

As there may be an increased risk of thromboembolic disease in the puerperium, anticoagulant prophylaxis should be considered. There are no published data on the effect of ECT on breastfeeding (Henshaw *et al*, 2009: p. 227).

The use of ECT in children and adolescents for the treatment of depression

The American Academy for Child and Adolescent Psychiatry (2004) has produced a practice parameter for the use of ECT with adolescents. This acknowledges that ECT may be an effective treatment for adolescents with severe mood disorders when other treatments have been unsuccessful. Practitioners working in child and adolescent mental health services may be unfamiliar with its use, but should consider ECT in appropriate clinical situations. The limited data available suggest that cognitive adverse effects are not disproportionately severe (Cohen *et al*, 2000; Ghaziuddin *et al*, 2001). The procedure seems to be acceptable to young people with severe psychiatric illness and to their parents (Walter *et al*, 1999).

As seizure threshold is likely to be low in young people, there may be an advantage in the use of propofol as the anaesthetic.

There are particular issues in obtaining consent in adolescents; specifically, there are legal requirements which must be met before giving ECT to minors in some jurisdictions (see Chapter 22).

Recommendations

Electroconvulsive therapy is a proven effective treatment for depression. It is a safe form of treatment even in the medically ill, the elderly and in pregnancy. There are benefits in using it in emergencies. It should not be relegated to a treatment of last resort.

We would recommend that ECT be used in the treatment of depression using the guidelines below.

- as a first-line treatment for:
  - the emergency treatment of depression where a rapid definitive response is needed
  - patients with high suicidal risk
  - patients with severe psychomotor retardation and associated problems of eating and drinking or physical deterioration
  - patients with treatment-resistant depression that have responded to ECT in a previous episode of illness

- patients who are pregnant, where there is concern about the teratogenic effects of psychotropic medications
- patients who prefer this form of treatment and for whom there are clinical indications for its use;
- as a second-line treatment for:
  - patients with treatment-resistant depression
  - patients who experience severe side-effects from medication
  - patients whose medical or psychiatric condition, in spite of other treatments, has deteriorated to an extent that raises concern.

References

American Academy for Child and Adolescent Psychiatry (2004) Practice parameter for use of electroconvulsive therapy with adolescents. *Journal of the American Academy for Child and Adolescent Psychiatry*, **43**, 1521–1539.

Anderson, E. L. & Reti, I. M. (2009) ECT in pregnancy: a review of the literature from 1941 to 2007. *Psychosomatic Medicine*, **71**, 235–242.

Cohen, D., Taieb, O., Flament, M., *et al* (2000) Absence of cognitive impairment at long term follow-up in adolescents treated with ECT for severe mood disorders. *American Journal of Psychiatry*, **157**, 460–462.

Dombrovski, A. Y., Mulsant, B. H., Hasket, R. F., *et al* (2005) Predictors of remission after electroconvulsive therapy in unipolar major depression. *Journal of Clinical Psychiatry*, **66**, 1043–1049.

Eschweiler, G. W., Vonthein, R., Bode, R., *et al* (2007) Clinical efficacy and cognitive side effects of bifrontal versus right unilateral electroconvulsive therapy (ECT): a short-term randomised controlled trial in pharmaco-resistant major depression. *Journal of Affective Disorders*, **101**, 149–157.

Freeman, C. P., Basson, J. V. & Crighton, A. (1978) Double-blind controlled trial of therapy (ECT) and simulated electroconvulsive ECT in depressive illness. *Lancet*, **i**, 738–740.

Gangadhar, B. N. & Thirthalli, J. (2010) Frequency of electroconvulsive therapy sessions in a course. *Journal of ECT*, **26**, 181–185.

Gangadhar, B. N., Janakiramaiah, N., Subbakrishna, D. K., *et al* (1993) Twice versus thrice weekly ECT in melancholia: a double-blind prospective comparison. *Journal of Affective Disorders*, **27**, 273–278.

Ghaziuddin, N., Laughrin, D. & Giordani, B. (2001) Cognitive side-effects of electroconvulsive therapy (ECT) in adolescents. *Journal of Child and Adolescent Psychopharmacology*, **10**, 269–276.

Gregory, S., Shawcross, C. R. & Gill, D. (1985) The Nottingham ECT Study. A double-blind comparison of bilateral, unilateral and simulated ECT in depressive illness. *British Journal of Psychiatry*, **146**, 520–524.

Hansen, P. E., Ravnkilde, B., Videbech, P., *et al* (2011) Low-frequency repetitive transcranial magnetic stimulation inferior to electroconvulsive therapy in treating depression. *Journal of ECT*, **27**, 26–32.

Heikman, P., Kalska, H., Katila, H., *et al* (2002) Right unilateral and bifrontal electroconvulsive therapy in the treatment of depression: a preliminary study. *Journal of ECT*, **18**, 26–30.

Henshaw, C., Cox, J. & Barton, J. (2009) *Modern Management of Perinatal Psychiatric Disorders*. RCPsych Publications.

Janakiramaiah, N., Motreja, S., Gangadhar, B. N., *et al* (1998) Once vs. three times weekly ECT in melancholia: a randomised control trial. *Acta Psychiatrica Scandinavica*, **98**, 316–320.

Johnstone, E. C., Deakin, J. F., Lawler, P., *et al* (1980) The Northwick Park electroconvulsive therapy trial. *Lancet*, **2**, 1317–1320.

Kellner, C. H., Monroe, J., Prichett, J., *et al* (1992) Weekly ECT in geriatric depression. *Convulsive Therapy*, **8**, 245–252.

Kellner, C. H., Knapp, R., Husain, M. M., *et al* (2010) Bifrontal, bitemporal and right unilateral electrode placement in ECT: randomised trial. *British Journal of Psychiatry*, **196**, 226–234.

Lambourn, J. & Gill, D. (1978) A controlled comparison of simulated and real ECT. *British Journal of Psychiatry*, **133**, 514–519.

Lerer, B., Shapira, B., Calev, A., *et al* (1995) Antidepressant and cognitive effects of twice- versus three-times weekly ECT. *American Journal of Psychiatry*, **152**, 564–570.

Martín, J. L., Barbanoj, J. M., Schlaepfer, T. E., *et al* (2002) Transcranial magnetic stimulation for treating depression. *Cochrane Database of Systematic Reviews*, **2**, CD003493.

McCall, W. V., Dunn, A., Rosenquist, P. B., *et al* (2002) Markedly suprathreshold right unilateral ECT versus minimally suprathreshold bilateral ECT: antidepressant and memory effects. *Journal of ECT*, **18**, 126–129.

McCormick, L. M., Brumm, M. C., Benede, A. K., *et al* (2009) Relative ineffectiveness of ultrabrief right unilateral versus bilateral electroconvulsive therapy in depression. *Journal of ECT*, **25**, 238–242.

National Collaborating Centre for Mental Health (2010) *Depression: The Treatment and Management of Depression in Adults* (update edn) (National Clinical Practice Guideline 90). British Psychological Society & Royal College of Psychiatrists.

National Institute for Health and Clinical Excellence (2006) *Interventional Procedure Overview of Transcranial Magnetic Stimulation for Severe Depression* (IP346). NICE.

Porter, R. & Ferrier, N. (1999) Emergency treatment of depression. *Advances in Psychiatric Treatment*, **5**, 3–10.

Prudic, J., Sackeim, H. A. & Devanand, D. P. (1990) Medication resistance and clinical response to ECT. *Psychiatry Research*, **31**, 287–296.

Prudic, J., Haskett, R. F., Mulsant, B., *et al* (1996) Resistance to antidepressant medications and short-term clinical response to ECT. *American Journal of Psychiatry*, **153**, 985–992.

Ranjkesh, F., Barekatain, M. & Akuchakian, S. (2005) Bifrontal versus right unilateral and bitemporal electroconvulsive therapy in major depressive disorder. *Journal of ECT*, **21**, 207–210.

Reed, P., Sermin, N., Appleby, L., *et al* (1999) A comparison of clinical response to electroconvulsive therapy in puerperal and non-puerperal psychoses. *Journal of Affective Disorders*, **54**, 255–260.

Sackeim, H. A., Prudic, J., Nobler, M. S., *et al* (2008) Effects of pulse width and electrode placement on the efficacy and cognitive effects of electroconvulsive therapy. *Brain Stimulation*, **1**, 71–83.

Scott, A. I. F. (ed.) (2005) *The ECT Handbook: The Third Report of the Royal College of Psychiatrists' Special Committee on ECT* (2nd edn) (Council Report CR128), pp. 9–24. Royal College of Psychiatrists.

Semkovska, M., Keane, D., Babalola, O., *et al* (2011) Unilateral brief-pulse electroconvulsive therapy and cognition: effects of electrode placement, stimulus dosage and time. *Journal of Psychiatric Research*, **45**, 770–780.

Shapira, B., Tubi, N., Drexler, H., *et al* (1998) Cost and benefit in the choice of ECT schedule. Twice versus three times weekly ECT. *British Journal of Psychiatry*, **172**, 44–48.

Sienaert, P., Vansteelandt, K., Demyttenaere, K., *et al* (2009) Randomized comparison of ultra-brief bifrontal and unilateral electroconvulsive therapy for major depression: clinical efficacy. *Journal of Affective Disorders*, **122**, 60–67.

Sobin, C., Prudic, J., Devanand, D. P., *et al* (1996) Who responds to electroconvulsive therapy? A comparison of effective and ineffective forms of treatment. *British Journal of Psychiatry*, **169**, 322–328.

Souery, D., Amsterdam, J., de Montigny, C., *et al* (1999) Treatment resistant depression: methodological overview and operational criteria. *European Psychopharmacology*, **9**, 83–91.

Stoppe, A., Louzã, M., Rosa, M., *et al* (2006) Fixed high-dose electroconvulsive therapy in the elderly with depression: a double-blind, randomized comparison of efficacy and tolerability between unilateral and bilateral electrode placement. *Journal of ECT*, **22**, 92–99.

Tew, J. D. J., Mulsant, B. H., Haskett, R. F., *et al* (2002) A randomized comparison of high-charge right unilateral electroconvulsive therapy and bilateral electroconvulsive therapy in older depressed patients who failed to respond to 5 to 8 moderate-charge right unilateral treatments. *Journal of Clinical Psychiatry*, **63**, 1102–1105.

Thase, M. E. & Rush, A. J. (1997) When at first you don't succeed: sequential strategies for antidepressant non-responders. *Journal of Clinical Psychiatry*, **58** (suppl. 13), 23–29.

UK ECT Review Group (2003) Efficacy and safety of electro-convulsive therapy in depressive disorders: a systematic review and meta-analysis. *Lancet*, **361**, 799–808.

Vieweg, R. & Shawcross, C. R. (1998) Trial to determine any difference between two and three times a week ECT in the rate of recovery from depression. *Journal of Mental Health*, **7**, 403–409.

Walter, G., Rey, J. M. & Mitchell, P. M. (1999) Practitioner preview: ECT use in adolescents. *Journal of Child Psychology and Psychiatry*, **38**, 594–599.

West, E. D. (1981) Electric convulsion therapy in depression: a double blind controlled trial. *BMJ*, **282**, 355–357.

Wilson, I. C., Vernon, J. T., Guin, T., *et al* (1963) A controlled study of treatments of depression. *Journal of Neuropsychiatry*, **4**, 331–337.

CHAPTER 15

The use of ECT in the treatment of mania

Andrew M. Whitehouse and Jonathan Waite

Some of the earliest case reports of the efficacy of convulsive therapy (both chemical and electrical) concerned patients with mania. In reviewing the early literature on ECT in mania, Mukherjee *et al* (1994) noted that the proportion of patients showing remission or marked clinical improvement varied between 63% and 84%.

Electroconvulsive therapy is no longer regularly considered in the UK for the treatment of mania. There is no mention of ECT for management of acute mania in the NICE guideline on bipolar disorder (2006). This was in spite of the acknowledgement by NICE that ECT is an effective treatment for mania (National Institute for Clinical Excellence, 2003). In contrast, both the American Psychiatric Association and World Federation of Societies of Biological Psychiatry treatment guidelines recommend the use of ECT in the treatment of acute manic episodes which are resistant to treatment with antipsychotic and mood-stabilising medication (American Psychiatric Association, 2002; Grunze *et al*, 2010).

Efficacy of ECT in acute mania

There have been no new randomised controlled studies of ECT in acute manic episodes since the previous edition of *The ECT Handbook*.

Retrospective studies

McCabe (1976) compared patients with mania treated with ECT against an untreated matched control group from a period when ECT was unavailable. The ECT-treated group had a better outcome and shorter hospital stay. These two groups were then compared with a matched group treated with chlorpromazine (McCabe & Norris, 1977). Of the 28 patients treated with chlorpromazine, 18 responded. The 10 patients who did not respond satisfactorily to chlorpromazine, recovered with ECT treatment. This is in comparison to the ECT-treated group, in which all 28 patients responded.

Thomas & Reddy (1982) found ECT, chlorpromazine and lithium to be equally effective. Black *et al* (1987) found that a significantly greater proportion of ECT-treated patients improved markedly than lithium-treated patients. Three other studies, with no comparison groups, found marked clinical improvement or remission in 56–78% of patients (Alexander *et al*, 1988; Stromgren, 1988; Mukherjee & Debsikdar, 1992).

Prospective studies

There have been three prospective studies of the efficacy of ECT in mania. Small *et al* (1988) randomised 34 patients admitted to hospital with mania to ECT or lithium carbonate. Unilateral ECT was initially prescribed but with the option of switching to bilateral ECT. The details of stimulus dosing were not provided. After the first six patients received unilateral ECT with little or no benefit, or even a worsening of their condition, the study design was changed so that bilateral ECT was administered from the beginning. Electroconvulsive therapy was given three times weekly. Both the ECT and lithium groups received concomitant antipsychotic medication. When the ECT treatment was completed, patients were prescribed prophylactic lithium carbonate. Over an 8-week period, ratings of observers indicated that the ECT-treated patients improved more than those treated with lithium carbonate.

Mukherjee *et al* (1988) examined the effectiveness of ECT in 20 patients with mania who had proved treatment resistant to pharmacotherapy of at least 3 weeks' duration. The patients were randomised to receive left unilateral ECT, right unilateral ECT, bilateral ECT or a lithium and haloperidol combination (five patients in each group). Empirical measurement of the seizure threshold was conducted at the start of ECT, and thereafter the stimulus exceeded the seizure threshold by 150%. Fifty-nine per cent of the ECT-treated patients were responders, compared with none of the small group of patients receiving pharmacotherapy. No difference in outcome was found between unilateral and bilateral ECT.

Sikdar *et al* (1994) were the only group to compare actual ECT with simulated ECT. In this double-blind, controlled study, 30 patients who fulfilled DSM–III–R criteria for a manic episode (American Psychiatric Association, 1987) were randomised to an experimental group (actual ECT) or a simulated group (control). The experimental group received eight bilateral ECT treatments in addition to chlorpromazine 600 mg/day. After a patient had received six ECT treatments, the dose of chlorpromazine could be changed or another antipsychotic could be prescribed in its place. The simulated group received eight simulated ECT treatments and their medication was managed in an identical way to that of the experimental group.

At the end of the study, 12 patients in the experimental group were completely recovered, compared with only 1 patient in the simulated group. There was a significantly greater decrease on the Mania Rating Scale (Bech *et al*, 1979) in the experimental group compared with the simulated group after the second, fourth, sixth and eighth ECT treatments ($P<0.001$).

Eleven patients in the simulated group required an increase in antipsychotic medication compared with two patients in the experimental group, which is a significant difference ($P<0.05$). The patients receiving real ECT also had a significantly shorter duration of illness than the simulated ECT group. Sikdar *et al* (1994) commented that their findings 'demonstrate that a combination of ECT and a moderate dose of a neuroleptic is extremely effective in rapidly aborting an acute episode of mania' (p. 809). They concluded that their results 'highlight the fact that ECT can be recommended for any manic patient, irrespective of the severity or the duration of the illness' (p. 809).

Kutcher & Robertson (1995) offered ECT to a group of 22 young people (aged 16−22) with resistant bipolar disorder (11 manic, 11 depressed). Sixteen accepted the offer of ECT and received a total of 166 treatments. Compared with the group who declined ECT, they had a much shorter mean hospital stay (74 days *v*. 176 days).

Incident mania

Please see Chapter 7 for information about the frequency with which manic episodes ensue after a course of ECT for the treatment of depression.

Electrode placement

Because of the small scale and methodological weaknesses of the studies of ECT in mania, there is little evidence on the optimal electrode placement for randomised controlled trials in mania.

Small *et al* (1985) concluded that 'patients who exhibit significant symptoms of mania and who do not respond to right unilateral ECT, can benefit from bilateral treatment. In all probability such patients should receive bilateral treatment from the beginning' (p. 132). Mukherjee *et al* (1988) found no difference between unilateral and bilateral ECT in patients with mania, but the study lacked the statistical power to compare the treatments because of the small sample size.

These studies of the efficacy of unilateral ECT were conducted before it was clearly established that electrical dose is an important determinant of the efficacy of unilateral ECT in depressive illness. There have been no controlled comparisons of high-dose unilateral ECT with moderately suprathreshold bilateral ECT.

Two small studies (Barekatain *et al*, 2008; Hiremani *et al*, 2008) have suggested that bifrontal electrode placement may produce comparable or more rapid improvement in manic symptoms to bitemporal ECT, with the same or fewer cognitive adverse effects. However, in view of the findings from more adequately powered studies of electrode placement in patients with depressive disorders, it is not possible to make a firm recommendation for bifrontal electrode placement for ECT in the treatment of mania. Where the speed of response is critical, for example in life-threatening illness, it may be advisable to use bitemporal ECT.

Recommendations

Electroconvulsive therapy has been shown to be an effective treatment in mania. The treatment of choice for mania is the use of mood-stabilising drugs plus an antipsychotic drug (American Psychiatric Association, 2002; National Institute for Health and Clinical Excellence, 2006; Grunze *et al*, 2010). Electroconvulsive therapy should be considered for the treatment of persistent or life-threatening symptoms in severe or prolonged manic episodes where there is inadequate response to first-line treatments.

References

Alexander, R. C., Salmon, M., Ionescu-Pioggia, M., *et al* (1988) Convulsive therapy in the treatment of mania: McLean Hospital 1973–1986. *Convulsive Therapy*, **4**, 115–125.

American Psychiatric Association (1987) *Diagnostic and Statistical Manual of Mental Disorders (3rd edn, revised) (DSM–III–R)*. APA.

American Psychiatric Association (2002) *Practice Guideline for the Treatment of Patients with Bipolar Disorder*. APA.

Barekatain, M., Jahangard, L., Haghighi, M., *et al* (2008) Bifrontal versus bitemporal electroconvulsive therapy in severe manic patients. *Journal of ECT*, **24**, 199–202.

Bech, P., Bolwig, T. G., Kramp, P., *et al* (1979) The Bech–Rafaelsen Mania Scale and Hamilton Depression Scale. *Acta Psychiatrica Scandinavica*, **59**, 420–430.

Black, D. W., Winokur, G. & Nasrallah, A. (1987) A naturalistic study of electroconvulsive therapy versus lithium in 460 patients. *Journal of Clinical Psychiatry*, **48**, 132–139.

Grunze, H., Vieta, E., Goodwin, G. M., *et al* (2010) The World Federation of Societies of Biological Psychiatry (WFSBP) Guidelines for the Biological Treatment of Bipolar Disorders: Update 2010 on the treatment of acute bipolar depression. *World Journal of Biological Psychiatry*, **11**, 81–109.

Hiremani, R. M., Thirthalli, J., Tharayil, B. S., *et al* (2008) Double-blind randomized controlled study comparing short-term efficacy of bifrontal and bitemporal electroconvulsive therapy in acute mania. *Bipolar Disorders*, **10**, 701–707.

Kutcher, S. & Robertson, H. A. (1995) Electroconvulsive therapy in treatment-resistant bipolar youth. *Journal of Child and Adolescent Psychopharmacology*, **5**, 167–175.

McCabe, M. S. (1976) ECT in the treatment of mania: a controlled study. *American Journal of Psychiatry*, **133**, 688–691.

McCabe, M. S. & Norris, B. (1977) ECT versus chlorpromazine in mania. *Biological Psychiatry*, **12**, 245–254.

Mukherjee, S. & Debsikdar, V. (1992) Unmodified electroconvulsive therapy of acute mania: a retrospective naturalistic study. *Convulsive Therapy*, **8**, 5–11.

Mukherjee, S., Sackheim, H. A. & Lee, C. (1988) Unilateral ECT in the treatment of manic episodes. *Convulsive Therapy*, **4**, 74–80.

Mukherjee, S., Sackheim, H. A. & Schnur, D. B. (1994) Electroconvulsive therapy of acute manic episodes: a review of 50 years' experience. *American Journal of Psychiatry*, **151**, 169–176.

National Institute for Clinical Excellence (2003) *Guidance on the Use of Electroconvulsive Therapy* (Technology Appraisal TA59). NICE.

National Institute for Health and Clinical Excellence (2006) *Bipolar Disorder: The Management of Bipolar Disorder in Adults, Children and Adolescents, in Primary and Secondary Care* (Clinical Guideline CG38). NICE.

Sikdar, S., Kulhara, P., Avasthi, A., *et al* (1994) Combined chlorpromazine and electroconvulsive therapy in mania. *British Journal of Psychiatry*, **164**, 806–810.

Small, J. G., Small, I. F., Milstein, V., *et al* (1985) Manic symptoms: an indication for bilateral ECT. *Biological Psychiatry*, **20**, 125–134.

Small, J. G., Klapper, M. H., Kellams, J. J., *et al* (1988) Electroconvulsive treatment compared with lithium in the management of manic states. *Archives of General Psychiatry*, **45**, 727–732.

Stromgren, L. S. (1988) Electroconvulsive therapy in Aarhus, Denmark, in 1984: its application in non-depressive disorders. *Convulsive Therapy*, **4**, 306–313.

Thomas, J. & Reddy, B. (1982) The treatment of mania: a retrospective evaluation of the effects of ECT, chlorpromazine, and lithium. *Journal of Affective Disorders*, **4**, 85–92.

CHAPTER 16

The use of ECT in the treatment of schizophrenia and catatonia

Christopher F. Fear, Ross A. Dunne and Declan M. McLoughlin

From its beginning in 1938 through to the 1950s, ECT enjoyed considerable popularity for the treatment of schizophrenia. As one of the very few available treatments, it appeared to offer rapid alleviation of psychotic symptoms, particularly in the acutely ill, and was said to be without significant risks. Nevertheless, the availability of antipsychotic drugs from 1953, together with increasing opposition to the use of ECT, led to its gradual decline through the 1960s and 1970s (Fink, 2001). A resurgence of interest in the 1980s in its use to augment the action of drugs in individuals resistant to antipsychotics was eclipsed with the arrival of atypical antipsychotics, particularly clozapine, for the pharmacotherapy of treatment-resistant schizophrenia. The finding that a proportion of patients have symptoms that fail to respond to clozapine has prompted investigation of combining this drug with ECT. In addition, many psychiatrists see ECT as the treatment of choice for catatonic schizophrenia.

It is remarkable that, despite being available for more than 60 years, there are few good-quality controlled trials of ECT for schizophrenia. This has not been rectified since the publication of the previous edition of *The ECT Handbook* (Scott, 2005), but a number of excellent reviews of the evidence is available (Johns & Thompson, 1995; Krueger & Sackeim, 1995; Fink & Sackeim, 1996; Lehman *et al*, 1998). These were supplemented by a systematic review as part of the Cochrane Collaboration (Tharyan & Adams, 2005). This chapter has been updated slightly to incorporate additions to the literature since the last edition of the *Handbook*.

Efficacy

A comparison of real ECT against 'sham' ECT is the most rigorous method of establishing efficacy, comparable to a pharmaceutical placebo-controlled trial. In sham ECT, the control group undergoes the full ECT procedure with the exception of the stimulus, controlling for all extraneous influences on outcome. The design was developed in the 1950s, and it often included a group who received a subconvulsive stimulus. These studies are fraught with ethical and methodological difficulties and few have been published since 1965. Moreover, a lack of operationalised diagnostic criteria, compounded by an overinclusive approach to schizophrenia in the USA, often resulted in the misdiagnosis of affective psychoses. This makes many of these early studies difficult to interpret. It is perhaps surprising, therefore, that it is primarily on the results of these early studies that the American Psychiatric Association's Work Group on Schizophrenia based its assertion that ECT treatment gives a 50–70% improvement in psychosis and return to work in patients who have been ill for less than 1 year (American Psychiatric Association, 1997).

Krueger & Sackeim (1995) reviewed all four studies of ECT *v.* sham or subconvulsive ECT published between 1953 and 1964, one of which demonstrated the benefit of ECT over subconvulsive therapy. None of the studies found a therapeutic advantage for ECT over general anaesthesia alone. These studies can reasonably be criticised for their lack of diagnostic criteria and use of mixed samples of both chronic and acute psychotic presentations. It was not until the 1980s that this area was re-examined using a more rigorous approach, perhaps because of the ethical issues involved, together with the complexity of the study design, reflected in smaller sample sizes. The later studies used the Present State Examination (Wing *et al*, 1967) or Research Diagnostic Criteria (Spitzer & Robins, 1978) to classify their patients, and all three of these studies found ECT to be superior to sham ECT. It seems likely that the exclusion of chronic schizophrenia explains the different findings from earlier studies. Further, concurrent antipsychotic medication may have improved outcomes by enhancing the efficacy of ECT (see 'ECT combined with antipsychotics', pp. 142–143). Sadly, none of the studies included medium- or long-term follow-up, so that the duration of improvement is not clear. Similar conclusions have been drawn by other authors (see Johns & Thompson, 1995; Fink & Sackeim, 1996; and Lehman *et al*, 1998).

Under the auspices of the Cochrane Schizophrenia Group, Tharyan & Adams (2005) reviewed all trials of ECT to determine whether treatment 'results in meaningful benefit with regard to global improvement, hospitalisation, changes in mental state, behaviour and functioning in those with schizophrenia' (p. 1). The review included only randomised controlled trials in which ECT was compared with placebo, sham ECT, antipsychotics and non-pharmacological interventions (psychotherapy, social casework, milieu therapy, etc.). The studies were examined by two reviewers, who assigned them to categories according to the *Cochrane Collaboration Handbook*, and only those that satisfied A or B quality standards were included. Of 36 studies considered, 12 were included, only 1 of which was assigned A quality. Exclusions were the result of inappropriate control groups ($n = 10$), lack of or improper randomisation ($n = 12$), both ($n = 1$) or mixed diagnostic groups ($n = 1$). All studies considered related either to schizophrenic or schizophreniform disorders. Data were extracted from the papers and subjected to statistical analyses, including odds ratios and confidence intervals for binary data, and numbers needed to treat. Non-parametric data were excluded. An advantage was found for ECT over placebo and sham ECT on the basis of ratings on the Clinical Global Impression (CGI) scale and BPRS. Electroconvulsive therapy resulted in earlier improvement in BPRS scores, which was maintained at 6 weeks after treatment. Limited data suggested that there were fewer relapses in the short term with ECT and that discharge from hospital was more likely, but 'sparse' data showed no evidence that the early improvement was maintained over 6–24 months.

In conclusion, there is evidence to support the efficacy of ECT in the short-term treatment of schizophrenic symptoms but no evidence to show that the effects are maintained in the medium to long term.

ECT *v.* antipsychotics

There is a signal lack of trial data comparing ECT with antipsychotics. Three studies included in the Cochrane review (Tharyan & Adams, 2005) compared ECT directly with antipsychotics. The results favour the medication group, ECT predicting failure to improve at the end of treatment (relative risk 2.18, 95% CI 1.13 – 3.63). One study that compared ECT with psychoanalytical psychotherapy gave equivocal results, with a trend favouring ECT in both the short and medium term. The addition of antipsychotics to the psychotherapy group resulted in a significant advantage over ECT in the short term, with a continued trend at 2-year follow-up.

The consensus view is that studies favour antipsychotic drug treatment over ECT in both the short and medium term (Johns & Thompson, 1995; Krueger & Sackeim, 1995; Fink & Sackeim, 1996; Lehman *et al*, 1998; Greenhalgh *et al*, 2005; Tharyan & Adams, 2005), although Krueger & Sackeim (1995: p. 514) assess these results as being limited 'in fundamental aspects of clinical trial methodology, particularly the reliability and validity of diagnosis, the nature of assignment to treatment groups, and the blindness and reliability of clinical evaluations.'

ECT combined with antipsychotics

Studies examining whether additional benefit is obtained from ECT plus antipsychotics compared with antipsychotics or ECT alone have again run into considerable methodological problems, including questionable adequacy of pharmacotherapy, masking and randomisation. Nine studies have been published to date, eight involving typical antipsychotics and considered in published reviews. The results suggest that the addition of ECT to antipsychotic treatment improves outcome in the short term in terms of number improved but without any evidence for an increased speed of response (Klapheke, 1993; Krueger & Sackeim, 1995). Four of these nine studies satisfied Cochrane inclusion criteria (Taylor & Fleminger, 1980; Brandon *et al*, 1985; Abraham & Kulhara, 1987; Wu *et al*, 1989), and these showed a non-significant trend in favour of ECT plus antipsychotics, with no data comparing discharge or relapse rates. Tharyan & Adams (2005) concluded that the 'results of trials most strongly favouring ECT in the short term do suggest a role for the addition of ECT in those who show a limited response to antipsychotic medication' (p. 19).

Using a more rigorous design, one study randomised 36 patients with operationally defined schizophrenia into three equal groups to receive thrice-weekly bilateral, unilateral non-dominant or sham ECT with concurrent haloperidol (Sarita *et al*, 1998). Patients were rated by an independent psychiatrist, masked to treatment group, using the BPRS, CGI and a rating scale for extrapyramidal side-effects. No therapeutic advantage was found for combined ECT and antipsychotics, whereas the ECT groups performed worse than the sham ECT group on memory tests 4 weeks after treatment. This study, despite its small sample size, is sounder in its design than many of those demonstrating a benefit for combined treatment and merits replication.

There is a single report of a case series in which the atypical antipsychotic risperidone was combined with ECT for the treatment of aggression in schizophrenia (Hirose *et al*, 2001). Ten male patients were given risperidone 5–9 mg daily together with 1 or 2 weeks of ECT five times per week. The authors claimed efficacy based on BPRS ratings but their data must be treated with circumspection because there were no controls or masking of the raters and the sample size was small.

Finally, a novel use for ECT in combination with clozapine for acute schizophrenia has been reported by James & Gray (1999), who gave a course of 12 ECT sessions to 6 patients with treatment-resistant schizophrenia at the start of a course of concomitant clozapine. A 32% improvement on the BPRS at week 6 was seen as a rapid treatment response in patients who by then had sufficient insight to comply with blood testing and tablet-taking.

Treatment resistance

Claims for the efficacy of ECT in treatment-resistant schizophrenia would perhaps best be described as a triumph of anecdote over empiricism. None of the studies considered by the Cochrane review met criteria for inclusion because, as asserted by Krueger & Sackeim (1995: p. 523):

> 'we have yet to have a double-blind, random assignment study contrasting the efficacy of ECT and antipsychotic treatment with continued antipsychotic treatment alone in medication-resistant schizophrenic patients.'

The eight papers reviewed by them (which reported 'largely impressionistic observations', p. 523) suggested that in a small minority of patients with chronic treatment-resistant schizophrenia there may be a dramatic improvement, probably in patients with an affective component to their illness. Whether these are simply patients whose concurrent acute depression has been lost within their negative symptoms or whether there is a benefit to the schizophrenia *per se* is impossible to untangle, but there is little evidence for ECT alone improving chronic schizophrenia (Christison *et al*, 1991). There may be a benefit for patients with relatively short-term resistant illness but the data do not bear close scrutiny.

With the advent of atypical antipsychotic treatments, there has been less interest in the possible benefits of adding ECT to conventional antipsychotic treatment. Most pharmacotherapeutic algorithms indicate clozapine treatment for patients who are deemed 'treatment resistant' to adequate trials of two different classes of antipsychotic drugs (Lehman *et al*, 1998). Over the past decade there has been a growth of interest in ECT given in addition to atypical antipsychotics for patients with schizophrenia that has proved resistant to treatment with both conventional antipsychotics and clozapine. There has been some work from a group of researchers at the Srinakharinwirot University, Thailand, who have undertaken comparatively large, open (Chanpattana *et al*, 1999*a*), randomised (Chanpattana, 2000) and randomised and masked (Chanpattana *et al*, 1999*b*) studies of ECT in combination with typical antipsychotics for medication-resistant schizophrenia. The studies suggest a benefit for combination therapy in the short term as well as for continuation and maintenance.

Electroconvulsive therapy was first recognised as a possible adjunct to clozapine treatment in 1991, with a case report of the administration of one treatment to a man with schizophrenia who was unresponsive to an 800 mg daily dose of clozapine (Masiar & Johns, 1991). Although the effects were not good, with two delayed seizures occurring 4 and 6 days after treatment and no clinical improvement, other case reports followed. Reviewers have interpreted the results in remarkably different ways. Considering the same studies, two reviews have found no evidence that ECT enhances or hastens the response to clozapine (Krueger & Sackeim, 1995; Barnes *et al*, 1996), and one has suggested beneficial outcomes (Fink, 1998). Case reports continue to appear, most of which are positive (Benatov *et al*, 1996; Bhatia *et al*, 1998; Kales *et al*, 1999). A review of the literature (Kupchik *et al*, 2000) found reports of a total of 36 patients treated with combined ECT and clozapine for antipsychotic-resistant schizophrenia. Of these, 24 patients (67%) responded, with a 16.6% incidence of adverse effects, including seizure prolongation, transient hypertension, sinus tachycardia and supraventricular tachycardia in 1 patient whose seizure induction had been augmented with caffeine. Sadly, the authors' conclusions that this combination is effective and safe cannot be supported by any form of clinical trial.

In summary, although there are a number of case reports, most of which suggest a benefit from combining ECT with antipsychotics for treatment-resistant schizophrenic symptoms, the evidence base is too small and unreliable to allow conclusions to be drawn regarding its benefit or otherwise. Resorting to this approach with patients for whom all other therapeutic opportunities have been exhausted is understandable and current evidence suggests that it is without major complications.

Maintenance ECT

The best time at which to end a course of ECT is uncertain and relapse is an ever-present concern. In a study of major depression, 50% of patients who responded to a course of ECT relapsed within a year, 79% of them within the first 4 months (Sackeim *et al*, 1990); no comparable data exist for schizophrenia. Early studies supported the use of maintenance ECT for patients with schizophrenia who had responded to acute treatment. In one study, 12% of 57 patients who agreed to have maintenance ECT relapsed over a 5-year period, compared with 79% of 153 patients who declined (Karliner & Wehrheim, 1965). These studies are unreliable as there are problems of design and diagnostic validity, as discussed previously. In considering recent studies, the distinction between continuation ECT, occurring within 6 months of acute treatment, and maintenance ECT, given beyond the 6-month point, as defined by the American Psychiatric Association Task Force on ECT (1990), has been disregarded. In practice, most studies blur this definition so that it seems of little value. Stiebel (1995) retrospectively examined the notes of nine patients with schizophrenia ($n = 3$), schizoaffective disorder ($n = 2$) or affective disorder ($n = 4$) who received maintenance ECT from the University of Minnesota Hospital. Patients in the schizophrenia/schizoaffective group received up to four maintenance ECT treatments per month for 9–17 months after acute treatment and were reported to have made substantial recoveries which were sustained during the maintenance period, but relapsed after cessation of maintenance ECT. No significant adverse effects were reported. A similar retrospective case review, this time at the University of Southern California, reported on 57 patients, 3 of whom had schizophrenia, who received maintenance ECT for 6–8 months (Kramer, 1999). The clinical characteristics of the patients are poorly reported but two patients were assessed as 'much improved' and one patient was 'partially improved'. The limitations of both studies are obvious and concurrent pharmacotherapies were not recorded.

Swoboda *et al* (2001) included eight patients with schizoaffective disorder in a trial of maintenance ECT. These patients had significantly longer remission than controls, although their response was not as good as patients with depressive disorder.

The only other prospective series was reported by Chanpattana and colleagues. In a pilot study of continuation ECT, 12 patients with schizophrenia who had responded to ECT were treated, antipsychotic free, with bilateral ECT for 6 months. The treatment regimen was weekly for 4 weeks, twice weekly for 4 weeks, then monthly; diazepam was used as required to control agitation. Eight patients completed the study period and they remained well throughout. Two patients continued beyond 6 months but relapsed at 8 and 9 months; no longer-term data were reported (Chanpattana, 1997). A second pilot followed a similar group for 12 months; it found that only 3 of 11 patients managed to remain well at 1 year after an acute ECT course (Chanpattana, 1998). In a controlled trial, 58 patients with medication-resistant schizophrenia, who had responded to acute treatment with bilateral ECT and flupenthixol, were randomised to three treatment groups: flupenthixol alone, continuation ECT alone or a combination (Chanpattana *et al*, 1999*b*). Ratings were conducted by trained raters, who were masked to treatment group, using the BPRS. Forty-five patients completed the trial. Out of 15 patients in the single treatment groups, 14 relapsed within 6 months compared with 6 of the 15 patients receiving flupenthixol plus continuation ECT. Of the nine remaining responders in this group, therapeutic benefits were sustained during maintenance ECT treatment lasting from 3 to 17 months. This is the most rigorous trial to date and appears to indicate beneficial effects for maintenance ECT combined with a antipsychotic. Although encouraging, the samples used were small, and it is not clear whether other treatment possibilities, such as atypical antipsychotics (including clozapine), had been tried in these patients. A further open study by these authors of continuation ECT for patients with schizophrenia concurrently receiving flupenthixol, adds little to the debate (Chanpattana & Chakrabhand, 2001).

With regard to cognitive side-effects of ECT, Rami *et al* (2004) compared ten patients with schizophrenia receiving ECT *v.* ten controls. The study failed to find a large difference in verbal or executive function tests and was underpowered to find smaller differences.

In summary, there is some evidence to suggest that, as in major depression, a few patients who respond to ECT treatment for schizophrenic symptoms may benefit from maintenance treatment. The characteristics of these patients, beyond initial response to ECT, are unclear, as are the optimal frequency and duration of treatment. Given that the efficacy of ECT for schizophrenia is unclear, however, considerable work in this area should be undertaken first to justify research into maintenance ECT. The American Psychiatric Association's Work Group on Schizophrenia (2004: p. 102) concluded:

> 'These findings supplement clinical observations of the benefits of maintenance ECT for some patients (Stiebel, 1995; Swoboda *et al*, 2001) and support the use of ECT for those responding to an acute course of ECT in whom pharmacological prophylaxis alone has been ineffective or cannot be tolerated.'

Catatonia

The behavioural neurological syndrome of catatonia has been associated with schizophrenia since its inclusion as a subtype of dementia praecox by Kraepelin in 1896 and, later, of schizophrenia by Bleuler (Hawkins *et al*, 1995). This is a misconception and catatonia would perhaps better now be considered as a non-specific syndrome of multiple aetiologies. Its nosological status was in doubt during the drafting of DSM–IV (American Psychiatric Association, 1994) but a move to create a separate diagnostic category did not prevail (Fink, 1994). Nevertheless, catatonic schizophrenia is well recognised, albeit rare. In one study of 55 patients admitted with catatonic symptoms, only 4 satisfied the diagnostic criteria for schizophrenia (Abrams & Taylor, 1976). A retrospective study found that, of 19 patients with diagnoses of catatonic schizophrenia on admission to hospital, only 7 were classified as having schizophrenia on discharge, the rest being rediagnosed with affective or organic disorders (Pataki *et al*, 1992). The physical seriousness of catatonia – which can present as psychomotor disturbances leading to extreme behaviour such as hyperkinesis, stupor, catalepsy, negativism and anomalies of voluntary movement, which in turn are associated with dehydration, malnutrition, hyperpyrexia and outbursts of violence – merits urgent physical treatment. In such circumstances ECT has long been considered the treatment of choice. A recent alternative approach has been the use of benzodiazepines.

The only trial of ECT in catatonic schizophrenia of sufficient methodological rigour to be considered by the Cochrane review (Tharyan & Adams, 2005) was that of Miller *et al* (1953), who studied ECT in patients with chronic catatonic schizophrenia and found no beneficial effects. Other literature comprises case reports of variable worth.

Despite this, the American Psychiatric Association (1990) endorsed ECT as an effective treatment for the catatonic subtype of schizophrenia. In Britain, NICE (2003) concluded that ECT could be used in individuals with catatonia to achieve rapid and short-term improvement of severe symptoms after an adequate trial of other treatment options has proven ineffective and/or when the condition is considered to be potentially life-threatening.

Hawkins *et al* (1995) reviewed all articles published over 10 years from 1985 to 1994, selecting 70 of a total of 87 papers on the basis that they were written in English, reported clinical symptoms that met two or more DSM–IV diagnostic criteria for catatonia (American Psychiatric Association, 1994), detailed treatment interventions and responses, and neuroleptic malignant syndrome was not suspected. The authors recorded 270 treatment episodes in 178 patients aged 13–90 years, 52% of whom were male. The aetiologies were diverse, including medical and psychiatric causes, and no single cause predominated. The most common intervention was with benzodiazepines (39%), mostly lorazepam. Seventy per cent of treatments with lorazepam alone resulted in a complete resolution of symptoms using a mean (s.d.) daily dose of 3.0 (2.8) mg. Other benzodiazepines (diazepam, clonazepam, midazolam, clorazepate, oxazepam) were used alone in 20 treatments, of which 16 produced complete resolution. Electroconvulsive therapy, used alone, comprised 20% of treatments, and it proved superior to benzodiazepines, in that it gave an 85% complete response rate. The authors reported that ECT 'demonstrated high efficacy' when used in combination with other treatments, although, in fact, the numbers are too small for such conclusions to be drawn with any confidence. Fifteen per cent ($n = 40$) of treatments were with antipsychotics alone, to which only 7.5% of patients responded completely. Moreover, four patients died, including two who had received antipsychotic treatment for catatonia; and four cases of neuroleptic malignant syndrome occurred in patients who had received antipsychotic treatment for their catatonia. There are many limitations to this work beyond the reporting bias considered by the authors in their discussion. The failure to consider response to treatment within different aetiologies of catatonia limits the applicability of the findings to any one clinical syndrome such as schizophrenia. At best, it is a review of case reports relating to a diverse syndrome of catatonia, without the methodological rigour of a clinical trial. Nevertheless, Hawkins *et al* conclude that catatonia (regardless of aetiology) should initially be treated with a benzodiazepine, proceeding to ECT if there is no improvement within 48–72 h, if the patient's condition worsens, or if malignant catatonia (see p. 149) is suspected.

In an attempt to relate the finding more clearly to schizophrenia, data were extracted from the paper by Hawkins *et al* (1995: Table 1, pp. 350–359) where the patients studied had clear diagnoses of schizophrenia, catatonic schizophrenia or schizophreniform disorder. Eight studies were identified (Walter-Ryan, 1985; Salam *et al*, 1987; Rankel & Rankel, 1988; Ripley & Millson, 1988; DeLisle, 1991; Smith & Lebegue, 1991; Van der Kelft *et al*, 1991; Martényi *et al*, 2001), which reported a total of 14 cases. Of these, 11 patients responded completely to benzodiazepine treatment, two following a failure of ECT and a variety of other treatments (Ripley & Millson, 1988; Smith & Lebegue, 1991). Only one patient showed a complete response to ECT, in combination with dantrolene following a failure of dantrolene alone (Van der Kelft *et al*, 1991), and one patient each responded to carbamazepine and bromocriptine.

A retrospective review of patients with catatonia between 1985 and 1990 by Pataki *et al* (1992) found seven patients who satisfied DSM criteria for schizophrenia, of whom four were treated with ECT: one had 'much improved/recovered', two had 'improved' and one remained unchanged. In a comparison group of seven patients with affective disorders, all five of the patients who were given ECT had 'much improved/recovered'. Although of interest, the picture is complicated by the variety of concurrent pharmacotherapies administered, including tricyclic antidepressants, benzodiazepines and antipsychotics. The results are supported by those of Abrams (1997), who found that patients with catatonia who fail to respond to ECT are more likely to have a primary diagnosis of schizophrenia, and by Escobar *et al* (2000), who showed a greater improvement among patients with catatonia associated with mood disorders than with schizophrenia. There has been a recent suggestion that catatonia in the context of schizophrenia responds more quickly to ECT than schizophrenia without catatonia (Thirthalli *et al*, 2009).

The *Journal of ECT* devoted the December 2010 issue to ECT and catatonia (Fink 2010). Van Waarde *et al* (2010) reported on 27 patients with catatonia over an 18-year period: medication was unsuccessful in 85%, but 59% responded to ECT. Consoli *et al* (2010) reviewed the literature on ECT for catatonia in adolescence.

Malignant (or 'lethal') catatonia

This is a variant of catatonia characterised by psychomotor abnormalities, delirium and hyperpyrexia, which, untreated, is rapidly fatal as a result of a combination of exhaustion and dehydration. The seminal review is that of Mann *et al* (1986), who identified 292 cases in the world literature from 1960, of which 117 were primarily schizophrenic. A further 71 cases were identified in a review of the literature from 1986 to 1992 (Singerman & Raheja, 1994), of which 50% had a diagnosis of schizophrenia. These articles indicate the seriousness of a condition with a mortality rate of 75–100% in the pre-antipsychotic era, 60% in the period 1960–1985 and 31% between 1986 and 1992. The use of antipsychotics to treat the condition may be harmful, not least because of the difficulty of distinguishing the symptoms from those of neuroleptic malignant syndrome, into which it has been suggested it may develop (White & Robbins, 1991). There is some evidence, in the form of case reports, for the efficacy of ECT (see Krueger & Sackeim, 1995), which led Singerman & Raheja (1994) to recommend it as the first-line treatment once the diagnosis of malignant catatonia has been made. Other treatments such as dantrolene or bromocriptine may also be effective. One case report has been published since 1992, concerning a 47-year-old man with acute schizophrenia and malignant catatonia who could not be treated with antipsychotics as he had previously experienced neuroleptic malignant syndrome. No improvement was obtained with dantrolene, bromocriptine or lorazepam, but the condition was relieved by 11 applications of bilateral ECT (Boyarsky *et al*, 1999). No accounts were found of the use of atypical antipsychotics for malignant catatonia occurring in patients with schizophrenia. There is one account of a patient with a bipolar affective disorder whose malignant catatonic features responded to olanzapine at a dose of 30 mg/day (Cassidy *et al*, 2001). Van Waarde *et al* (2010) recommend daily ECT for the treatment of malignant catatonia.

Summary

Studies of ECT for the treatment of catatonia are confined largely to single case reports, although there are also a few small series. Most studies consider catatonia as a clinical syndrome in its own right and fail to examine the differential response of underlying conditions such as schizophrenia, or affective or organic disorders. When these factors are taken into consideration, the evidence for the beneficial effect of ECT in catatonic schizophrenia would appear to be less than that in affective disorders. Benzodiazepines and barbiturates have also been found to be effective, and it seems that benzodiazepines offer a safe alternative to ECT and one that is less invasive. Indeed, the absence of randomised clinical trials, particularly studies of sham ECT *v.* true ECT in catatonic schizophrenia, has led one author to suggest that the barbiturate anaesthetic induction agent may be the effective element in ECT for catatonia (DeLisle, 1992). There is clearly a need for more research, but, on the basis of the available evidence, the first-line treatment should be benzodiazepines before proceeding to ECT in uncomplicated cases of catatonia. For malignant catatonia, or in circumstances where use of benzodiazepines is contraindicated, ECT should be the first-line treatment. Conventional antipsychotics may be harmful: their use is cautioned, and contraindicated in malignant catatonia.

Schizoaffective disorder

Little recent attention has been paid to schizoaffective disorder, despite observations that the presence of affective symptoms in schizophrenia may predict a good response to ECT (World Health Organization, 1979).

No conclusions could be drawn by the Cochrane review since only one study containing patients with schizoaffective disorder met the criteria for inclusion and these patients were in any case excluded as they could not be separated from a heterogeneous group of patients with affective disorders (Tharyan & Adams, 2005). Only one study has looked exclusively at the response of schizoaffective disorders to ECT, and it reported a strong response in nine patients who had failed to respond to two different antipsychotic medications (Ries *et al*, 1981). Nevertheless, there are a number of case reports of a favourable response on the part of patients with a depressed type of schizoaffective disorder, who have been said to respond as well as patients with psychotic depression (Lapensée, 1992). There is a single study of maintenance ECT in patients with schizoaffective disorder (Swoboda *et al*, 2001).

Schizoaffective disorder is a heterogeneous condition of uncertain nosological affiliation and there is little clarity in the research as to which symptoms respond to ECT. It is unclear whether the affective and schizophrenic symptoms are equally responsive or whether manic and depressive subtypes respond similarly. Indeed, it is possible that the improvement seen in case reports represents a short-term relief of affective symptoms alone and that the schizoaffective disorder, *per se*, is relatively unchanged. Much research is needed and the most that can be concluded at present is that ECT may provide relief for some symptoms experienced by patients with schizoaffective disorder.

Schizophreniform disorder

Schizophrenic symptoms of brief onset associated with good social functioning are included as a separate category of DSM–IV (American Psychiatric Association, 1994) but not ICD–10 (World Health Organization, 1992). Although it has been included as a purist diagnosis in some studies of acute schizophrenia, neither the Cochrane review (Tharyan & Adams, 2005) nor the authors of this chapter found studies that looked specifically at this group. Given the evidence for acute schizophrenia, there is no indication for the use of ECT in this disorder.

Delusional disorder

Although delusional disorder is probably unrelated, nosologically, to schizophrenia (Fear *et al*, 1998), it is convenient to consider the few case reports of ECT in delusional disorder in this chapter. Fink (1995) suggested that ECT was an 'antidelusional agent', given its reported efficacy for a variety of conditions in which delusions feature as a symptom. The supporting evidence consists of only two reports of delusional infestation (Hopkinson, 1973; Bebbington, 1976) and one reporting erotomanic delusions (Remington & Jeffries, 1994). It is likely that response in these cases was attributable to an improvement of underlying mood disorders.

ECT technique in schizophrenia

Most of the research into the effect of electrode placement on efficacy in schizophrenia was conducted more than 30 years ago and is of uncertain relevance to contemporary practice; substantial, but unexplained, discontinuation of treatment was another methodological problem that complicates interpretation of the findings (see Sackeim, 2003). There is preliminary evidence that the extent to which the electrical dose exceeds the seizure threshold is correlated with the rate of improvement, but not final efficacy, in patients with schizophrenia who respond to bilateral ECT (Sackeim, 2003). Many contradictory assertions have been made concerning the frequency of treatments and length of course, with some authors suggesting courses of 20 treatments or more (e.g. Fink, 1979). In fact, there is no good evidence to support these views and more recent studies have tended towards an identical approach to that used in treating depression, with a course of 6–12 treatments.

Adverse effects

There is no evidence of particular adverse effects being more common in patients with schizophrenia than those, for example, with depression who are given ECT.

Discussion

Schizophrenia was one of the first indications given for ECT and since 1938 a vast literature has explored many aspects of its use. Sadly, the majority of these publications consist of case reports and anecdotes, so that there is a dearth of good-quality clinical trials based on sound methods.

Most of the work on ECT as the sole intervention dates from before antipsychotics were widely available, and although there is some evidence to support its efficacy for patients with acute schizophrenia, antipsychotic drugs appear to be superior. The studies on which this view is based relate only to typical antipsychotics and it is likely that, given the variety of atypicals now available, the advantage of pharmacotherapy over ECT will be assured. There is currently no research to support this, however, and in countries with more limited therapeutic options, ECT is likely to remain an important intervention (Agarwal et al, 1992; Daradkeh et al, 1998; Tang & Ungvari, 2001). There is no evidence to suggest that the beneficial effects of ECT persist beyond the short term.

Recent attention has turned towards adding ECT to antipsychotic treatment in patients who have failed to respond fully to antipsychotics. There are no good-quality studies to support this approach, but neither is there any information to suggest that the combination of ECT with antipsychotics, including clozapine, is intrinsically harmful. Approximately a third of patients with schizophrenia have symptoms that are resistant to all antipsychotics, including clozapine (Meltzer, 1995), and in this group a trial of ECT is an option and relatively safe. There is a need for good-quality research in this area. Even if effective, ECT appears to offer only short-term relief of symptoms and there is some evidence to support the use of maintenance ECT as an adjunct to antipsychotics for prophylaxis in this group.

It is impossible to examine the evidence on the effect of ECT on catatonic schizophrenia in isolation from other causes of catatonia. No clinical trials have been conducted but evidence from case studies suggests that benzodiazepines, particularly lorazepam, provide a safe alternative which is at least as effective as ECT in alleviating acute symptoms. Antipsychotics appear ineffective and may be harmful in malignant catatonia, which is often indistinguishable from neuroleptic malignant syndrome. It is recommended that, unless contraindicated, a trial of benzodiazepines is undertaken for up to 72 h, before proceeding to ECT in the event of a partial response or non-response. For malignant catatonia, ECT is the treatment of choice.

There is some evidence to support the relief of affective symptoms in schizoaffective disorder and ECT is a therapeutic option when pharmacological interventions have failed. In the case of severe depressive or manic symptoms, it is recommended that treatment accords with the recommendations applying to major depression and hypomania (see Chapter 14). Electroconvulsive therapy is not indicated in schizophreniform psychosis. In delusional disorder it may be effective as a treatment of last resort, but evidence is scanty and ECT is probably most effective where affective symptoms are present.

No recommendations can be made with regard to technique and a standard bitemporal electrode placement and twice-weekly applications given as clinically indicated offer the best results. There are no particular problems or adverse effects specific to ECT in schizophrenia.

Recommendations

Schizophrenia

The treatment of choice for acute schizophrenia is antipsychotic drug treatment. Electroconvulsive therapy may be considered as an option for treatment-resistant schizophrenia, where treatment with clozapine has already proven ineffective or intolerable. There is presently no evidence to support the use of ECT as a maintenance treatment in schizophrenia.

Catatonia

Catatonia is a syndrome that may complicate several psychiatric and medical conditions. Electroconvulsive therapy may be considered as a first-line treatment in life-threatening malignant catatonia. In less severe cases, the treatment of choice is a benzodiazepine drug; most experience is with lorazepam – ECT may be indicated when treatment with lorazepam has been ineffective.

Acknowledgements

Dr Christopher F. Fear thanks Bill Evans of the Gloucestershire Partnership Trust library service, and Alex Celini, research assistant at the Royal College of Psychiatrists, for their assistance with the initial version of this chapter.

References

Abraham, K. & Kulhara, P. (1987) The efficacy of electroconvulsive therapy in the treatment of schizophrenia. A comparative study. *British Journal of Psychiatry*, **151**, 152–155.

Abrams, R. (ed.) (1997) Technique of electro-convulsive therapy: theory. In *Electroconvulsive Therapy*, pp. 185–189. Oxford University Press.

Abrams, R. & Taylor, M. A. (1976) Catatonia. A prospective clinical study. *Archives of General Psychiatry*, **33**, 579–581.

Agarwal, A. K., Andrade, C. & Reddy, M. C. (1992) The practice of ECT in India: issues relating to the administration of ECT. *Indian Journal of Psychiatry*, **34**, 285–297.

American Psychiatric Association (1994) *Diagnostic and Statistical Manual of Mental Disorders (4th edn) (DSM–IV)*. APA.

Amercan Psychiatic Association (1997) *Practice Guideline for the Treatment of Patients with Schizophrenia*. APA.

American Psychiatric Association (2004) *Practice Guideline for the Treatment of Patients with Schizophrenia* (2nd edn). APA.

American Psychiatric Association Task Force on ECT (1990) *The Practice of ECT: Recommendations for Treatment, Training and Priviledging*. APA.

Barnes, T. R. E., McEvedy, C. J. B. & Nelson, H. E. (1996) Management of treatment resistant schizophrenia unresponsive to clozapine. *British Journal of Psychiatry*, **169 (suppl. 31)**, 31–40.

Bebbington, P. E. (1976) Monosymptomatic hypochondriasis, abnormal illness behaviour and suicide. *British Journal of Psychiatry*, **128**, 475–478.

Benatov, R., Sirota, P. & Megged, S. (1996) Neuroleptic-resistant schizophrenia treated with clozapine and ECT. *Convulsive Therapy*, **12**, 117–121.

Bhatia, S. C., Bhatia, S. K. & Gupta, S. (1998) Concurrent administration of clozapine and ECT: a successful treatment strategy for a patient with treatment-resistant schizophrenia. *Journal of ECT*, **14**, 280–283.

Boyarsky, B. K., Fuller, M., Early, T., *et al* (1999) Malignant catatonia-induced respiratory failure with response to ECT. *Journal of ECT*, **15**, 232–236.

Brandon, S., Cowley, P., McDonald, C., *et al* (1985) Leicester ECT trial: results in schizophrenia. *British Journal of Psychiatry*, **146**, 177–183.

Cassidy, E. M., O'Brien, M., Osman, M. F., *et al* (2001) Lethal catatonia responding to high-dose olanzapine therapy. *Journal of Psychopharmacology*, **15**, 302–304.

Chanpattana, W. (1997) Continuation electroconvulsive therapy in schizophrenia: a pilot study. *Journal of the Medical Association of Thailand*, **80**, 311–318.

Chanpattana, W. (1998) Maintenance ECT in schizophrenia: a pilot study. *Journal of the Medical Association of Thailand*, **81**, 17–24.

Chanpattana, W. (2000) Maintenance ECT in treatment-resistant schizophrenia. *Journal of the Medical Association of Thailand*, **83**, 657–662.

Chanpattana, W. & Chakrabhand, M. L. S. (2001) Factors influencing treatment frequency of ECT in schizophrenia. *Journal of ECT*, **17**, 190–194.

Chanpattana, W., Chakrabhand, M. L. S., Kongsakon, R., *et al* (1999*a*) Short-term effect of combined ECT and neuroleptic therapy in treatment-resistant schizophrenia. *Journal of ECT*, **15**, 129–139.

Chanpattana, W., Chakrabhand, M. L., Sackeim, H. A., *et al* (1999*b*) Continuation ECT in treatment-resistant schizophrenia: a controlled study. *Journal of ECT*, **15**, 178–192.

Christison, G. W., Kirch, D. G. & Wyatt, R. J. (1991) When symptoms persist: choosing among alternative somatic treatments for schizophrenia. *Schizophrenia Bulletin*, **17**, 217–245.

Consoli, A., Benmiloud, M., Wachtel, L., *et al* (2010) Electroconvulsive therapy in adolescents with catatonic syndrome: efficacy and ethics. *Journal of ECT*, **26**, 259–265.

Daradkeh, T. K., Saad, A. & Younis, Y. (1998) Contemporary status of electroconvulsive therapy in a teaching psychiatric unit in the United Arab Emirates. *Nordisk Psykiatrisk Tidsskrift*, **52**, 481–485.

DeLisle, J. D. (1991) Catatonia unexpectedly reversed by midazolam. *American Journal of Psychiatry*, **148**, 809–809.

DeLisle, J. D. (1992) Failure to use ECT in treatment of catatonia. *American Journal of Psychiatry*, **149**, 145–146.

Escobar, R., Rios, A., Montoya, I. D., *et al* (2000) Clinical and cerebral blood flow changes in catatonic patients treated with ECT. *Journal of Psychosomatic Research*, **49**, 423–429.

Fear, C. F., McMonagle, T. & Healy, D. (1998) Delusional disorder: boundaries of a syndrome. *European Psychiatry*, **13**, 210–218.

Fink, M. (1979) *Convulsive Therapy: Theory and Practice*. Raven Press.

Fink, M. (1994) Catatonia in DSM–IV. *Biological Psychiatry*, **36**, 431–433.

Fink, M. (1995) Electroconvulsive therapy in delusional disorders. *Psychiatric Clinics of North America*, **18**, 393–406.

Fink, M. (1998) ECT and clozapine in schizophrenia. *Journal of ECT*, **14**, 223–226.

Fink, M. (2001) Convulsive therapy: a review of the first 55 years. *Journal of Affective Disorders*, **63**, 1–15.

Fink, M. (2010) The intimate relationship between catatonia and convulsive therapy. *Journal of ECT*, **26**, 243–245.

Fink, M. & Sackeim H. A. (1996) Convulsive therapy in schizophrenia? *Schizophrenia Bulletin*, **22**, 27–39.

Greenhalgh, J., Knight, C., Hind, D., *et al.* (2005) Clinical and cost-effectiveness of electro-convulsive therapy for depressive illness, schizophrenia, catatonia and mania: systematic reviews and economic modelling studies. *Health Technology Assessment*, **9**, 1–156, iii–iv.

Hawkins, J. M., Archer, K. J., Strakowski, S. M., *et al* (1995) Somatic treatment of catatonia. *International Journal of Psychiatry in Medicine*, **25**, 345–369.

Hirose, S., Ashby Jr, C. R. & Mills, M. J. (2001) The effectiveness of ECT combined with risperidone against aggression in schizophrenia. *Journal of ECT*, **17**, 22–26.

Hopkinson, G. (1973) The psychiatric syndrome of infestation. *Psychiatric Clinics of North America*, **6**, 330–345.

James, D. V. & Gray, N. S. (1999) Elective combined electroconvulsive and clozaril therapy. *International Clinical Psychopharmacology*, **14**, 69–72.

Johns, C. A. & Thompson, J. W. (1995) Adjunctive treatments in schizophrenia: pharmacotherapies and electroconvulsive therapy. *Schizophrenia Bulletin*, **21**, 607–619.

Kales, H. C., Dequardo, J. R. & Tandon, R. (1999) Combined electroconvulsive therapy and clozapine in treatment-resistant schizophrenia. *Progress in Neuropsychopharmacology and Biological Psychiatry*, **23**, 547–556.

Karliner, W. & Wehrheim, H. (1965) Maintenance convulsive treatments. *American Journal of Psychiatry*, **121**, 1113–1115.

Klapheke, M. M. (1993) Combining ECT and antipsychotic agents: benefits and risks. *Convulsive Therapy*, **9**, 241–255.

Kramer, B. A. (1999) A naturalistic review of maintenance ECT at a university setting. *Journal of ECT*, **15**, 262–269.

Krueger, R. B. & Sackeim, H. A. (1995) Electroconvulsive therapy and schizophrenia. In *Schizophrenia* (eds S. R. Hirsch & D. R. Weinberger), pp. 503–545. Blackwell.

Kupchik, M., Spivak, B., Mester, R., *et al* (2000) Combined electroconvulsive–clozapine therapy. *Clinical Neuropharmacology*, **23**, 14–16.

Lapensée, M. A. (1992) A review of schizoaffective disorder: II. Somatic treatment. *Canadian Journal of Psychiatry*, **37**, 347–349.

Lehman, A. F., Steinwachs, D. M., Dixon, L. B., *et al* (1998) Translating research into practice: the Schizophrenia Patient Outcomes Research Team (PORT) treatment recommendations. *Schizophrenia Bulletin*, **24**, 1–10.

Mann, S. C., Caroff, S. N., Bleier, H. R., *et al* (1986) Lethal catatonia. *American Journal of Psychiatry*, **143**, 1374–1381.

Martényi, F., Metcalfe, S., Schausberger, B., *et al* (2001) An efficacy analysis of olanzapine treatment data in schizophrenia patients with catatonic signs and symptoms. *Journal of Clinical Psychiatry*, **62** (suppl. 2), 225–227.

Masiar, S. J. & Johns, C. A. (1991) ECT following clozapine. *British Journal of Psychiatry*, **158**, 135–136.

Meltzer, H. Y. (1995) Atypical antipsychotic drug therapy for treatment-resistant schizo-phrenia. In *Schizophrenia* (eds S. R. Hirsch & D. R. Weinberger), pp. 485–502. Blackwell.

Miller, D. H., Clancy, J. & Cumming, E. (1953) A comparison between unidirectional current nonconvulsive electrical stimulation given with Reiters machine, standard alternating current electroshock (Cerletti method), and Pentothal in chronic schizophrenia. *American Journal of Psychiatry*, **109**, 617–620.

National Institute for Clinical Excellence (2003) *Guidance on the Use of Electroconvulsive Therapy* (Technical Appraisal TA59). NICE.

Pataki, J., Zervas, I. M. & Jandorf, L. (1992) Catatonia in a university inpatient service (1985–1990). *Convulsive Therapy*, **8**, 163–173.

Rami, L., Bernardo, M., Valdes, M., *et al* (2004) Absence of additional cognitive impairment in schizophrenia patients during maintenance electroconvulsive therapy. *Schizophrenia Bulletin*, **30**, 185–189.

Rankel, H. W. & Rankel, L. E. (1988) Carbamazepine in the treatment of catatonia. *American Journal of Psychiatry*, **145**, 361–362.

Remington, G. J. & Jeffries, J. J. (1994) Erotomanic delusions and electroconvulsive therapy: a case series. *Journal of Clinical Psychiatry*, **55**, 306–308.

Ries, R. K., Wilson, L., Bokan, J. A., *et al* (1981) ECT in medication resistant schizoaffective disorder. *Comprehensive Psychiatry*, **22**, 167–173.

Ripley, T. L. & Millson, R. C. (1988) Psychogenic catatonia treated with lorazepam. *American Journal of Psychiatry*, **145**, 764–765.

Sackeim, H. A. (2003) Electroconvulsive therapy and schizophrenia. In *Schizophrenia* (2nd edn) (eds S. R. Hirsch & D. R. Weinberger), pp. 517–551. Blackwell.

Sackeim, H. A., Prudic, J., Devanand, D. P., *et al* (1990) The impact of medication resistance and continuation pharmacotherapy on relapse following response to electroconvulsive therapy in major depression. *Journal of Clinical Psychopharmacology*, **10**, 96–104.

Salam, S. A., Pillai, A. K. & Beresford, T. P. (1987) Lorazepam for psychogenic catatonia. *American Journal of Psychiatry*, **144**, 1082–1083.

Sarita, E. P., Janakiramaiah, N., Gangadhar, B. N., *et al* (1998) Efficacy of combined ECT after two weeks of neuroleptics in schizophrenia: a double blind controlled study. *National Institute of Mental Health and Neurosciences Journal*, **16**, 243–251.

Scott, A. I. F. (ed.) (2005) *The ECT Handbook: The Third Report of the Royal College of Psychiatrists' Special Committee on ECT* (2nd edn) (Council Report CR128), pp. 9–24. Royal College of Psychiatrists.

Singerman, B. & Raheja, R. (1994) Malignant catatonia – a continuing reality. *Annals of Clinical Psychiatry*, **6**, 259–266.

Smith, M. & Lebegue, B. (1991) Lorazepam in the treatment of catatonia. *American Journal of Psychiatry*, **148**, 1265.

Spitzer, R. L. & Robins, E. (1978) Research diagnostic criteria: rationale and reliability. *Archives of General Psychiatry*, **35**, 773–782.

Stiebel, V. G. (1995) Maintenance electroconvulsive therapy for chronic mentally ill patients: a case series. *Psychiatric Services*, **46**, 265–268.

Swoboda, E., Conca, A., Konig, P., *et al* (2001) Maintenance electroconvulsive therapy in affective and schizoaffective disorder. *Neuropsychobiology*, **43**, 23–28.

Tang, K.-W. & Ungvari, G. S. (2001) Electroconvulsive therapy in rehabilitation: the Hong Kong experience. *Psychiatric Services*, **52**, 303–306.

Taylor, P. & Fleminger, J. J. (1980) ECT for schizophrenia. *Lancet*, **1**, 1380–1383.

Tharyan, P. & C. E. Adams (2005) Electroconvulsive therapy for schizophrenia. *Cochrane Database of Systematic Reviews*, **2**, CD000076.

Thirthalli, J., Phutane, V. H., Muralidharan, K., *et al* (2009) Does catatonic schizophrenia improve faster with electroconvulsive therapy than other subtypes of schizophrenia? *World Journal of Biological Psychiatry*, **10**, 772–777.

Van der Kelft, E., De Hert, M., Hayten, L., *et al* (1991) Management of lethal catatonia with dantrolene sodium. *Critical Care Medicine*, **19**, 1449–1451.

van Waarde, J. A., Tuerlings, J. H., Verwey, B., *et al* (2010) Electroconvulsive therapy for catatonia: treatment characteristics and outcome in 27 patients. *Journal of ECT*, **26**, 248–252.

Walter-Ryan, W. G. (1985) Treatment for catatonic symptoms with intra-muscular lorazepam. *Journal of Clinical Psychopharmacology*, **5**, 123–124.

White, D. A. C. & Robbins, A. H. (1991) Catatonia: harbinger of the neuroleptic syndrome. *British Journal of Psychiatry*, **158**, 419–421.

Wing, J. K., Birley, J. L. T. & Cooper, J. E. (1967) Reliability of a procedure for measuring and classifying 'present psychiatric state'. *British Journal of Psychiatry*, **113**, 499–515.

World Health Organization (1979) *Schizophrenia: An International Follow-Up Study*. Wiley.

World Health Organization (1992) *International Classification of Diseases (Tenth Revision) (ICD–10)*. Wiley.

Wu, D., She, C. W., She, C. W., *et al* (1989) Using BPRS and serial numbers and picture recall to test the effectiveness of ECT versus chlorpromazine versus chlorpromazine alone in the treatment of schizophrenia: 40 cases, single blind observations. *Chinese Journal of Nervous and Mental Disorders*, **15**, 26–28.

CHAPTER 17

The use of ECT in neuropsychiatric disorders

Ennapadam S. Krishnamoorthy

Electroconvulsive therapy has come a long way from Meduna's early theory of antagonism between epilepsy and schizophrenia to its application today in a range of neuropsychiatric disorders. Meduna (1935) postulated that epilepsy and psychosis were antagonistic, and that seizures therefore could be used to treat schizophrenia. Although this idea is in the broad sense no longer the basis for the use of ECT *per se*, the antagonism between seizures and behavioural disorders, also seen in another clinical setting, the so-called 'forced normalisation and alternative psychosis' of epilepsy (Krishnamoorthy & Trimble, 1999), is but one example of antagonisms in clinical neuropsychiatry. Other examples include: the creation of brain lesions to treat psychiatric conditions such as depression and obsessive–compulsive disorders (psychosurgery); the treatment of schizophrenia with antipsychotics, leading in turn to convulsions; the treatment of Parkinsonism with L-dopa, leading to improvement in the symptoms of that disease but also psychotic symptoms; and temporal lobectomy for patients with epilepsy, producing seizure freedom but also associated with psychiatric disorders such as depression and psychosis (Trimble, 1996).

Rooted in such a background of biological antagonism one would expect ECT to have established itself, or alternatively been eliminated, as a form of treatment in neurology and neuropsychiatry. In this chapter we examine the objective evidence for the use of ECT in neurological and neuropsychiatric disorders.

Parkinson's disease

Parkinson's disease is a neurodegenerative disorder characterised by akinesia, tremor, rigidity, postural instability and disturbances in mood and cognition. Its medical management is complicated by 'on–off' syndrome (abrupt changes in motor function, ranging from excessive dyskinetic movements to freezing instability) and debilitating (often drug-induced) psychotic symptoms, such as delusions and hallucinations (Kellner & Bernstein, 1993). Electroconvulsive therapy is known to enhance dopaminergic function in both animals and humans (see Chapter 1). The role of ECT as a treatment for Parkinson's disease, without some of these side-effects, indeed with improvement in some of the behavioural features, has been the source of considerable debate. Comprehensive reviews have looked at the efficacy of ECT as a modality of treatment in Parkinson's disease. Faber & Trimble (1991) concluded in their review of the early literature and all 27 modern reports published by then as follows:

> 'approximately half of patients with severe Parkinson's disease might be expected to have a meaningful response of sufficient duration to make ECT a worthwhile adjunctive consideration when current therapies are unsatisfactory, especially if maintenance ECT can be continued when warranted.'

Other reviewers, for example Kennedy *et al* (2003), have also concluded that ECT is a safe adjunctive treatment for both motor and affective symptoms in patients with Parkinson's disease who do not respond well to drugs. It has been pointed out that future research must focus on optimal ECT techniques in Parkinson's disease.

Reviewing the literature, the overwhelming number of single and multiple case reports contrast with the paucity of well-designed clinical trials. The vast majority of these case reports have shown positive results, with very few studies failing to demonstrate a response to ECT among patients with Parkinson's disease, but the possibility of publication bias favouring the publication of positive results must be considered.

Following on from earlier prospective research examining patients with on–off syndrome (Balldin *et al*, 1980, 1981), Andersen *et al* (1987) conducted a double-blind trial of ECT in 11 patients with Parkinson's disease. The patients were aged between 51 and 81 years, had on–off syndrome, and were described as without depression and without dementia. Patients were randomly allocated to either active ECT or 'sham' ECT. The patients given active ECT had significantly ($P<0.05$) longer 'on' phases after ECT than the sham ECT group. We could find no other controlled trials in a detailed review of several standard databases.

A prospective clinical trial of bilateral ECT in Parkinson's disease in seven patients, carried out by Douyon *et al* (1989), also showed very positive results. Mean (s.d.) scores on the New York University Parkinson's Disease Scale fell from 65 (15) to 32 (6), with all five subscales showing a roughly equal response.

Moellentine *et al* (1998), in a retrospective study of 25 patients with Parkinson's disease matched for age and gender with 25 patients receiving ECT for psychiatric symptoms, found ECT to improve psychiatric symptoms in both groups, as expected, but also, at least transiently, motor symptoms, in 14 of 25 patients in the Parkinson's disease group.

Pridmore & Pollard (1996) studied 14 patients with Parkinson's disease without comorbid psychiatric illness, who were given ECT for motor symptoms and followed up over 30 months (although data were incomplete for 2 patients). About a third had either no benefit or mild benefit that lasted 2 weeks or less, a third had mild benefit that lasted from 4 weeks to 30 months, and a third had marked benefit that lasted from 10 weeks to 35 months.

Thus there is some evidence that suggests a role for ECT as an adjunctive treatment for the motor symptoms of Parkinson's disease. In addition, ECT can be given safely for comorbid affective disorder in these patients, if clinically warranted. Several reviewers have examined issues such as electrode placement, type of ECT, frequency, dosing, continuation of levodopa and other Parkinson's disease drugs and duration of response. There is little evidence that would help one make firm recommendations. It has been opined, however, that continuous and maintenance therapy with ambulatory ECT will allow improvement to be maintained in both motor disorder and mood disorder (Krystal & Coffey, 1997).

Other movement disorders in neuropsychiatry

The use of ECT in many other movement disorders has been the subject of case reports and some reviews (e.g. Kennedy *et al*, 2003), although there have been no controlled clinical trials of note.

It has been used with some success in antipsycotic-induced Parkinsonism, where it has been reported to improve motor function quite significantly (Gangadhar *et al*, 1983; Goswami *et al*, 1989).

Multisystem atrophy

Multisystem atrophy is a neurodegenerative disorder which may be manifest by Parkinsonian, autonomic, cerebellar or pyramidal signs. There have been several case reports of patients with multisystem atrophy showing improvement in motor function and mood after ECT (Roane *et al*, 2000; Shioda *et al*, 2006).

Tardive dyskinesia

There is considerable literature on the use of ECT in tardive dyskinesia, much of it surprisingly contradictory and inconclusive: several case reports suggest that ECT improves this condition, while several others report that tardive dyskinesia worsens with ECT (Kennedy *et al*, 2003). Similarly, contradictory reports and the absence of clinical trials characterise the literature relating to ECT and other antipsychotic-induced movement disorders, such as tardive dystonia, and also conditions such as Tourette syndrome and other tic disorders (see Faber & Trimble (1991) for a review). The reason for such variability in response in tardive dyskinesia and allied disorders may be the heterogeneous nature of these disorders. Other conditions in which the utility of ECT is unclear include Huntingdon's disease, progressive supranuclear palsy and Wilson's disease.

Neuroleptic malignant syndrome

Neuroleptic malignant syndrome can follow exposure to antipsychotic drugs and is attributed to abnormal dopaminergic activity in the brain. It constitutes a medical emergency, as it has considerable morbidity and mortality, even in the best settings. It may be difficult to differentiate from catatonia (see Chapters 16 and 18). In a review of 45 reported cases and 9 new cases of neuroleptic malignant syndrome treated with ECT, Trollor & Sachdev (1999) concluded that ECT is the preferred treatment in severe neuroleptic malignant syndrome. Electroconvulsive therapy should be considered where the condition does not respond to withdrawal of antipsychotic medication, supportive theory and treatment with a dopamine agonist and muscle relaxant (Strawn et al, 2007). The use of suxamethonium in these patients may be hazardous – a non-depolarising muscle relaxant may be preferred (Chapter 3). However, no controlled trials of ECT in neuroleptic malignant syndrome have been carried out.

Other disorders at the interface between neurology and psychiatry

Catatonia

Catatonia is a syndrome associated with a variety of medical and neurological conditions, including diffuse brain injury, status epilepticus, thyroid and parathyroid disorders and encephalopathy (metabolic and infectious). The psychiatric causes of catatonia include affective disorders, schizophrenia and even hysteria, and in this context it is important to remember that catatonia is a clinical syndrome caused more often by medical disorders rather than an independent disease entity (Gelenberg, 1976). The evidence for the efficacy of ECT in catatonia is reviewed in Chapter 4. When considering the cost–benefit analysis of the use of ECT in catatonia, it is important to remember the cautionary note of Krystal & Coffey (1997); they pointed out that 'when administering ECT to such patients, it is important to carry out a careful evaluation of the etiology of the catatonia in order to determine whether the underlying process increases the risks of ECT' (pp. 285–286).

Dementia with depression

As the differential diagnosis of dementia and depression is complicated because individuals are often unable to report classic symptoms of depression such as anhedonia, there is much to be said in favour of a therapeutic trial of ECT for patients who have dementia and depression in tandem (see Kellner & Bernstein (1993) for a review). It is noteworthy that studies have suggested unilateral non-dominant ECT rather than bilateral ECT to reduce cognitive blunting and post-seizure confusion.

Post-stroke depression

Post-stroke depression is a frequent and disabling condition that is considered to be a direct consequence of brain injury. In a review of the records of 193 patients with stroke and depression, treated at the Massachusetts General Hospital, Murray *et al* (1986) found 14 to have had ECT, 12 of whom showed improvement, and none showed deterioration. Interestingly, cognition was found to improve in five out of six patients with 'cognitive impairment'. Coffey *et al* (1989) have reported that older patients with white matter lesions (hyperintensity) on magnetic resonance scans showed an excellent response to ECT. That these white matter hyperintensity lesions have been attributed to vascular disease is of interest.

Seizures

It is common experience that repeated ECT administration leads to an increase in seizure threshold, with progressive treatments requiring larger doses. Animal studies show that electroconvulsive seizures have anticonvulsant properties in that they raise seizure threshold and block kindling. The elegant work of Sackeim *et al* (1987a,b) on the effects of ECT on seizure threshold has led to an understanding of the potent anticonvulsant properties of ECT. Sackeim *et al* (1983) have also demonstrated a reduction in cerebral flow after ECT, using the xenon inhalation technique, and postulated that the neural hypometabolic state and anticonvulsant effect may be due to the effects of ECT on GABA.

Probably the only clinical study of the anticonvulsant effects of ECT has been in children. Two children with intractable epilepsy were treated with ECT for seizure control. One child showed a change in seizure pattern with treatment, which at greater intensity was also effective in stopping non-convulsive status epilepticus. The other child showed a decrease in spontaneous seizure frequency during short-term treatment. These findings suggest a role for ECT in the management of intractable epilepsy in children who are not candidates for epilepsy surgery (Griesemer *et al*, 1997).

It has been argued that ECT, a relatively benign and non-invasive treatment, may be preferred to radical methods such as epilepsy surgery (Kellner & Bernstein, 1993). Electroconvulsive therapy continues to be used in the management of resistant epilepsy (Kamel *et al*, 2010) but there have been no controlled trials of ECT in refractory epilepsy. It has been used for the treatment of non-epileptic seizure disorder (Blumer *et al*, 2009).

Cerebral tumours

Although the presence of a space-occupying cerebral lesion and raised intracranial tension due to this and any other cause are conventionally considered to be contraindications for ECT, there are a number of case reports that suggest the relative safety and utility of ECT in patients with cerebral tumours and comorbid psychopathology, even following craniotomy (see Chapter 19).

Delirium

Electroconvulsive therapy has also been used successfully in delirium that has resulted from a number of conditions. It has been argued that ECT is effective for the treatment of neuropsychiatric symptoms of delirium, and should be considered when other treatments fail (Krystal & Coffey, 1997). It must be noted, however, that ECT is known to cause delirium in a number of individuals, particularly those with lesions of the basal ganglia (Figiel *et al*, 1990), and caution therefore needs to be exercised in adopting it as a treatment for refractory delirium, particularly in the absence of clinical trials.

Other neurological disorders

Electroconvulsive therapy has also been used with varying effects in patients with a number of other neurological disorders and comorbid neuropsychiatric conditions, including cerebral aneurysm, multiple sclerosis, cerebral lupus, neurosyphilis, traumatic brain injury, brain infections, myasthenia gravis and muscular dystrophy (Kellner & Bernstein, 1993; Krystal & Coffey, 1997). The vast majority of these are individual case reports, and no significant adverse effects have been consistently reported.

Discussion

It is evident from this review that although ECT has been used extensively in a number of neurological and neuropsychiatric disorders, there is little by way of empirical evidence to recommend its routine use in these conditions. The one disorder in which ECT has been used successfully to ameliorate both neurological (motor) and neuropsychiatric (affective and psychotic) symptoms is Parkinson's disease. It is also the only disorder in this group in which some clinical trials have been performed, including a double-blind controlled study (Andersen *et al*, 1987). Although a number of issues with regard to the use of ECT in Parkinson's disease remain unresolved, it seems fair to conclude that it can be used safely for the treatment of Parkinson's disease, provided the recommendations made here are followed. The only other neuropsychiatric disorder in which ECT has been shown to be consistently helpful is catatonia. In this condition, however, the evidence has largely been drawn from case series and individual case reports, and prospective clinical trials are indicated.

There are other conditions, such as dementia with depression and post-stroke depression, where case series and individual reports seem to indicate that ECT is relatively safe and efficacious, provided it is used judiciously.

Then there are disorders such as the antipsychotic-induced movement disorders (e.g. drug-induced Parkinsonism, tardive dyskinesia), where ECT may be tried, although there is no hard evidence for its use.

Finally, there are disorders such as epilepsy, neuroleptic malignant syndrome and cerebral tumours with comorbid psychopathology, where a trial of ECT may lead to beneficial effects, provided a great deal of caution is exercised and a careful risk analysis undertaken in each case.

Recommendations

- Electroconvulsive therapy is a safe, adjunctive treatment for both motor and affective symptoms in people with Parkinson's disease with severe disability despite medical treatment.
- Catatonia is a syndrome that may complicate several psychiatric and medical conditions. The treatment of choice is a benzodiazepine drug; most experience is with lorazepam. Electroconvulsive therapy may be indicated when treatment with lorazepam has been ineffective.
- The use of ECT remains an experimental treatment for neuropsychiatric disorders such as neuroleptic malignant syndrome, Huntingdon's disease and treatment-resistant epilepsy.

Acknowledgement

Professor Michael Trimble contributed to the original draft of this chapter, but has not been involved in its revision for this edition of *The ECT Handbook*.

References

Andersen, K., Balldin, J., Gottfries, C. G., *et al* (1987) A double-blind evaluation of electroconvulsive therapy in Parkinson's disease with 'on–off' phenomena. *Acta Neurologica Scandinavica*, **76**, 191–199.

Balldin, J., Eden, S., Granerus, A. K., *et al* (1980) Electroconvulsive therapy in Parkinson's syndrome with 'on–off' phenomenon. *Journal of Neural Transmission*, **47**, 11–21.

Balldin, J., Granerus, A. K., Lindstedt, G., *et al* (1981) Predictors for improvement after electroconvulsive therapy in parkinsonian patients with 'on–off' symptoms. *Journal of Neural Transmission*, **52**, 199–211.

Blumer, D., Rice, S. & Adamolekun, B. (2009) Electroconvulsive treatment for nonepileptic seizure disorders. *Epilepsy and Behavior*, **15**, 382–387.

Coffey, C. E., Figiel, G. S., Djang, W. T., *et al* (1989) White matter hyperintensity on magnetic resonance imaging: clinical and neuroanatomic correlates in the depressed elderly. *Journal of Neuropsychiatry*, **1**, 135–144.

Douyon, R., Serby, M., Klutchko, B., *et al* (1989) ECT and Parkinson's disease revisited: a 'naturalistic' study. *American Journal of Psychiatry*, **146**, 1451–1455.

Faber, R. & Trimble, M. R. (1991) Electroconvulsive therapy in Parkinson's disease and other movement disorders. *Movement Disorders*, **6**, 293–303.

Figiel, G. S., Coffey, C. E., Djang, W. T., *et al* (1990) Brain magnetic resonance imaging findings in ECT-induced delirium. *Journal of Neuropsychiatry and Clinical Neurosciences*, **2**, 53–58.

Gangadhar, B. N., Roychowdhury, J. & Channabasavanna, S. M. (1983) ECT and drug induced parkinsonism. *Indian Journal of Psychiatry*, **25**, 212–213.

Gelenberg, A. (1976) The catatonic syndrome. *Lancet*, **i**, 1339–1341.

Goswami, U., Dutta, S., Kuruvilla, K., *et al* (1989) Electroconvulsive therapy in neuroleptic-induced parkinsonism. *Biological Psychiatry*, **26**, 234–238.

Griesemer, D. A., Kellner, C. H., Beale, M. D., *et al* (1997) Electroconvulsive therapy for the treatment of intractable seizures. Initial findings in two children. *Neurology*, **49**, 1389–1392.

Kamel, H., Cornes, S. B., Hegde, M., *et al* (2010) Electroconvulsive therapy for refractory status epilepticus: a case series. *Neurocritical Care*, **12**, 204–210.

Kellner, C. H. & Bernstein, H. J. (1993) ECT as a treatment for neurologic illness. In *The Clinical Science of Electroconvulsive Therapy* (ed. C. E. Coffey), pp. 183–212. American Psychiatric Press.

Kennedy, R., Mittal, D. & O'Jile, J. (2003) Electroconvulsive therapy in movement disorders: an update. *Journal of Neuropsychiatry and Clinical Neuroscience*, **15**, 407–421.

Krishnamoorthy, E. S. & Trimble, M. R. (1999) Forced normalization: clinical and therapeutic relevance. *Epilepsia*, **40** (suppl. 10), S57–S64.

Krystal, A. D. & Coffey, C. E. (1997) Neuropsychiatric considerations in the use of electroconvulsive therapy. *Journal of Neuropsychiatry and Clinical Neurosciences*, **9**, 283–292.

Meduna, L. (1935) Verushe uber die biologische Beeinflussung des Ablaufes der Schizophrenic. I. Campher- und Cardiazol-Krampfe. *Zeitschrift für die gesamte Neurologie und Psychiatrie*, **152**, 235–262.

Moellentine, C., Rummans, T., Ahlskog, J. E., *et al* (1998) Effectiveness of ECT in patients with parkinsonism. *Journal of Neuropsychiatry and Clinical Neurosciences*, **10**, 187–193.

Murray, G., Shea, V. & Conn, D. (1986) Electroconvulsive therapy for post-stroke depression. *Journal of Clinical Psychiatry*, **47**, 258–260.

Pridmore, S. & Pollard, C. (1996) Electroconvulsive therapy in Parkinson's disease: 30 month follow up. *Journal of Neurology, Neurosurgery and Psychiatry*, **61**, 693.

Roane, D. M., Rogers, J. D., Helew, L., *et al* (2000) Electroconvulsive therapy for elderly patients with multiple system atrophy: a case series. *American Journal of Geriatric Psychiatry*, **8**, 171–174.

Sackeim, H., Decina, P., Provohnik, I., *et al* (1983) Anticonvulsant and antidepressant properties of electroconvulsive therapy: a proposed mechanism of action. *Biological Psychiatry*, **18**, 1301–1309.

Sackeim, H., Decina, P., Provohnik, I., *et al* (1987a) Seizure threshold in electroconvulsive therapy: effects of age, sex, electrode placement, and number of treatments. *Archives of General Psychiatry*, **44**, 355–360.

Sackeim, H., Decina, P., Portnoy, S., *et al* (1987b) Studies of dosage, seizure threshold, and seizure duration in ECT. *Biological Psychiatry*, **22**, 249–268.

Shioda, K., Nisijima, K. & Kato, S. (2006) Electroconvulsive therapy for the treatment of multiple system atrophy with major depression. *General Hospital Psychiatry*, **28**, 81–83.

Strawn, J. R., Keck Jr, P. E. & Caroff, S. N. (2007) Neuroleptic malignant syndrome. *American Journal of Psychiatry*, **164**, 870–876.

Trimble, M. R. (1996) *Biological Psychiatry* (2nd edn). Wiley.

Trollor, J. N. & Sachdev, P. S. (1999) Electroconvulsive treatment of neuroleptic malignant syndrome: a review and report of cases. *Australian and New Zealand Journal of Psychiatry*, **33**, 650–659.

CHAPTER 18

The use of ECT in people with intellectual disability

Peter Cutajar, Jo Jones and Walter J. Muir

Intellectual disability is a descriptive term not a condition in itself and although the number of identifiable disorders that alter neurodevelopment and create an associated intellectual disability is steadily increasing, we are only beginning to understand the many ways in which the altered neural substrate modifies the course and presentation of coexisting psychiatric disorders. Save in the case of relatively common conditions, such as Down syndrome or fragile-X syndrome, studies in intellectual disability usually involve patients with ill-defined, heterogeneous aetiologies grouped on the basis of their degree of intellectual impairment rather than aetiology. It is clear, however, that adults with intellectual disability are susceptible to the whole range of psychiatric disorders seen in the general population. In addition, our understanding of behaviour phenotypes has developed over recent years; this concept has helped us understand some of the links between genetics and behaviour (O'Brien & Yule, 1995).

The term intellectual disability is used throughout this chapter because it has been adopted by the Royal College of Psychiatrists and is used internationally.

The evidence base in this area of ECT use is composed almost entirely of case reports. The limited nature of this evidence, compounded with specific issues regarding diagnosis and consent, partially explains why ECT seems to be used rarely in people with intellectual disability.

Diagnostic issues

Principles of psychiatric assessment in this population are similar to those in general adult and child psychiatry; particular attention is given to the person's level of communication and understanding, developmental history, direct observation and information from informants, as well as the exploration of associated disabilities.

The predominant view is that psychiatric disorder can be reliably diagnosed using standard diagnostic classifications in people with mild intellectual disability (Meins, 1995; Hurley, 2006). However, diagnosis is more difficult in those with a more severe level of intellectual disability. Diagnostic criteria are very much language-based, so they are less relevant to people with significant communication difficulties. It is then much more difficult, if not impossible, to assess cardinal features of psychiatric disorder such as low self-esteem, guilt (Hemmings, 2007), delusions or hallucinations. The presence of intellectual disability will alter the way that signs of psychiatric disorder manifest themselves. Psychiatric diagnosis can be difficult because of the frequent assumption that symptoms could be part of the presentation of the intellectual disability because of 'diagnostic overshadowing' (Santosh & Baird, 1999).

The *Diagnostic Criteria for Psychiatric Disorders for Use with Adults with Learning Disabilities/Mental Retardation* (DC-LD; Royal College of Psychiatrists, 2001) can be useful in standardising the diagnosis of psychiatric disorder in those with moderate to severe intellectual disability. It is based on a consensus of current practice among psychiatrists working with people with intellectual disability. Other specific instruments used in the diagnosis of psychiatric disorder in people with intellectual disability include the Psychiatric Assessment Schedules for Adults with Developmental Disabilities (PAS-ADD) (Moss *et al*, 1993) and the Psychopathology Instrument for Mentally Retarded Adults (PIMRA) (Matson *et al*, 1984).

Epidemiology of psychiatric disorders in people with intellectual disability

A number of studies have demonstrated an increased prevalence of psychiatric disorders in people with intellectual disability compared with the general population (Cooper *et al*, 2007; Smiley *et al*, 2007). Bailey (2007) found a prevalence rate of psychiatric disorders (including autism and problem behaviour) in a sample population of people with moderate to profound intellectual disability of 57% (DC-LD diagnoses); this is over three times the rate found in a similar study of the general population (Meltzer *et al*, 1995). Cooper & Bailey (2001) found an overall psychiatric disorder prevalence rate of 49.2% in a population-based study; those with more severe intellectual disability had a higher prevalence of psychiatric disorder. Deb *et al* (2001) found an overall rate of psychiatric disorders of 14.4% in a sample of 90 adults with mild intellectual disability, and Gostason (1985) described an overall rate of 33.9% in a sample of 115 adults with intellectual disability. Corbett's (1979) Camberwell study found a prevalence rate of all psychiatric disorders (including behaviour problems but excluding dementia) of 46% in a London population of adults in contact with learning disability services. Cooper *et al* (2008) described a high prevalence of affective disorders in people with intellectual disability. The prevalence of DC-LD depression was 3.8%. Depression was associated with female gender, smoking, number of general practitioner appointments, and preceding life events.

Whitaker & Read (2006) reviewed the literature on the prevalence of psychiatric disorders in people with intellectual disability. They argued that although the prevalence is higher in adults with severe intellectual disability, there is no sound evidence that the prevalence is higher in those with mild intellectual disability compared with the general population. They also concluded that children with intellectual disability are more likely to have psychiatric disorders than children with normal intelligence. They discussed the relevance of 'administrative prevalence' and the possibility that the presence of psychiatric disorder brings people with intellectual disability to the attention of services, thereby influencing measured prevalence. People with intellectual disability also have a higher prevalence of chronic physical illnesses and conditions, as well as syndrome-related illnesses (Cooper *et al*, 2006; Bhaumik *et al*, 2008; van Schrojenstein Lantman-de Valk & Noonan Walsh, 2008).

It is recognised that people with intellectual disability tend to have a higher frequency of life events (Hatton & Emerson, 2004). Studies have shown that, as in the general population, life events have a causal relationship with psychological problems in this population. However, further research is needed to understand the mechanism of this effect (Hulbert-Williams & Hastings, 2008).

Although recognising the limitations of the evidence, we can conclude that people with intellectual disability have more chronic physical illness, poorer coping strategies in the face of increased life events and impoverished social networks, all of which are associated with higher psychiatric morbidity.

History of the use of ECT in people with intellectual disability

In spite of the scarcity of reports, ECT has a long history of use in people with intellectual disability. Bender (1970, 1973) conducted a long-term outcome study on 100 children with 'childhood schizophrenia' who were patients of the Bellevue Hospital in New York during the period 1935–1952. This group would now be regarded as having a mixture of unrelated disorders, including autism spectrum disorder. A large proportion of the 63 most chronically institutionalised children had intellectual disability, ranging from mild to very severe. In total, 59 received ECT and a further 28 had metrazol-induced convulsive therapy. The reports of subsequent clinical improvement are unfortunately difficult to interpret. Payne (1968) and Reid (1972) gave an insight into early/mid-20th-century descriptions of patients with intellectual disability and psychiatric disorder, and also mentioned the use of ECT in some of their cases.

Research in this area has remained sparse; the rest of this chapter considers the available evidence in respect of specific psychiatric disorders in this population.

ECT in people with intellectual disability and mood disorders

In the diagnosis of mood disorders, as much reliance is placed on observable features – such as cyclical mood swings or behavioural/psychomotor change, reduction in the use of speech (mutism in some cases), disturbance of sleep pattern, weight change, apparent loss of day-to-day living skills or decrease in self-care (including continence) and obvious low mood and crying – as on subjective symptoms such as self-expressed low mood and guilt. It is known that people with intellectual disability are much less likely to complain directly of psychological symptoms, although they often somatise their complaints; observations of change by carers are crucial to diagnosis. People with mild intellectual disability tend to have a similar presentation of depression to the general population. Those with more severe intellectual disability tend to present with somatic and behavioural changes, including energy level changes, sleep and appetite changes and social withdrawal (Davis *et al*, 1997; Clarke & Gomez, 1999; Evans *et al*, 1999; Matson *et al*, 1999; Vanstraelen *et al*, 2003). The DC-LD suggests that mixed affective episodes are more common in adults with intellectual disability than in the general population (Royal College of Psychiatrists, 2001). The following are case series and case reports about the use of ECT in mood disorders in this population.

Friedlander & Solomons (2002) retrospectively reviewed the clinical details of ten patients receiving bilateral ECT who had intellectual disability and psychiatric disorders of varying severity. Retrospective scores on the Clinical Global Impression (CGI) scale were used to judge outcome. It was noted that good responders (seven out of ten) tended to have a response within the first few treatments, sometimes noted after the first treatment. Two patients whose schizoaffective disorder was accompanied by catatonia responded less well. Three patients with bipolar disorder, either manic or mixed type, showed a good response, as did the two patients with a depressive disorder.

Reinblatt *et al* (2004) carried out a retrospective review of 20 in-patients who received ECT. Seven had mild, five had moderate, one had severe and seven had profound intellectual disability. Twelve had a mood disorder (bipolar or depressive disorder), six had a psychotic disorder and two had intermittent explosive disorder (both had profound intellectual disability). There was an improvement in symptoms in those with a mood disorder, but not in those with intermittent explosive disorder. Reinblatt *et al*'s data indicated that the presence of hyperactivity and irritability in those with treatment-resistant mood disorders or psychosis might predict likelihood of response to ECT.

Kessler (2004) concluded from a literature review that ECT is as safe for people with intellectual disability as it is for the general population.

He described four cases (depression, rapid-cycling bipolar disorder, schizoaffective disorder and mania) where ECT was used with positive results and provided extensive follow-up information. All four patients had mild intellectual disability. In spite of the chronicity of their illness and the lack of response to pharmacotherapy, in three of the four cases ECT had not been considered previously.

Cutajar & Wilson (1999) reported that the best responses were obtained when biological features of depression and psychotic features predominated. They reported on eight people, seven of whom had depression; one person went into status epilepticus after ECT, requiring intravenous treatment, and a second relapsed soon after the course of ECT. Five responded to ECT, including a woman with mild intellectual disability who developed depression with psychotic features after childbirth. She responded remarkably well to six applications of ECT (Cutajar *et al*, 1998).

Judicial approval was required for the use of unilateral ECT in a patient with bipolar disorder, cerebral palsy and mild intellectual disability (Guze *et al*, 1987), who subsequently had a manic episode questionably related to the therapy (6 weeks after ECT). Delusions may be a prominent feature in patients with depression and mild to moderate intellectual disability who have the required communication skills and, as in the general population, psychotic features may predict a better response to ECT (Kearns, 1987).

Other case reports pertaining to the successful use of ECT in mood disorders in intellectual disability include those by Karvounis *et al* (1992), Jancar & Gunaratne (1994), Snowdon *et al* (1994) and van Waarde *et al* (2001).

One of the criticisms that can be made of the majority of reports is that there is little use of outcome scales or measures. Examples of scales used include the Hamilton Rating Scale for Depression (Hamilton, 1960), Adaptive Behaviour Scale (Nihira *et al*, 1974), Brief Psychiatric Rating Scale (BPRS; Overall & Gorham, 1962), the Global Assessment of Functioning (Luborsky, 1962) and the Mini-Mental State Examination (Folstein *et al*, 1975), although they have been used in the minority of cases. In their review, van Waarde *et al* (2001) found that these scales were used in 11% of the cases they looked at. In their comprehensive review they tabulate all the case reports (which is a useful reference source) and conclude that further studies are needed to firmly establish the efficacy of ECT in people with intellectual disability and severe psychiatric disorders.

In the case of depression, consideration must be given to the whole range of available treatment in the non-acute stage. For example, cognitive–behavioural therapy can be used in people with intellectual disability; they can deal with abstract concepts, providing their knowledge and understanding are assessed and the therapist is prepared to take on a didactic role (Stenfert Kroese *et al*, 2006). Taylor *et al* (2008) described in detail the emerging evidence, which is sparse but deemed promising, of the use of adapted cognitive–behavioural therapy in people with intellectual disability. Some studies demonstrate how ECT can be used in conjunction with other therapies: Mackay & Wilson (2007) described a woman with intellectual disability who experienced a major depressive disorder and who responded to ECT in combination with other treatments including cognitive–behavioural therapy. Clinical guidelines include ECT as part of the range of treatments available depending on clinical need (e.g. The Frith Prescribing Guidelines for Adults with Learning Disability; Bhaumik & Branford, 2005).

In most case reports, ECT was the treatment of last resort. It was used most frequently in medication-resistant, psychotic depression associated with a serious risk to the physical condition of the patient.

The use of ECT in bipolar disorder presenting with mania is described in Chapter 15.

Some of the case reports outlined include people with intellectual disability and mania or bipolar disorder. In addition, a report described ECT (laterality not stated) used to control treatment-resistant mania in a patient with mild intellectual disability (Everman & Stoudemire, 1994). Another case report described the successful use of ECT to treat a woman with intellectual disability, bipolar disorder and catatonic features (Ligas *et al*, 2009). Fink (1999) described a patient with moderate intellectual disability where catatonia coexisted with bipolar (mixed affective) disorder. Electroconvulsive therapy followed by maintenance ECT produced symptom alleviation without the need for continuation of psychotropic drugs.

Some reports, however, group all mood disorders in one study category, making it difficult to distinguish response by diagnosis. It is important to note that these case reports and series tend to describe only the positive effect of ECT in people with intellectual disability and mood disorders. Although case series do include some patients who have not responded to ECT in this group, there is likely to be some publication bias.

ECT used in people with intellectual disability and catatonia in autism

Catatonia is a syndrome of specific motor abnormalities, principally mutism, immobility, negativism, posturing, stereotypy and echophenomena in association with psychiatric disorder (Fink & Taylor, 2003). Fink & Taylor additionally refer to 'catatonic spectrum' behaviours. These more subtle behaviours – although not by themselves catatonic – can be suggestive of it (Box 18.1).

Autism spectrum disorder is a developmental condition in which there is impairment of social interaction, communication and imagination, including a narrow range of repetitive interests and other language and movement abnormalities, with or without intellectual disability. A number of these catatonic spectrum behaviours, as well as those classically associated with catatonia, can also occur in people with autism. Severe forms of catatonia are less common. Wing & Shah (2000) found that a

---

Box 18.1 Catatonic spectrum behaviours

- Tiptoe walking
- Skipping and hopping
- Repeating questions
- Manneristic hand movements
- Inconspicuous repetitive actions
- Oddities of speech
- Holding head in odd positions
- Rocking
- Rituals

Reproduced with permission from Fink & Taylor (2003)

---

severe exacerbation of catatonic features had occurred in 17% of patients over 15 years of age referred to their national specialist clinic for autism spectrum disorders. Given the nature of the clinic, the numbers are likely to be atypical of the population of people with autism, but nevertheless the milder, subtler forms of catatonic spectrum movement disorder referred to by Fink & Taylor (2003) are regularly seen in the autism population. This begs the question of potentially undiagnosed autism spectrum disorder in some cases of catatonia, or an overlap between the phenomena – particularly motor phenomena. Wing & Shah (2000) discussed the potential relationship between catatonia and autism, but not the treatment of catatonia in autism.

Fink & Taylor (2003) discussed how the diagnosis and aetiology of catatonia can be established. They referred to catatonia in childhood and adolescence – including those with developmental disorder – and reviewed the existing case reports and studies. There are only a few reports of catatonia with intellectual disability or autism. There are some accounts of the efficacy of benzodiazepines and/or ECT (Fink *et al*, 2006). There have also been concerns that the use of antipsychotic medication for disruptive behaviour in this group could lead to neuroleptic malignant syndrome, which requires urgent treatment (Fink & Taylor, 2003).

Zaw *et al* (1999) treated a 14-year-old boy with moderate intellectual disability, autism and catatonic stupor that required him to have nasogastric nutrition and fluid replacement. There were affective components to his illness but standard antidepressant treatment had not helped and zolpidem produced only a temporary improvement in the catatonia. Bilateral ECT produced a significant response after the third treatment, and progressive improvement to the end of the course of 13 sessions. Successful maintenance on an antipsychotic–lithium combination and previous episodes of catatonic excitement are suggestive of an underlying bipolar disorder in this case.

A case of malignant catatonia (characterised by catatonia, bradycardia and hypothermia) in a 14 year-old boy who had mild intellectual disability was described by Wachtel *et al* (2010*a*). The boy responded to bilateral ECT after a course of ten unilateral ECT applications proved ineffective, and he continued to improve with weekly maintenance ECT. One of Cutajar & Wilson's (1999) patients had autism and received ECT for catatonia without effect. In that case there was no clear diagnosis of depression, neither were antidepressants effective. However, subsequently a combination of low-dose haloperidol and lorazepam relieved the symptoms (J. Jones, personal communication, 1999).

Wachtel *et al* (2010*b*) described the use of maintenance ECT for three people with autism who developed catatonia. They also reported a case of a 19-year-old man with mild intellectual disability and autism who developed severe depression and life-threatening self-injurious behaviour as well as symptoms of catatonia. He responded to bilateral ECT after other treatments (medication and behaviour interventions) had failed (Wachtel *et al*, 2010*c*).

In conclusion, there is considerable overlap in the motor symptoms of autism spectrum disorders and the catatonic spectrum. There are only a few reported cases of severe catatonia and autism where ECT has been tried and was successful. Electroconvulsive therapy was used where the condition was severe or life-threatening or where other interventions were unsuccessful.

There is therefore limited evidence of the therapeutic effect of ECT, but it may be important to consider its use where other interventions have failed and the clinical presentation necessitates further intervention.

ECT in people with intellectual disability and self-injurious behaviour

The interaction between psychiatric disorder, intellectual disability and challenging behaviour is a complex one. Not all challenging behaviour is an expression of psychiatric disorder; however, untreated psychiatric disorder in people with intellectual disability may be an important contributory factor in the manifestation of challenging behaviours (Hemmings, 2007). Challenging behaviour needs to be assessed in order to implement appropriate treatment plans that can be audited (Deb *et al*, 2006). One has to exercise caution in using the term challenging behaviour, which is a loose descriptive term and can hide undiagnosed psychiatric disorders, including autism spectrum disorder.

Persistent self-injurious behaviour can be difficult to manage in this population. This behaviour can persist for several years; one study showed that 84% of a sample population was still showing self-injurious behaviour almost 20 years later (Taylor *et al*, 2010). McClintock *et al* (2003) found that self-injury is more common in people with more severe intellectual disability, autism or communication deficits. Numerous psychopharmacological treatments have been suggested for the management of self-injury occurring in people with intellectual disability or autism. These include antipsychotics, antidepressants, mood stabilisers, anxiolytics and opioid antagonists. The lack of consensus indicates how difficult effective management can be and the paucity of evidence. There are some data to support the use of benzodiazepines and/or ECT in the management of self-injury associated with features of catatonia. Wachtel *et al* (2009) described the use of ECT in a boy who had autism and associated self-injurious behaviour. He did not have classic signs of catatonia. There was only a limited, transient response to behaviour management and psychotropic medication. His rate of self-injury improved after bilateral ECT.

Other reports include Bates & Smeltzer (1982) who used bilateral ECT in a patient with severe intellectual disability, pervasive developmental disorder (autism spectrum disorder) and a family history of bipolar disorder. Life-threatening self-injury, which might have been a manifestation of an underlying depressive illness, responded to a course of six sessions of ECT, followed by maintenance with lithium. Fink (1999) reported success in treating severe repetitive self-injurious behaviour in a child of 14 years with moderate intellectual disability. Twice-weekly maintenance therapy was continued to a total of 16 treatments. Merrill (1990) reported the case of a treatment-refractory patient who had severe intellectual disability with cycles of severe agitated behaviour, including self-injury. A course of six sessions of ECT resulted in marked improvement.

There are problems in using ECT in these cases: self-injurious behaviour is not a diagnosis. These cases of reported response to ECT raise the possibility that the underlying condition might have been a mood disorder or catatonia. However, these case reports show that in some instances of severe persistent self-injury where other pharmacological or psychological interventions have failed, a trial of ECT could be considered.

ECT in syndromes associated with intellectual disability

Adults with Down syndrome are at increased risk of medical and psychological conditions (such as hypothyroidism and depression) and whose symptoms can mimic cognitive impairment, as well as having a predisposition to develop early dementia. Of five patients aged 17–38 years with Down syndrome referred to Warren *et al* (1989) for evaluation of apparent dementia, all had major depressive disorder, and psychotic features were present in four. Electroconvulsive therapy was used successfully in three patients who had either failed to respond to or developed unacceptable side-effects from medication. Lazarus *et al* (1990) described two women with Down syndrome who had mild intellectual disability as well as treatment-refractory/recurrent major depression. Both responded to bilateral ECT;

one went on to have maintenance ECT and the other had received this in the past.

People with Down syndrome are at increased risk of atlanto-axial instability. The anaesthetist performing ECT should be aware of these risks, especially relating to intubation and muscle relaxation.

Very little has been published about the use of ECT in people with other syndromes that have intellectual disability as a component.

Gothelf et al (1999) noted that the psychotic symptoms of two patients with mild intellectual disability, chronic schizophrenia and the velocardiofacial syndrome (microdeletion within the long arm of chromosome 22) did not respond to repeated courses of ECT.

The co-occurrence of intellectual disability in a man who developed the extremely rare adult-onset form of Tay–Sach's disease (GM2 gangliosidosis) was described by Renshaw et al (1992). His severe depression responded to unilateral ECT and fluoxetine.

These cases illustrate the complexity in terms of aetiology, presentation, treatment response and comorbidity within this population. It is difficult to draw any firm conclusions about the use of ECT in these clinical situations, other than stating that a full consideration of underlying aetiological factors must be undertaken.

ECT for other psychiatric disorders in people with intellectual disability

In addition to mood disorders, catatonia in autism and self-injurious behaviour, ECT has been used in other psychiatric disorders in people with intellectual disability. The following reports give examples of ECT used in people with intellectual disability and challenging behaviours, catatonia, schizophrenia or schizoaffective disorder.

In Thuppal & Fink's series (1999), one man with moderate intellectual disability had behavioural symptoms of decreased sleep, agitation and periods of excitability with assaults on staff. These symptoms were unresponsive to a variety of antipsychotics, including clozapine, and mood stabilisers, including carbamazepine and sodium valproate. A course of 13 sessions of bilateral ECT produced a marked improvement. Four sessions of out-patient continuation ECT were given after discharge. Clozapine was continued throughout. Thuppal & Fink (1999) also described a man with mild intellectual disability and schizophrenia with catatonia who required intravenous fluids. The catatonia responded to six sessions of bilateral ECT, but he required a further 45 sessions as maintenance therapy over 7 months. Another patient with moderate intellectual disability and bipolar disorder poorly controlled by medication was treated with bilateral ECT during a depressed phase with marked lorazepam-responsive catatonic features. Again, maintenance therapy was used (31 sessions over 9 months).

Aziz *et al* (2001) reported the case of a woman aged 39 years with moderate intellectual disability who had schizoaffective disorder with marked catatonic features. A marked improvement was seen in the catatonic symptoms after 5 sessions of bilateral ECT in an eventual course of 11 treatments. Their paper includes a review of other relevant case reports.

Jyoti Rao *et al* (1993) reported the case of an 18-year-old man with moderate intellectual disability where treatment for a non-organic psychosis (diagnosis not further specified) with a course of ECT incurred the rare complication of non-convulsive status epilepticus during the ninth treatment. The authors argued for intratreatment EEG monitoring, which would seem a sensible general precaution.

Symptoms of schizophrenia in people with intellectual disability have also been treated with ECT. Chanpattana (1999) described three cases of ECT use in people with schizophrenia: one had severe intellectual disability, schizophrenia and epilepsy. She improved after six ECT sessions and this improvement was maintained by weekly ECT for 4 months. The second case was a man with moderate intellectual disability and paranoid schizophrenia. He improved after 21 treatments, and he then received weekly maintenance ECT. The third case was a man with moderate intellectual disability and schizophrenia. He improved after four ECT sessions, and then he received maintenance ECT for 6 months.

Electroconvulsive therapy has also been used in the treatment of people with intellectual disability where neuroleptic malignant syndrome has complicated treatment with medication (McKinney & Kellner, 1997; Aziz *et al*, 2001); some authors (see Caroff *et al*, 2004) suggest that neuroleptic malignant syndrome and catatonia could be part of a unitary syndrome.

Although these cases appear to have different and varied presentations, it could be that the response to ECT was primarily due to an effect on the affective or catatonic symptoms; as often is the case in people with intellectual disability, there is difficulty in establishing a definitive diagnosis of the underlying condition.

ECT as maintenance therapy

In some of these case reports the initial phase of treatment with ECT has been followed by maintenance ECT. In addition to some reports mentioned above (e.g. Chanpattana, 1999; Thuppal & Fink, 1999; Wachtel, 2010*a,b*), Puri *et al* (1992) described maintenance bilateral ECT (given every 3 weeks for over a year), which was useful in treating relapsing depression with psychotic features in a man with mild intellectual disability. In another case, a woman with mild intellectual disability and recurrent psychotic depression improved with a course of ECT followed by another seven after a relapse (Ruedrich & Alamir, 1999); monthly maintenance ECT was then instigated over a 2-year period. Gabriel (1998) used maintenance ECT in a woman aged 65 who had chronic, treatment-refractory schizophrenia and moderate intellectual disability. Twice-weekly ECT (30 treatments) was followed by maintenance on a 7- to 10-day interval schedule. The patient's score on the BPRS decreased and the Global Assessment of Functioning score increased significantly from baseline.

Bebchuk *et al* (1996) described problems in differential diagnosis (between major depressive disorder, bipolar disorder and dementia) in a man with profound intellectual disability. Episodic self-injury was a feature of his condition. The early rapid response to unilateral ECT and monthly maintenance ECT was followed by a relapse. A course of bilateral ECT and twice-weekly maintenance out-patient therapy was successful.

Observations on reported use of ECT by psychiatrists working with people with intellectual disability

Cutajar & Wilson (1999) studied the use of ECT by consultant psychiatrists working with people with intellectual disability in the East Midlands, UK (population 4.7 million), during the years 1990–1995. Of the 26 questionnaires sent out, 24 were returned. The use of ECT was low compared with general adult psychiatry; the suggested reasons for this included:

- some people with intellectual disability might have been treated by general adult psychiatrists
- diagnostic difficulties
- problems in obtaining consent
- ECT being considered as a treatment of last resort.

Sayal & Bernard (1998) reported that trainee psychiatrists were less likely to suggest ECT for depressive illness in vignettes of cases of mild intellectual disability, even though they diagnosed psychotic depression more frequently in this group.

Another issue that might prevent psychiatrists prescribing ECT in this population is the apprehension of causing or contributing to further organic or memory change. This subject is discussed fully in Chapter 8.

In their review of the use of ECT in people with intellectual disability and concurrent psychiatric disorder, Little *et al* (2002) concluded that there was a delay in the use of ECT, yet when there is a positive response to ECT, this is often reported as rapid. They discussed the possible ethical issues that could explain this reluctance in using ECT, which could be related to the paucity of the available evidence base; ECT is then used as a treatment of last resort. This situation raises the ethical issue of giving ECT to people who do not have the capacity to consent; carers can feel uneasy about the administration of ECT to this population. The authors also described three people with intellectual disability who received ECT; all had a depressive episode with psychotic features, and all responded to ECT.

The literature relevant to this topic indicates that ECT is used relatively less in people with intellectual disability than in the general population. There are some reasons for this, including the fact that the literature is limited to case studies, as well as consent issues. This area of capacity and consent is considered in Chapter 22.

Discussion

Overall, the evidence base for the use of ECT in this population is limited. There have been no randomised controlled trials specifically in people with intellectual disability. Case reports about the use of ECT in people with intellectual disability often lack information about concomitant medication, psychological intervention or social changes happening during the course of ECT. There is also the inherent problem of cases generally being published mainly when positive responses to treatment are described.

The literature available is generally lacking in outcome measures that quantify response to ECT. Although some papers describe the use of scales, outcome is often described in terms of resolution of presenting symptoms, rather than the use of standardised outcome scales.

In the case reports referenced, the most common level of disability is mild intellectual disability. There is no evidence that adverse effects from ECT are more likely in those with more severe intellectual disability. Among reported cases, the use of maintenance ECT has been frequent; could this reflect the severity and refractory nature of the underlying psychiatric disorder?

Where laterality is stated, bilateral ECT is the most frequently used. As is the case in the general population, its use has not been restricted to the treatment of depressive disorders. Most case descriptions are of patients whose psychiatric disorder has failed to respond to medication or of patients who exhibit life-threatening behaviour.

The use of ECT seems to be much less frequent in adults with intellectual disability than among the general population. The presence of intellectual disability of any degree is not a contraindication to the use of ECT. Many of the case reports indicate that ECT is considered as a treatment of last resort; the evidence shows that ECT can be effective when it is indicated (e.g. depression with psychotic features). So why do we seem reluctant to use it in people with intellectual disability? It could be that where there are well-developed learning disability psychiatric service networks, psychiatric disorder in this population is diagnosed and treated in other ways before ECT is considered. Collins *et al* (2012) reviewed the relevant literature published prior to March 2010. They outline a number of clinical implications and make the case for prompt treatment with ECT in this population where indicated.

Consideration of the use of ECT is sometimes delayed due to the complexity of consent issues. These can be resolved through multidisciplinary decision-making; a second psychiatric opinion would be useful even if not obligatory. The Mental Capacity Act 2005 may have altered practice in the use of ECT by clarifying the decision-making process for people who do not have capacity to consent to ECT. This would be a productive area to research.

In addition to the psychiatric indications for ECT, the presence of physical illness needs to be considered as well as its relevance to the preparation for, and administration of, ECT.

When a decision is made to prescribe ECT for people with intellectual disability, care must be taken to prepare the person and carers for this treatment, regardless of their capacity to consent to treatment. Information is available on the Royal College of Psychiatrists' website (www.rcpsych. ac.uk/mentalhealthinfoforall/treatments/ect.aspx). Pre-treatment visits to the ECT suite, or the use of photos or videos of the ECT suite, may also be helpful in the preparation process.

Recommendations

- Electroconvulsive therapy should be considered in carefully selected cases where clinically indicated: where the psychiatric disorder has proved refractory to medical treatment, where there are intolerable adverse effects of medication, or where the clinical condition of the patient has deteriorated severely or becomes life-threatening.
- Intellectual disability of any severity is not a contraindication to the use of ECT.
- Concerns about consent issues should not be a barrier to the use of ECT where this is clinically indicated.
- Outcome measures relevant to the condition being treated should be used to assess the efficacy of ECT.
- The use of ECT in this population, and related issues, continue to be a fertile ground for further research.
- Given the complexity of the issues described, it would be best practice to ensure that the decision to prescribe ECT includes assessment and advice by a specialist in the psychiatry of intellectual disability.

Acknowledgements

The authors thank Dr Richard Lansdall-Welfare, Consultant Psychiatrist, Learning Disabilities, Nottinghamshire Healthcare NHS Trust, for his insight and advice during the preparation of this chapter, and the staff of the Duncan MacMillan House Staff Library, Nottingham, for their help with sourcing information and references. The authors also thank Dr Jonathan Waite, Consultant Psychiatrist, Old Age Psychiatry, and Mr Michael Sergeant, Mental Capacity Act Lead, Nottinghamshire Healthcare NHS Trust, for their help and advice.

References

Aziz, M., Maixner, D. F., DeQuardo, J., *et al* (2001) ECT and mental retardation: a review and case reports. *Journal of ECT*, **17**, 149–152.

Bailey, N. M. (2007) Prevalence of psychiatric disorders in adults with moderate to profound learning disabilities. *Advances in Mental Health and Learning Disabilities*, **1**, 36–44.

Bates, W. J. & Smeltzer, M. A. (1982) Electroconvulsive treatment of psychotic self-injurious behavior in a patient with severe mental retardation. *American Journal of Psychiatry*, **139**, 1355–1356.

Bebchuk, J. M., Barnhill, J. & Dawkins, K. (1996) ECT and mental retardation. *American Journal of Psychiatry*, **153**, 1231.

Bender, L. (1970) The life course of schizophrenic children. *Biological Psychiatry*, **2**, 165–172.

Bender, L. (1973) The life course of children with schizophrenia. *American Journal of Psychiatry*, **130**, 783–786.

Bhaumik, S. & Blanford, D. (2005) *The Frith Prescribing Guidelines for Adults with Learning Disability*. Taylor & Francis.

Bhaumik, S., Watson, J. M., Thorp, C. F., *et al* (2008) Body mass index in adults with intellectual disability: distribution, associations and service implications: a population-based prevalence study. *Journal of Intellectual Disability Research*, **52**, 287–298.

Caroff, S. N., Mann, S. C., Francis, A., *et al* (2004) *Catatonia: From Psychopathology to Neurobiology*. American Psychiatric Publishing.

Chanpattana, W. (1999) Maintenance ECT in mentally retarded, treatment-resistant schizophrenic patients. *Journal of ECT*, **15**, 150–153.

Clarke, D. J. & Gomez, G. A. (1999) Utility of modified DCR-10 criteria in the diagnosis of depression associated with intellectual disability. *Journal of Intellectual Disability Research*, **43**, 413–420.

Collins, J., Halder, N. & Chaudhry, N. (2012) Use of ECT in patients with an intellectual disability: review. *The Psychiatrist*, **36**, 55–60.

Cooper, S. A. & Bailey, N. M. (2001) Psychiatric disorders amongst adults with learning disabilities – prevalence and relationship to ability level. *Irish Journal of Psychological Medicine*, **18**, 45–53.

Cooper, S. A., Morrison J., Melville C., *et al* (2006) Improving the health of people with intellectual disabilities: outcomes of a health screening programme after 1 year. *Journal of Intellectual Disability Research*, **50**, 667–677.

Cooper, S.-A., Smiley, E., Morrison, J., *et al* (2007) Mental ill-health in adults with intellectual disabilities: prevalence and associated factors. *British Journal of Psychiatry*, **190**, 27–35.

Cooper, S. A., Smiley, E., Allan, L., *et al* (2008) Prevalence and incidence of affective disorders and related factors: observational study. *Journal of Intellectual Disability Research*, **52**, 725.

Corbett, J. A. (1979) Psychiatric morbidity and mental retardation. In *Psychiatric Illness and Mental Handicap* (eds F. E. James & R. P. Snaith), pp. 11–25. Gaskell.

Cutajar, P. & Wilson, D. (1999) The use of ECT in intellectual disability. *Journal of Intellectual Disability Research*, **43**, 421–427.

Cutajar, P., Wilson, D. N. & Mukherjee, T. (1998) ECT used in depression following childbirth, in a woman with learning disabilities. *British Journal of Learning Disabilities*, **26**, 115–117.

Davis, J. P., Judd, F. K. & Herrman, H. (1997) Depression in adults with intellectual disability. Part 2: A pilot study. *Australian and New Zealand Journal of Psychiatry*, **31**, 232–242.

Deb, S., Thomas, M. & Bright, C. (2001) Mental disorder in adults with intellectual disability. 1: Prevalence of functional psychiatric illness among a community based sample population aged between 16 and 64 years. *Journal of Intellectual Disability Research*, **45**, 495–505.

Deb, S., Clarke, D. & Unwin, G. (2006) *Using Medication to Manage Behaviour Problems Among Adults with a Learning Disability*. University of Birmingham.

Evans, K. M., Cotton, M. M., Einfield, S. L., *et al* (1999) Assessment of depression in adults with severe or profound intellectual disability. *Journal of Intellectual Disability Research*, **24**, 147–160.

Everman, D. B. & Stoudemire, A. (1994) Bipolar disorder associated with Klinefelter's syndrome and other chromosomal abnormalities. *Psychosomatics*, **35**, 35–40.

Fink, M. (1999) *Electroshock, Restoring the Mind*. Oxford University Press.

Fink, M. & Taylor, M. A. (2003) *Catatonia: A Clinician's Guide to Diagnosis and Treatment*. Cambridge University Press.

Fink M., Taylor, M. A. & Ghaziuddin, N. (2006) Catatonia in autistic spectrum disorders: A medical treatment algorithm. *International Review of Neurobiology*, **72**, 233–244.

Folstein, M. F., Folstein, S. E. & McHugh, P. R. (1975) 'Mini-mental state': a practical method for grading the cognitive state of patients for the clinician. *Journal of Psychiatric Research*, **12**, 189–198.

Friedlander, R. I. & Solomons, K. (2002) ECT: use in individuals with mental retardation. *Journal of ECT*, **18**, 38–42.

Gabriel, A. (1998) ECT continuation and maintenance in a patient with psychosis and mental disability. *Canadian Journal of Psychiatry*, **43**, 305–306.

Gostason, R. (1985) Psychiatric illness among the mentally retarded: a Swedish population study. *Acta Psychiatrica Scandinavica*, **71** (suppl. 381), 1–117.

Gothelf, D., Frisch, A., Munitz, H., *et al* (1999) Clinical characteristics of schizophrenia associated with velo-cardio-facial syndrome. *Schizophrenia Research*, **35**, 105–112.

Guze, B. H., Weinman, B. & Diamond, R. P. (1987) Use of ECT to treat bipolar depression in a mental retardate with cerebral palsy. *Convulsive Therapy*, **3**, 60–64.

Hamilton, M. (1960) A rating scale for depression. *Journal of Neurology. Neurosurgery and Psychiatry*, **23**, 56–62.

Hatton, C. & Emerson, E. (2004) The relationship between life events and psychopathology amongst children with intellectual disabilities. *Journal of Applied Research in Intellectual Disabilities*, **17**, 109–117.

Hemmings, C. (2007) The relationships between challenging behaviours and psychiatric disorders in people with severe intellectual disabilities. In *Psychiatric and Behavioural Disorders in Intellectual and Developmental Disabilities* (eds N. Bouras & G. Holt), pp 62–75. Cambridge University Press.

Hulbert-Williams, L. & Hastings, R. (2008) Life events as a risk factor for psychological problems in individuals with intellectual disabilities: a critical review. *Journal of Intellectual Disability Research*, **52**, 883–895.

Hurley, A. D. (2006) Mood disorders in intellectual disabilities. *Current Opinion in Psychiatry*, **19**, 465–469.

Jancar, J. & Gunaratne, I. J. (1994) Dysthymia and mental handicap. *British Journal of Psychiatry*, **164**, 691–693.

Jyoti Rao, K. M. J., Gandahar, B. N. & Janakirmaiah, N. (1993) Nonconvulsive status epilepticus after the ninth electroconvulsive therapy. *Convulsive Therapy*, **9**, 128–129.

Karvounis, S., Holt, G. & Hodgkiss, A. (1992) Out-patient ECT for depression in a man with moderate learning disability. *British Journal of Psychiatry*, **161**, 426–427.

Kearns, A. (1987) Cotard's syndrome in a mentally handicapped man. *British Journal of Psychiatry*, **150**, 112–114.

Kessler, R. (2004) Electroconvulsive therapy for affective disorders in persons with mental retardation. *Psychiatric Quarterly*, **75**, 99–104.

Lazarus, A., Jaffe, R. L. & Dubin, W. R. (1990) Electroconvulsive therapy and major depression in Down's syndrome. *Journal of Clinical Psychiatry*, **51**, 422–425.

Ligas, A., Petrides, G., Istafanous, R., *et al* (2009) Successful electroconvulsive therapy in a patient with intellectual disability and bipolar disorder, and catatonic features misdiagnosed as encephalopathy. *Journal of ECT*, **25**, 202–204.

Little, J. D., McFarlane, J. & Ducharme, H. M. (2002) ECT use delayed in the presence of comorbid mental retardation: a review of clinical and ethical issues. *Journal of ECT*, **18**, 218–222.

Luborsky, L. (1962) Clinicians judgements of mental health. *Archive of General Psychiatry*, **7**, 407–417.

Mackay, F. & Wilson, C. (2007) Successful multi-disciplinary and multi-treatment working for a person with learning disability who experienced major depressive disorder. *Learning Disability Review*, **12**, 39–47.

Matson, J. L., Senatore, V. & Kazdin, A. E. (1984) Psychometric properties of the psychopathology instrument for mentally retarded adults. *Applied Research in Mental Retardation*, **5**, 81–89.

Matson, J. L., Rush, K. S., Hamilton, M., *et al* (1999) Characteristics of depression as assessed by the Diagnostic Assessment for the Severely Handicapped – II (DASH-II). *Research in Developmental Disabilities*, **20**, 305–313.

McClintock, K., Hall, S. & Oliver, C. (2003) Risk markers associated with challenging behaviours in people with intellectual disabilities: a meta-analytic study. *Journal of Intellectual Disability Research*, **47**, 405–416.

McKinney, P. & Kellner, C. (1997) Multiple ECT late in the course of neuroleptic malignant syndrome. *Convulsive Therapy*, **13**, 269–273.

Meins, W. (1995) Symptoms of major depression in mentally retarded adults. *Journal of Intellectual Disability Research*, **39**, 41–45.

Meltzer, H., Gill, B., Peeticrew, M., *et al* (1995) *OPCS Survey of Psychiatric Morbidity in Great Britain. Report 1. The Prevalence of Psychiatric Morbidity Among Adults Living in Private Households*. HMSO.

Merrill, R. D. (1990) ECT for a patient with profound mental retardation. *American Journal of Psychiatry*, **147**, 256–257.

Moss, S. C., Patel, P., Prosser, H., *et al* (1993) Psychiatric morbidity in older people with moderate and severe learning disability. I: Development and reliability of the patient interview (PAS-ADD). *British Journal of Psychiatry*, **163**, 471–480.

Nihira, K., Foster, R., Shellhaas, M., *et al* (1974) *AAMD Adaptive Behavior Scale*. American Association on Mental Deficiency.

O'Brien, G. & Yule, W. (eds) (1995) *Behavioural Phenotypes. Clinics in Developmental Medicine No. 138*. Mac Keith Press.

Overall, J. E. & Gorham, D. R. (1962) The Brief Psychiatric Rating Scale. *Psychological Reports*, **10**, 790–812.

Payne, R. (1968) The psychotic subnormal. *Journal of Mental Subnormality*, **139**, 1355–1356.

Puri, B. K., Langa, A., Coleman, R. M., *et al* (1992) The clinical efficacy of maintenance electroconvulsive therapy in a patient with a mild mental handicap. *British Journal of Psychiatry*, **161**, 707–709.

Reid, A. H. (1972) Psychoses in adult mental defectives. I: Manic depressive psychosis. *British Journal of Psychiatry*, **120**, 205–212.

Reinblatt, S. P., Rifkin, A. & Freeman, J. (2004) The efficacy of ECT in adults with mental retardation experiencing psychiatric disorders. *Journal of ECT*, **20**, 208–212.

Renshaw, P. R., Stern, T. A., Welch, C., *et al* (1992) Electroconvulsive therapy treatment of depression in a patient with adult GM2 gangliosidosis. *Annals of Neurology*, **31**, 342–344.

Royal College of Psychiatrists (2001) *DC-LD: Diagnostic Criteria for Psychiatric Disorders for Use with Adults with Learning Disabilities/Mental Retardation*. Gaskell.

Ruedrich, S. L. & Alamir, S. (1999) Electroconvulsive therapy for persons with developmental disabilities: review, case report and recommendations. *Mental Health Aspects of Developmental Disability*, **2**, 83–91.

Santosh, P. J. & Baird, G. (1999) Psychopharmacotherapy in children and adults with intellectual disability. *Lancet*, **354**, 233–242.

Sayal, K. & Bernard, S. (1998) Trainees' assessment and management of mental illness in adults with mild learning disabilities. *Psychiatric Bulletin*, **22**, 571–572.

Smiley, E., Cooper, S. A., Finlayson, J., *et al* (2007) Incidence and predictors of mental ill-health in adults with intellectual disabilities. Prospective study. *British Journal of Psychiatry*, **191**, 313–319.

Snowdon, J., Meehan, T. & Halpin, R. (1994) Continuous screaming controlled by electroconvulsive therapy: a case study. *International Journal of Geriatric Psychiatry*, **9**, 929–932.

Stenfert Kroese, B., Dagnan, D. & Loumidis, K. (2006) *Cognitive–Behaviour Therapy for People with Learning Disabilities*. Routledge.

Taylor, J. L, Lindsay, W. R. & Willner, P. (2008) CBT for people with intellectual disabilities: Emerging evidence, cognitive ability and IQ effects. *Behavioural and Cognitive Psychotherapy*, **36**, 723–733.

Taylor, L., Oliver, C. & Murphy, G. (2010) The chronicity of self-injurious behaviour: a long-term follow-up of a total population study. *Journal of Applied Research in Intellectual Disabilities*, **24**, 105–117.

Thuppal, M. & Fink, M. (1999) Electroconvulsive therapy and mental retardation. *Journal of ECT*, **15**, 140–149.

van Schrojenstein Lantman-de Valk, H. M. J. & Noonan Walsh, P. (2008) Managing health problems in people with intellectual disabilities. *BMJ*, **337**, 1408–1412.

van Waarde, J. A., Stolker, J. J. & van der Mast, R. C. (2001) ECT in mental retardation: a review. *Journal of ECT*, **17**, 236–243.

Vanstraelen, M., Holt, G. & Bouras, N. (2003) Adults with learning disabilities and psychiatric problems. In *Seminars in the Psychiatry of Learning Disabilities* (eds W. Fraser & M. Kerr), pp. 155–169. Gaskell.

Wachtel, L., Contrucci-Kuhn, S., Griffin, M., *et al* (2009) ECT for self-injury in an autistic boy. *European Journal of Child and Adolescent Psychiatry*, **18**, 458–463.

Wachtel, L., Griffin, M., Dhossche, D., *et al* (2010a) Brief report: electroconvulsive therapy for malignant catatonia in an autistic adolescent. *Autism*, **14**, 349–358.

Wachtel, L., Hermida, A. & Dhossche, D. (2010b) Maintenance electroconvulsive therapy in autistic catatonia. *Progress in Neuro-Psychopharmacology and Biological Psychiatry*, **34**, 581–587.

Wachtel, L., Griffin, M. & Reti, I. (2010c) Electroconvulsive therapy in a man with autism experiencing severe depression, catatonia and self-injury. *Journal of ECT*, **26**, 70–73.

Warren, A. C., Holroyd, S. & Folstein, M. F. (1989) Major depression in Down's syndrome. *British Journal of Psychiatry*, **155**, 202–205.

Whitaker, S. & Read, S. (2006) The prevalence of psychiatric disorders among people with intellectual disabilities: an analysis of the literature. *Journal of Applied Research in Intellectual Disabilities*, **19**, 330–345.

Wing, L. & Shah, A. (2000) Catatonia in autistic spectrum disorders. *British Journal of Psychiatry*, **176**, 357–362.

Zaw, F. K. M., Bates, G. D. L., Murali, V., *et al* (1999) Catatonia, autism and ECT. *Developmental Medicine and Child Neurology*, **41**, 843–845.

CHAPTER 19

Safe ECT practice in people with a physical illness

Susan M. Benbow and Jonathan Waite

Possible medical contraindications to ECT

People with a wide range of physical illnesses are successfully treated with ECT (Fink, 1999; American Psychiatric Association, 2001). Abrams (1997) pointed out that the death rate associated with ECT is lower than the spontaneous death rate in the general US population. Some medical problems may cause particular concern, however, especially cardiovascular and neurological problems.

During the passage of the electrical stimulus, both blood pressure and heart rate fall and then rise rapidly. There is a sudden, short-lived rise in intracranial pressure and cerebral blood flow, and cerebrovascular permeability increases. Vagal stimulation leads to a sinus bradycardia, sometimes with periods of asystole or electrical silence. This is rapidly replaced by a sympathetically mediated tachycardia, which, by decreasing the oxygen supply to the myocardium and increasing its oxygen consumption, increases cardiac work and can result in ischaemia. Subconvulsive stimuli are known to produce longer periods of bradycardia; this may be a concern when people with established heart disease are being treated using a dose-titration protocol to determine seizure threshold (Abrams, 1991; Dolinski & Zvara, 1997). Another risk factor for longer periods of asystole during ECT is the use of beta-blockers (McCall, 1996). Vagolytic drugs, such as glycopyrrolate and atropine, are sometimes used to attenuate the bradycardia (Applegate, 1997). It is not surprising that there is evidence that people with cardiovascular disease are more at risk of cardiac complications during ECT. Burke *et al* (1987) reported more complications in people on a greater total number of medications and in those on a greater number of cardiovascular medications. Complications during ECT may also increase as the age of the person being treated increases, although, in a naturalistic study, Brodaty *et al* (2000) found that the number and severity of adverse events were not associated with age.

Most cardiovascular complications are transient and do not prevent successful completion of an ECT course and so Zielinski *et al* (1998) concluded that ECT can still be used relatively safely for people with severe cardiac disease. The American Psychiatric Association (2001) also states that, in general, people with cardiovascular disease can be safely treated with ECT. Abrams (2002) has reviewed the use of ECT in people with previous cardiac surgery, myocardial infarction, cardiac pacemakers, aortic aneurysms and intracardiac thrombi, and who were taking drug treatments to reduce blood pressure, prevent arrhythmias or reduce heart rate. He noted that the 'detection and management of significant cardiovascular disease before administering EC is [...] the most important factor in reducing [...] cardiovascular morbidity and mortality' (p. 73).

Coexisting medical or surgical conditions

Since many medical illnesses could increase the risk associated with ECT, it is important that all people for whom ECT is being considered are fully evaluated before treatment. Any physical illness will need to be investigated and treated or at least stabilised as far as possible before ECT is begun (Tess & Smetana, 2009). The important principles here are as follows:

- When a person who is being considered for treatment with ECT is thought to present high risk, an appropriate medical opinion should be sought to clarify the degree of risk and ways of minimising that risk.
- Any underlying disorder will be fully assessed and treated before ECT.
- An anaesthetic opinion may also be sought at this stage and, in liaison with the anaesthetist, treatment technique may be modified to minimise the risks involved.
- During the consent process, patient and family should be informed of the increased risk and any recommendations for minimising it. Risk may need to be reassessed following cardiological or anaesthetic opinion or investigation.
- High-risk patients will not normally be treated at remote sites, or as day patients or out-patients.

Cardiovascular disease

Electroconvulsive therapy is classed as a low-risk procedure (Applegate 1997) but, although it is quite unlike other procedures for which a general anaesthetic is administered, the conditions that may present higher cardiac risks during treatment are likely to be similar to those that elevate the risks associated with surgical interventions (Dolinski & Zvara, 1997), and include:

- recent myocardial infarct (Magid et al, 2005)
- severe valvular heart disease (Rayburn, 1997; Mueller et al, 2007)
- clinically significant cardiac dysrhythmias (Applegate, 1997)
- unstable angina (Applegate, 1997)

- uncompensated congestive cardiac failure (Rayburn, 1997)
- some aneurysms: left ventricular aneurysm (Gardner *et al*, 1997); aortic aneurysm (Mueller *et al*, 2009)
- uncontrolled or poorly controlled hypertension, although blood pressure has been shown not to change during a course of ECT (Albin *et al*, 2007)
- patients on warfarin (Mehta *et al*, 2004).

Patients with implanted cardiac pacemakers can be safely treated with ECT. The device should be checked by an appropriately trained technician to ensure that it is functioning correctly prior to a course of ECT; if it is, no special precautions are required. Where a patient with an automated implanted cardiac defibrillator is being given ECT, a cardiology technician must be present in the ECT suite to inactivate the device prior to ECT and re-start it once treatment is complete (Davis *et al*, 2009).

Neurological conditions

Electroconvulsive therapy has been used safely for people with small, slow-growing cerebral tumours without raised intracranial pressure, but people who have space-occupying lesions of the brain are at high risk of neurological deterioration if treated with ECT (Krystal & Coffey, 1997). The aggravation of already raised intracranial pressure is thought to account for the risk (Abrams, 2002). Nevertheless, people with a wide range of neurological conditions have been treated successfully with ECT. This includes the following groups:

- People with cerebrovascular disease (Miller & Isenberg, 1998; van Herck *et al*, 2009); there are, however, no adequate trials of ECT for depression after stroke (Hackett *et al*, 2008).
- People with Parkinson's disease who do not respond well to drugs. Kennedy *et al* (2003) conclude that ECT is a safe adjunctive treatment for both motor and affective symptoms, and that future research must focus on optimal ECT techniques in Parkinson's disease. Reviewing the literature, the overwhelming number of single and multiple case reports contrast with the paucity of well-designed clinical trials. The vast majority of these case reports have shown positive results, with very few studies failing to demonstrate a response to ECT among patients with Parkinson's disease, but the possibility of publication bias favouring the publication of positive results must be considered.
- People with multisystem atrophy, a neurodegenerative disorder which may be manifest by Parkinsonian, autonomic, cerebellar or pyramidal signs. There have been several case reports of patients with multisystem atrophy showing improvement in motor function and mood after ECT (Roane *et al*, 2000; Shioda *et al*, 2006).
- People with tardive dyskinesia. There is considerable literature on the use of ECT in tardive dyskinesia, which is contradictory and

inconclusive: several case reports suggest that ECT improves this condition, while several others report that tardive dyskinesia worsens with ECT (Kennedy *et al*, 2003).

- People with implanted neurostimulators, see Chapter 13.
- People with epilepsy (for a review, see Hsiao *et al*, 1987).
- People with cerebral lupus (for a review, see Hsiao *et al*, 1987).
- People with dementia, including advanced dementia (for a case report, see Weintraub & Lippmann, 2001; and for a report of a retrospective series, see Rao & Lyketsos, 2000).
- People with intellectual disability (Chapter 18).
- Those who have had a stroke (for a review, see Gustafson *et al*, 1995).
- Those who have undergone craniotomy (Gursky *et al*, 2000).

Other medical conditions

The anaesthetist should be informed of all relevant medical and surgical conditions before treatment and of any conditions developing or diagnosed during treatment. The anaesthetist will advise on any special precautions; for example, since oesophageal reflux is associated with an increased risk of aspiration during ECT, measures to decrease or neutralise gastric acidity may be necessary, as may modifications to anaesthetic technique (Chapter 3). The patient's management of diabetes may need to be modified, although ECT does not greatly affect insulin requirements or glycaemic control (Weiner & Sibert, 1996, Netzel *et al*, 2002). Electroconvulsive therapy may exacerbate bronchospasm in patients with asthma, but serious adverse effects have not been reported (Mueller *et al*, 2006). Electroconvulsive therapy has been used successfully to treat severe depression complicating chronic renal failure requiring haemodialysis (Pearlman *et al*, 1988; Williams & Ostroff, 2005).

People with bone or joint disease may need an increased dose of muscle relaxant, although fracture during ECT has been virtually eliminated with the use of muscle-relaxant drugs (American Psychiatric Association, 2001). The use of the Hamilton cuff technique to monitor seizure duration should be avoided in patients with osteoporosis (Baethge & Bshor, 2003).

Ophthalmological advice should be sought in people with advanced glaucoma (Abrams, 2002) in view of the transient rise in intra-ocular pressure during ECT.

The American Psychiatric Association (2001) gave detailed advice regarding cardiovascular, neurological and other disorders, but the principles of good practice are common to all.

Minimising risk

When a person is thought to be at greater risk because of a coexisting medical or surgical condition, consideration should always be given to ways of minimising risk by modifying medical management or ECT technique. High-risk patients should not be treated at remote sites or as out-patients. Modifications to medical treatment or ECT technique will require liaison between anaesthetist, psychiatrist and any other specialist involved. Some people at high risk may best be treated in a cardiac care unit, with ECG monitoring before, during and after the treatment and with specialist staff to hand who are trained in cardiopulmonary resuscitation and the emergency treatment of arrhythmias.

Balance of risks and benefits

The balance of risks and benefits to physical and mental health must be considered for each individual. The risk–benefit analysis will include:

- the severity of the psychiatric illness and the risks it poses to the individual
- the likelihood of the psychiatric illness responding to ECT
- the medical risks of ECT and the extent to which they can be minimised or controlled
- options for alternative treatments, the likely response to and adverse effects of those treatments, and the likely outcome if the person opts for no treatment.

The patient and family will normally be fully involved in discussions about the treatment, the risk–benefit analysis and alternative treatments. Where the risk of ECT remains high, the patient and, where appropriate, the family should be informed and then involved in the careful balancing of risks and benefits. Where a person is detained under the Mental Health Act 1983 or being given treatment under mental capacity legislation and is unable to give consent, it is good practice to involve the relatives fully during assessment and before invoking the 'second opinion' procedure (see also Chapter 22).

Recommendations

- All coexisting medical or surgical conditions should be assessed and, where possible, treated or stabilised before ECT is administered.
- When a patient is thought to be at greater risk during ECT, consideration should always be given to ways of minimising risk by modifying medical management or ECT technique (or both).
- The balance of risks and benefits to physical and mental health must be considered for each individual.
- As far as possible, patients and, where appropriate, their families should be involved in discussions about the treatment, its risks, its possible benefits and any alternative treatments.
- On the occasions when ECT is prescribed to save life, there may be no absolute contraindications to it.

References

Abrams, R. (1991) Electroconvulsive therapy in the medically compromised patient. *Psychiatric Clinics of North America*, **14**, 871–885.

Abrams, R. (1997) The mortality rate with ECT. *Convulsive Therapy*, **13**, 125–127.

Abrams, R. (2002) Electroconvulsive therapy in the high-risk patient. In *Electroconvulsive Therapy* (4th edn), pp. 72–100. Oxford University Press.

Albin, S. M., Stevens, S. R. & Rasmussen, K. G. (2007) Blood pressure before and after electroconvulsive therapy in hypertensive and nonhypertensive patients. *Journal of ECT*, **23**, 9–10.

American Psychiatric Association (2001) *The Practice of Electroconvulsive Therapy: Recommendations for Treatment, Training and Privileging* (2nd edn). APA.

Applegate, R. J. (1997) Diagnosis and management of ischaemic heart disease in the patient scheduled to undergo electroconvulsive therapy. *Convulsive Therapy*, **13**, 128–144.

Baethge, C. & Bshor, T. (2003) Wrist fracture in a patient undergoing electroconvulsive treatment monitored using the 'cuff' method. *European Archives of Psychiatry and Clinical Neuroscience*, **253**, 160–162.

Brodaty, H., Hickie, I., Mason, C., *et al* (2000) A prospective follow-up study of ECT outcome in older depressed patients. *Journal of Affective Disorders*, **60**, 101–111.

Burke, W. J., Rubin, E. H., Zorumski, C. F., *et al* (1987) The safety of ECT in geriatric psychiatry. *Journal of the American Geriatrics Society*, **35**, 516–521.

Davis, A., Zisselman, M., Simmons, T., *et al* (2009) Electroconvulsive therapy in the setting of implantable cardioverter-defibrillators. *Journal of ECT*, **25**, 198–201.

Dolinski, S. Y. & Zvara, D. A. (1997) Anesthetic considerations of cardiovascular risk during electroconvulsive therapy. *Convulsive Therapy*, **13**, 157–164.

Fink, M. (1999) *Electroshock: Restoring the Mind*. Oxford University Press.

Gardner, M. W., Kellner, C. H., Hood, D. E., *et al* (1997) Safe administration of ECT in a patient with a cardiac aneurysm and multiple cardiac risk factors. *Convulsive Therapy*, **13**, 200–203.

Gursky, J. T., Rummans, T. A. & Black, J. L. (2000) ECT administration in a patient after craniotomy and gamma knife surgery: a case report and review. *Journal of ECT*, **16**, 295–299.

Gustafson, Y., Nilsson, I., Mattsson, M., *et al* (1995) Epidemiology and treatment of post-stroke depression. *Drugs and Aging*, **7**, 298–309.

Hackett, M. L., Anderson, C. S., House. A., *et al* (2008) Interventions for treating depression after stroke. *Cochrane Database of Systematic Reviews*, **4**, CD003437.

Hsiao, J. K., Messenheimer, J. A. & Evans, D. L. (1987) ECT and neurological disorders. *Convulsive Therapy*, **3**, 121–136.

Kennedy, R., Mittal, D. & O'Jile, J. (2003) Electroconvulsive therapy in movement disorders: an update. *Journal of Neuropsychiatry and Clinical Neuroscience*, **15**, 407–421.

Krystal, A. D. & Coffey, C. E. (1997) Neuropsychiatric considerations in the use of electroconvulsive therapy. *Journal of Neuropsychiatry and Clinical Neurosciences*, **9**, 283–292.

Magid, M., Lapid, M. I., Sampson, S. M., *et al* (2005) Use of electroconvulsive therapy in a patient 10 days after myocardial infarction. *Journal of ECT*, **21**, 182–185.

McCall, W. V. (1996) Asystole in electroconvulsive therapy: report of four cases. *Journal of Clinical Psychiatry*, **5**, 199–203.

Mehta, V., Mueller, P. S., Gonzalez-Arriada, H. L., *et al* (2004) Safety of electro-convulsive therapy in patients receiving long-term warfarin therapy. *Mayo Clinic Proceedings*, **79**, 1396–1401.

Miller, A. R. & Isenberg, K. E. (1998) Reversible ischemic neurologic deficit after ECT. *Journal of ECT*, **14**, 42–48.

Mueller, P. S., Schak, K. M., Barnes, R. D., *et al* (2006) Safety of electroconvulsive therapy in patients with asthma. *Netherlands Journal of Medicine*, **64**, 417–421.

Mueller, P. S., Barnes, R. D., Varghese, R., *et al* (2007) The safety of electroconvulsive therapy in patients with severe aortic stenosis. *Mayo Clinic Proceedings*, **82**, 1360–1363.

Mueller, P. S., Albin, S. M., Barnes, R. D., *et al* (2009) Safety of electroconvulsive therapy in patients with unrepaired abdominal aortic aneurysm: report of 8 patients. *Journal of ECT*, **25**, 165–169.

Netzel, P. J., Mueller, P. S., Rummans, T. A., *et al* (2002) Safety, efficacy and effects on glycemic control of electroconvulsive therapy in insulin requiring type 2 diabetic patients. *Journal of ECT*, **18**, 16–21.

Pearlman, C., Carson, W. & Metz, A. (1988) Hemodialysis, chronic renal failure, and ECT. *Convulsive Therapy*, **4**, 332–333.

Rao, V. & Lyketsos, C. G. (2000) The benefits and risks of ECT for patients with primary dementia who also suffer from depression. *International Journal of Geriatric Psychiatry*, **15**, 729–735.

Rayburn, B. K. (1997) Electroconvulsive therapy in patients with heart failure or valvular heart disease. *Convulsive Therapy*, **13**, 145–156.

Roane, D. M., Rogers, J. D., Helew, L., *et al* (2000) Electroconvulsive therapy for elderly patients with multiple system atrophy: a case series. *American Journal of Geriatric Psychiatry*, **8**, 171–174.

Shioda, K., Nisijima, K. & Kato, S. (2006) Electroconvulsive therapy for the treatment of multiple system atrophy with major depression. *General Hospital Psychiatry*, **28**, 81–83.

Tess, A. V. & Smetana, G. W. (2009) Medical evaluation of patients undergoing electroconvulsive therapy. *New England Journal of Medicine*, **360**, 1437–1444.

van Herck, E., Sienaert, P. & Hagon, A. (2009) Electroconvulsive therapy for patients with intracranial aneurysms: a case study and literature review [in Dutch]. *Tijdschrift voor Psychiatrie*, **51**, 43–51.

Weiner, R. D. & Sibert, T. E. (1996) Use of ECT in treatment of depression in patients with diabetes mellitus. *Journal of Clinical Psychiatry*, **57**, 138.

Weintraub, D. & Lippmann, S. B. (2001) ECT for major depression and mania with advanced dementia. *Journal of ECT*, **17**, 65–67.

Williams, S. & Ostroff, R. (2005) Chronic renal failure, hemodialysis, and electroconvulsive therapy: a case report. *Journal of ECT*, **21**, 41–42.

Zielinski, R. J., Roose, S. P., Devanand, D. P., *et al* (1998) Cardiovascular complications of ECT in depressed patients with cardiac disease. *American Journal of Psychiatry*, **150**, 904–909.

CHAPTER 20

ECT for older adults

Susan M. Benbow

A survey of old age psychiatrists in the early 1990s found that they regarded the main indication for ECT in older people to be severe depressive illness (Benbow, 1991), but they also rated the treatment as often or sometimes useful in schizoaffective disorder and depressive illness with dementia. Similarly, ECT was regarded as the treatment of choice for people with depressive illness:

- that has failed to respond to antidepressant drugs
- in which previous episodes responded to ECT but not to antidepressant drugs
- with psychotic symptoms
- with severe agitation and those with high suicidal risk.

These clinical views are compatible with literature reporting favourable outcomes for older people treated with ECT (Damm *et al*, 2010) and for depressive psychosis (Birkenhager *et al*, 2004). Van der Wurff *et al* (2003) reviewed efficacy in older adults and found immediate response rates of between 55% and 85% in 10 naturalistic prospective studies and immediate response rates ranging from 48% complete recovery to 92% improvement in 14 retrospective studies. They concluded that immediate response rates are 'impressive', although based on non-randomised evidence. Many studies have reported response rates of around 70% or more among older adults (Fraser & Glass, 1980; Gaspar & Samarasinghe, 1982; Karlinsky & Shulman, 1984; Benbow, 1987; Godber *et al*, 1987; Rubin *et al*, 1991; Casey & Davies, 1996; Tomac *et al*, 1997).

The NICE (2003: p. 5) technology appraisal of ECT recommends that ECT only be used 'to achieve rapid and short-term improvement of severe symptoms after an adequate trial of other treatment options has proven ineffective and/or when the condition is considered to be life-threatening, in individuals with:

- severe depressive illness
- catatonia
- a prolonged or severe manic episode.'

The technology appraisal was reviewed in May 2010: the recommendations on ECT in catatonia and mania were unchanged, and guidance on ECT in depression has been updated by the clinical guideline CG90 (National Institute for Health and Excellence, 2009), which states that 'the risks associated with ECT may be greater in older people; exercise particular caution when considering ECT treatment in this group' (p. 41). This is in the context of evidence that older people have been major users of ECT services in the past (Pippard & Ellam, 1981; Duffett *et al*, 1999).

The evidence is that age in itself does not contraindicate the use of ECT. Indeed, older people appear to tolerate and respond to ECT relatively well. Flint & Gagnon (2002) went further and stated that there is a positive association between advancing age and the efficacy of ECT, which they related to clinical factors in later-life depressive illnesses. There are other possibilities. For example, it may be that concern about comorbid medical conditions might lead to preferential use of ECT in some groups of older adults in order to take advantage of the more rapid response to ECT compared with drug treatments, or that older people find ECT a more acceptable treatment option (Benbow, 2008).

Access to ECT among older people

Older people who might benefit from ECT ought not to be denied treatment solely on the grounds of age. It is reasonable to conclude that older people are no less likely to respond to ECT than younger people and are entitled to have access to a treatment that might benefit them when it is appropriate. The *National Service Framework for Older People* (Department of Health, 2001) stated that services should be provided, regardless of age, on the basis of clinical need alone, and that older people should have access to a full range of psychological and physical treatments. Since then there have been efforts to eradicate age discrimination from healthcare (Care Services Improvement Partnership, 2009; Royal College of Psychiatrists, 2009). This would include access to ECT where appropriate.

Coexisting medical and surgical conditions

When ECT is being considered for an older person, all coexisting medical and surgical conditions should be assessed and, where possible, stabilised or treated before ECT (see Chapters 3 and 19). It is important to note that such conditions tend to accumulate with increasing age.

Technical aspects of treating older adults

There is an increased likelihood of a high seizure threshold in an elderly person, particularly an older man. This may increase the difficulty of eliciting effective seizures (Sackeim *et al*, 1987; Coffey *et al*, 1995; Boylan *et al*, 2000). Clinics should agree local protocols regarding the choice of anaesthetic agent and other age-related factors (Benbow *et al*, 2002). Scrupulous attention should be paid to the sites where treatment electrodes will be placed. This should include removing traces of grease and applying electrode gel in good time to hydrate dry skin to reduce skin impedance and increase the chances of successful treatment without having to resort to high-stimulus doses.

Adverse effects

Zervas *et al* (1993) found that among people aged 20–65 years, 24–72 h after ECT, memory deficits were more severe in older people. The authors concluded that older people treated with ECT are more vulnerable to the development of cognitive side-effects during treatment and at risk of these effects lasting longer. Although this study excluded people aged over 65 years, it may be reasonable to conclude that they would be at even greater risk of cognitive adverse effects. People who have pre-existing memory problems should likewise be regarded as at higher risk of developing cognitive adverse effects during treatment. In either case, modifications to treatment technique may be indicated, such as choice of anaesthetic drug, consideration of unilateral treatment, changes to concurrent medication or reducing frequency of treatment. Any factors which place an individual at greater risk during treatment with ECT should be identified during the pre-ECT assessment, and should be discussed with the person concerned and family members as appropriate. For example, an individual with concurrent dementia would be regarded as at increased risk of cognitive side-effects during a course of ECT: they might be advised to have unilateral rather than bilateral ECT, and their concurrent medication should be reviewed. Alternatively, bilateral ECT in a cardiac care unit might be advised for an older adult with established cardiac disease, in order to minimise the number of anaesthetics required over the course of treatment.

Burke *et al* (1987) retrospectively reviewed the charts of 136 people treated with ECT and found that complications increased with age and were also related to health status and number of medications. Similar findings have been reported by other authors (e.g. Fraser & Glass, 1978, 1980; Gaspar & Samarasinghe, 1982; Alexopoulos *et al*, 1984; Tomac *et al*, 1997). Sobin *et al* (1995) found a similar relationship between pre-existing cognitive impairment and ratings of memory impairment after treatment.

For older adults, close monitoring of physical and cognitive states is recommended throughout a course of ECT. Clinic procedures will need to allow for regular routine exchange of information between the clinical team caring for a person who is being treated with ECT and the ECT team.

Recommendations

- Age does not by itself constitute a contraindication for ECT.
- People should not be denied access to ECT solely on the grounds of age.
- All coexisting medical or surgical conditions should be assessed and, where possible, stabilised or treated prior to ECT.
- The ECT clinic's treatment protocols (such as choice of anaesthetic agent) should take account of the increased likelihood of high seizure thresholds among older adults.
- The monitoring of older people who are receiving ECT should include attention to possible changes in their physical state and cognitive function during a course of treatment.
- Electroconvulsive therapy technique should be modified as necessary to minimise any cognitive adverse effects during ECT in those people deemed to be at higher risk.

References

Alexopoulos, G. S., Shamoian, C. J., Lucas, J., et al (1984) Medical problems of geriatric psychiatric patients and younger controls during electroconvulsive therapy. Journal of the American Geriatrics Society, 32, 651–654.

Benbow, S. M. (1987) The use of electroconvulsive therapy in old age psychiatry. International Journal of Geriatric Psychiatry, 2, 25–30.

Benbow, S. M. (1991) Old age psychiatrists' views on the use of ECT. International Journal of Geriatric Psychiatry, 6, 317–322.

Benbow, S. M. (2008) Electricity, magnetism and mood. In Practical Management of Affective Disorders in Older People: A Multi-professional Approach (eds S. Curran & J. P. Wattis), pp. 94–107. Radcliffe.

Benbow, S. M., Shah, P. & Crentsil, J. (2002) Anaesthesia for electroconvulsive therapy: a role for etomidate. Psychiatric Bulletin, 26, 351–353.

Birkenhager, T. K., Renes, J-W. & Pluijms, E. M. (2004) One-year follow-up after successful ECT: a naturalistic study in depressed inpatients. Journal of Clinical Psychiatry, 65, 87–91.

Boylan, L. S., Haskett, R. F., Mulsant, B. F., et al (2000) Determinants of seizure threshold in ECT: benzodiazepine use, anesthetic dosage and other factors. Journal of ECT, 16, 3–18.

Burke, W. J., Rubin, E. H., Zorumski, C. F., et al (1987) The safety of ECT in geriatric psychiatry. Journal of the American Geriatrics Society, 35, 516–521.

Care Services Improvement Partnership (2009) Age Equality: What Does it Mean for Older People's Mental Health Services? Guidance Note – Everybody's Business. Integrated Mental Health Services for Older Adults: A Service Development Guide. CSIP.

Casey, D. A. & Davies, M. H. (1996) Electroconvulsive therapy in the very old. General Hospital Psychiatry, 18, 436–439.

Coffey, C. E., Lucke, J., Weiner, R. D., et al (1995) Seizure threshold in electroconvulsive therapy 1: initial seizure threshold. Biological Psychiatry, 37, 713–720.

Damm, J., Eser, D., Schüle, C., et al (2010) Influence of age on effectiveness and tolerability of electroconvulsive therapy. Journal of ECT, 26, 282–288.

Department of Health (2001) National Service Framework for Older People. Department of Health.

Duffett, R., Siegert, D. R. & Lelliott, P. (1999) Electroconvulsive therapy in Wales. Psychiatric Bulletin, 23, 597–601.

Flint, A. J. & Gagnon, N. (2002) Effective use of electroconvulsive therapy in late-life depression. *Canadian Journal of Psychiatry*, **47**, 734–741.

Fraser, R. M. & Glass, I. B. (1978) Recovery from ECT in elderly patients. *British Journal of Psychiatry*, **133**, 524–528.

Fraser, R. M. & Glass, I. B. (1980) Unilateral and bilateral ECT in elderly patients: a comparative study. *Acta Psychiatrica Scandinavica*, **62**, 13–31.

Gaspar, D. & Samarasinghe, L. A. (1982) ECT in psychogeriatric practice – a sudy of risk factors, indications and outcome. *Comprehensive Psychiatry*, **23**, 170–175.

Godber, C., Rosenvinge, H., Wilkinson, D., *et al* (1987) Depression in old age: prognosis after ECT. *International Journal of Geriatric Psychiatry*, **2**, 19–24.

Karlinsky, H. & Shulman, K. T. (1984) The clinical use of electroconvulsive therapy in old age. *Journal of the American Geriatrics Society*, **32**, 183–186.

National Institute for Clinical Excellence (2003) *Guidance on the Use of Electroconvulsive Therapy* (Technology Appraisal TA59). NICE.

National Institute for Health and Clinical Excellence (2009) *Depression: The Treatment and Management of Depression in Adults* (Clinical Guideline CG90). NICE.

Pippard, J. & Ellam, L. (1981) *Electroconvulsive Treatment in Great Britain, 1980*. Gaskell.

Royal College of Psychiatrists (2009) *Age Discrimination in Mental Health Services: Making Equality a Reality* (Position Statement PS2/2009). Royal College of Psychiatrists.

Rubin, E. H., Kinscherf, D. A. & Wehrman, S. A. (1991) Response to treatment of depression in the old and the very old. *Journal of Geriatric Psychiatry and Neurology*, **4**, 65–70.

Sackeim, H. A., Decina, P., Prohovnik, I., *et al* (1987) Seizure threshold in electroconvulsive therapy: effects of sex, age, electrode placement and number of treatments. *Archives of General Psychiatry*, **44**, 355–360.

Sobin, C., Sackeim, H. A., Prudic, J., *et al* (1995) Predictors of retrograde amnesia following ECT. *American Journal of Psychiatry*, **152**, 995–1001.

Tomac, T. A., Rummans, T. A., Pileggi, T. S., *et al* (1997) Safety and efficacy of electroconvulsive therapy in patients over age 85. *American Journal of Geriatric Psychiatry*, **5**, 126–130.

van der Wurff, F. B., Stek, M. L., Hoogendijk, W. J. G., *et al* (2003) The efficacy and safety of ECT in depressed older adults: a literature review. *International Journal of Geriatric Psychiatry*, **18**, 894–904.

Zervas, I. M., Calev, A., Jandorf, L., *et al* (1993) Age-dependent effects of electroconvulsive therapy on memory. *Convulsive Therapy*, **9**, 39–42.

CHAPTER 21

The use of ECT as continuation or maintenance treatment

Richard Barnes

Electroconvulsive therapy is an effective treatment for depression and other psychiatric conditions, but relapse rates at the end of the course may be as high as 50% (Bourgon & Kellner, 2000) unless some form of prophylactic treatment – generally medication, singly or in combination – is used. However, a small proportion of patients relapse despite these methods and such patients may require a further course of ECT in order to recover. Recently, interest has returned to the use of ECT as a prophylactic treatment in these cases, where illness may be severe and frequently recurrent. For a patient who has already responded to ECT, continuation therapy – if given at sufficient intervals – can reduce the overall number of treatments given in a 12-month period.

Before the advent of effective drug treatments, ECT was often used as a prophylaxis and although developments in pharmacotherapy have reduced its popularity, evidence suggests it is still used widely (Gupta *et al*, 2011). Indeed, for those patients who appear to respond only to ECT, continuation or maintenance ECT may be the treatment of choice. The American Psychiatric Association (2001) recommends that ECT facilities offer continuation ECT as a treatment option.

There is a lack of clarity about the terminology used with regard to continuation and maintenance ECT. In keeping with current practice regarding antidepressant prophylaxis, we would suggest the term continuation ECT for treatments designed to prevent relapse of an index episode of illness, and maintenance ECT to be applied to ECT usage as a prevention of further episodes or recurrence of illness. By custom, continuation ECT has been defined as prophylactic treatment over the first 6 months of remission.

Evidence for the efficacy of continuation ECT

In May 2003, NICE published its first guidance on ECT for depressive illness, schizophrenia, catatonia and mania, and in these guidelines recommended that 'as the longer-term benefits and risks of ECT have not been clearly established, it is not recommended as a maintenance therapy in depressive illness' (p. 6). In October 2009, however, the updated NICE guidelines on the management of depression in adults changed these recommendations (although only with regard to the use of ECT in depression). These guidelines have removed the former advice against continuation and maintenance ECT and have taken a neutral position. The guidelines include a thorough and helpful review of the evidence for continuation/maintenance ECT and also give recommendations on future research. A further evaluation of the current understanding of continuation ECT has been published by Trevino *et al* (2010).

Kellner *et al* (2006) published the only prospective randomised controlled trial of continuation ECT, which compared it with continuation antidepressants after a successful course of ECT treatment. The ECT was administered bilaterally and dose titrated – treatment dose being 1.5 times seizure threshold – under EEG monitoring. Treatment frequency began at three times a week, reducing to weekly, biweekly and then monthly. The comparison group received nortriptyline and lithium in titrated doses. Both groups showed very similar relapse rates (ECT group: 37.1% relapse, 46.1% in remission, 16.8% withdrew from study; antidepressant group: 31.6% relapse, 46.3% in remission, 22.1% withdrew from study), which compared favourably with historical placebo-controlled results from a similarly designed study (Sackeim *et al*, 2001). The MMSE scores in both groups also improved after the acute ECT phase, and although the group in continuation ECT treatment improved less that the antidepressant group, this did not reach statistical significance. The study noted that the randomising element of the study meant that schedules were not individualised to each patient's requirements, and suggested that more flexibility could potentially further decrease the likelihood of relapse. Further improvements might also be achieved by combining continuation ECT and antidepressant therapies.

In a randomised controlled trial, Smith *et al* (2010) compared the memory effects of continuation ECT against continuation pharmacotherapy (nortriptyline and lithium). Although they showed an initial difference in autobiographical memory favouring pharmacotherapy after an initial 12 weeks, at 24 weeks there were no differences detected on a variety of memory scales in patients who had not relapsed.

Russell *et al* (2003) conducted a retrospective review of efficacy and cognitive outcome in patients receiving ECT for unipolar depression, depressive illness associated with bipolar disorder or depressive illness associated with schizoaffective disorder. The patients were on a variety of pharmacological treatments and had high levels of physical comorbidity. Their data showed a sustained improvement in post-treatment depression ratings and no long-term cognitive deterioration. They concluded that long-term ECT can be safe and effective for highly medicated patients with chronic depression.

Vothknecht *et al* (2003) – in a non-randomised, naturalistic, comparative study of 11 patients receiving maintenance ECT and 13 control patients treated with maintenance pharmacotherapy after index ECT – reported no significant differences in patient characteristics and effects of index ECT between the two groups. The maintenance pharmacotherapy group showed no change in cognitive function or depression ratings during 6-month follow-up, whereas the maintenance ECT group showed slight (but not statistically significant) improvements in neuropsychological tests and depression ratings over the same time period. However, in a cross-sectional study of 11 patients receiving maintenance ECT (Rami-Gonzalez et al, 2003), impairments were found in encoding new information and frontal lobe tests compared with a matched control group. Delayed recall showed no difference.

There have also been a number of individual case reports and brief case series supporting the view that maintenance ECT does not appear to cause cognitive deterioration (Barnes et al, 1997; Wijkstra & Nolen, 2005; Zisselman et al, 2007).

Practical provision of continuation ECT

Appropriate prescription of continuation and maintenance ECT will require a properly documented assessment of the potential risks and benefits of treatment for which valid informed consent has been obtained (see Chapter 22). Patients who are considering continuation treatment will have the personal experience of previous ECT, which will help them weigh the potential benefits and adverse effects of treatment. Evidence-based guidelines for continuation ECT are not currently available, but the following protocol is put forward to promote discussion of best practice.

Protocol for continuation ECT

Continuation ECT should be considered for patients who have a relapsing or refractory depression that has previously responded well to ECT, but for whom standard pharmacological and psychological continuation treatment is ineffective or inappropriate. Such patients might include those:

- who have had early (0–6 months) post-ECT relapse not controlled by medication
- with later recurrence (6–12 months) not controlled by medication
- who cannot tolerate prophylactic medication
- who repeatedly relapse because of poor adherence
- who request it.

Maintenance ECT is usually reserved for those whose illness recurs after continuation ECT. Either may also be considered for patients who express a preference for it.

Assessment

Before commencing continuation ECT, a full review of the case should be undertaken in a similar manner to any case of refractory or relapsing depression. Consideration should be given to ensuring the diagnosis is correct, that ECT has been proven to be of benefit and that alternative options have been adequately explored. The patient's informed consent will need to be sought after provision of a separate information sheet. If the patient is currently unwell, discussing continuation ECT should be deferred until they are sufficiently improved to allow a full understanding of the proposed plan. A specific consent form for continuation/maintenance ECT should be considered.

Once the decision to proceed has been made, the patient should have a full routine medical screening and examination, ideally performed in collaboration with an experienced anaesthetist. Electrocardiogram and chest radiography may be needed. Baseline standardised assessment of illness severity should also be performed (e.g. Hamilton Rating Scale for Depression (Hamilton, 1960), Montgomery–Åsberg Depression Rating Scale (Montgomery & Åsberg, 1979)). It would seem wise to seek a second opinion about continuation ECT from a consultant colleague, preferably one with experience in ECT. This is not a statutory requirement for an informal patient.

Exclusion criteria

Exclusion criteria for continuation ECT are the same as for acute ECT – recent myocardial infarction or cerebrovascular accident, raised intracranial pressure or the presence of an acute respiratory infection. One should, however, be more cautious when the use of acute ECT is of higher risk, for example with patients who have in the past shown significant post-ECT confusion or who have a depressive illness in the context of a progressive neurodegenerative disorder.

Treatment plan

Before starting continuation treatment, consideration should be given to the intended length of the course. The team should also agree on which symptoms would indicate deterioration in the mental state such that relapse would seem likely. This information can be used in determining frequency of treatment. Once completed, the plan should be clearly and explicitly documented in the notes.

A full discussion with the patient and family must be conducted to address treatment purpose, benefits and adverse effects, and details of this similarly recorded.

ECT procedure

The administration of ECT should proceed as recommended in Chapter 4, in either an in-patient or out-patient setting. The goals of continuation ECT are such that out-patient treatment would be the normal pattern once recovery is achieved. Separate protocols will be needed for this locally. Electrode placement will generally be the same as that used in the acute phase, although clinicians may wish to consider a change to unilateral ECT for the continuation phase if cognitive side-effects are a concern.

A stimulus dosing paradigm should be employed with the goal of inducing a seizure between 20 and 50 s in length. During longer courses of ECT, seizure threshold may rise, so a slight increase in dose may be required; however, experience suggests that clinical response is a more important indicator of efficacy than seizure duration and shorter seizures can be acceptable if the patient remains well. Once the clinical recovery has occurred with ECT being given twice weekly, the goal should be to reduce the frequency of ECT to the minimum required to maintain clinical response. Physical and psychological factors will influence how this is approached in each individual, so a rigid structure to treatment is inappropriate, although typically the following frequency reduction has been employed:

- twice weekly until clinical response is achieved
- reduce to weekly
- reduce to every 10 days
- reduce to every 2 weeks
- reduce to every 3 weeks
- reduce to monthly.

Administration of treatments less frequently than monthly may be possible in certain cases.

It has been suggested that a more flexible approach – where frequency of treatment is determined by a balance between clinical response and side-effects – may be a more appropriate strategy (see Lisanby et al, 2008). At the time of writing, this approach has yet to be fully evaluated.

For patients who are not commencing continuation ECT immediately after acute ECT, it may be possible to begin at a lower frequency of about every 2 weeks. Routine review of efficacy should be undertaken after every two sessions in the first instance and review of frequency monthly. Once a regimen is established, review may be possible less often as for patients on other forms of prophylaxis.

Consideration should be given to concurrent medication that may interfere with longer-term treatment (see Chapter 5). Since ECT is being used as a prophylaxis, it may be possible to reduce or withdraw psychotropics completely, although given the severity of illness in patients on continuation ECT, a 'pure' ECT prophylaxis is often not achieved. If possible, benzodiazepines and anticonvulsants should be stopped as they interfere with seizure activity. The majority of antipsychotics are proconvulsant. Lithium can contribute to post-ECT confusion and should be used with caution. Non-psychiatric medication should be discussed with the anaesthetists or other relevant clinicians.

Before each change in the frequency of ECT a full review should take place. For those patients who are in an out-patient setting, objective information will be needed from the patient, family and community staff. Feedback from carers, either formal or informal, is essential. Deterioration in mental state that suggests the return of a depressive disorder at any treatment frequency should result in a return to the previous level until improvement is re-established.

Review during the course of ECT

Once initial recovery – assessed clinically and/or by significant reduction in rating scale score – has been achieved, full baseline psychometric assessment should be performed. This should allow assessment of current and past functioning and also be able to detect change. There are no specific rating scales available, but we would suggest tests that establish premorbid intelligence, memory and language at the very least. Routine monthly cognitive assessment should be done as a rough guide to cognitive performance, although there is a need to be aware of practice effects. Again, there is no specific test available, and a generic assessment such as the MMSE (Folstein *et al*, 1975) may well suffice, perhaps supplemented with some frontal-executive tasks. At each review, information about side-effects should be sought, particularly subjective cognitive problems: this is most helpfully done by allowing the patient to talk freely about any perceived concerns/experiences before asking more directed questions about particular side-effects. It may be that for practical purposes the regular review can be undertaken by a senior psychiatrist on the day of the treatment (before its administration).

There should be a full anaesthetic review by a senior anaesthetist (with laboratory tests as appropriate) every 6 months and full repeat of all psychometric assessments every 12 months.

Regular review by nursing and medical staff is essential and it is advisable to update the general practitioner at intervals. Informal verbal consent should be sought before each treatment. Written consent should be attained at regular intervals, perhaps every 6 months or every six treatments.

Stopping continuation ECT

Reduction in the frequency of ECT should continue until a stable state is reached, where there is a maximum space between treatments without return of symptoms. Allowing for individual variation, monthly is an appropriate goal. Since relapse of major depression is most likely within the first 12 months of recovery, it is wise to employ continuation ECT for at least 1 year after recovery with reviews as mentioned earlier. At the end of this period, a full review of the need for long-term ECT should take place.

If the course was begun to prevent relapse (continuation ECT) it is reasonable to consider terminating the course at this stage. With maintenance ECT, however, the goal is to prevent further episodes, suggesting the course might continue longer or even indefinitely. Even so, a full review annually must be considered advisable with reaffirmation of consent. Further maintenance treatment should be monitored as stated previously.

There is currently no way of predicting how likely a relapse or recurrence is following the withdrawal of continuation ECT. Clinical predictors of relapse will be idiosyncratic to the individual patient, hence the need for careful documenting of each patient's particular symptoms initially. We would suggest that close clinical supervision is maintained in the period after a course, and that return of symptoms would indicate consideration of maintenance ECT.

References

American Psychiatric Association (2001) *The Practice of Electroconvulsive Therapy: Recommendations for Treatment, Training and Privileging* (2nd edn). APA.

Barnes, R. C., Hussein, A., Anderson, D. N., *et al* (1997) Maintenance electroconvulsive therapy and cognitive function. *British Journal of Psychiatry*, **170**, 285–287.

Bourgon, L. N. & Kellner, C. H. (2000) Relapse of depression after ECT: a review. *Journal of ECT*, **16**, 19–31.

Folstein, M. F., Folstein, S. E. & McHugh, P. R. (1975) 'Mini-mental state': a practical method for grading the cognitive state of patients for the clinician. *Journal of Psychiatric Research*, **12**, 189–198.

Gupta, S., Hood, C. & Chaplin, R. (2011) Use of continuation and maintenance electroconvulsive therapy: UK national trends. *Journal of ECT*, **27**, 77–80.

Hamilton, M. (1960) A rating scale for depression. *Journal of Neurological and Neurosurgical Psychiatry*, **23**, 56–62.

Kellner, C. H., Knapp, R. G., Petrides, G., *et al* (2006) Continuation electroconvulsive therapy vs pharmacotherapy for relapse prevention in major depression: a multisite study from the Consortium for Research in Electroconvulsive Therapy (CORE). *Archives of General Psychiatry*, **63**, 1337–1344.

Lisanby, S. H., Sampson, S., Husain, M. M., *et al* (2008) Toward individualised post-electroconvulsive therapy care: piloting the Symptom-Titrated, Algorithm-Based Longitudinal ECT (STABLE) intervention. *Journal of ECT*, **24**, 179–182.

Montgomery, S. A. & Åsberg, M. (1979) A new depression scale designed to be sensitive to change. *British Journal of Psychiatry*, **134**, 382–389.

National Institute for Clinical Excellence (2003) *Guidance on the Use of Electroconvulsive Therapy* (Technology Appraisal TA59). NICE.

National Institute for Health and Clinical Excellence (2009) *Depression: The Treatment and Management of Depression in Adults (Update)* (Clinical Guidance CG90). NICE.

Rami-Gonzalez, L., Salamero, M., Boget, T., *et al* (2003) Pattern of cognitive dysfunction in depressive patients during maintenance electroconvulsive therapy. *Psychological Medicine*, **33**, 345–350.

Russell, J. C., Rasmussen, K. G., O'Connor, M. K., *et al* (2003) Long-term maintenance ECT: a retrospective review of efficacy and cognitive outcome. *Journal of ECT*, **19**, 4–9.

Sackeim, H. A., Haskett, R. F., Mulsant, B. H., *et al* (2001) Continuation pharmocotherapy in the prevention of relapse following electroconvulsive therapy: a randomised controlled trial. *JAMA*, **285**, 1299–1307.

Smith, G. E., Rasmussen Jr, K. G., Cullum, C. M., *et al* (2010) A randomized controlled trial comparing the memory effects of continuation electroconvulsive therapy versus continuation pharmacotherapy: results from the Consortium For Research In ECT (CORE) study. *Journal of Clinical Psychiatry*, **71**, 185–193.

Trevino, K., McClintock, S. M. & Husain, M. M. (2010) A review of continuation electroconvulsive therapy: application, safety and efficacy. *Journal of ECT*, **26**, 186–195.

Vothknecht, S., Kho, K. H., van Schaick, H. W., *et al* (2003) Effects of maintenance electroconvulsive therapy on cognitive functions. *Journal of ECT*, **19**, 151–157.

Wijkstra, J. & Nolen, W. (2005) Successful maintenance electroconvulsive therapy for more than seven years. *Journal of ECT*, **21**, 171–173.

Zisselman, M. H., Rosenquist, P. B. & Curlick, S. M. (2007) Long-term weekly electroconvulsive therapy: a case series. *Journal of ECT*, **23**, 274–277.

CHAPTER 22

Consent, capacity and the law

Jonathan Waite, Richard Barnes, Daniel M. Bennett,
Donald Lyons, Declan M. McLoughlin and Hugh Series

All medical procedures, be they therapeutic or investigative, touch on the issue of consent – that is a measure of willingness on the part of the patient to undertake the procedure proposed. In this, ECT is no different to other therapeutic interventions. However, ECT has a particular status both within psychiatry and within the law that makes specific discussion of issues with regard to consent necessary.

General issues regarding consent

Electroconvulsive therapy is unusual in that consent obtained is for a course of treatments rather than for an individual procedure. It is also customary that the person seeking the consent will not be the person giving the treatment. The fact that the person receiving treatment has a psychiatric disorder sufficiently severe for ECT to be considered raises questions about their capacity; this makes it particularly important that consent is properly obtained and valid. It is unlawful and unethical to treat a patient who is capable of understanding the nature of any procedure, its purpose and implications, the anticipated benefits and any reasonably foreseeable adverse effects without first explaining it. The patient must then agree. Even if patients choose not to be informed of the full details of their diagnosis and treatment, they must be given the option of receiving this information. Guidance on good practice in consent can be found in publications from the Department of Health in England and Wales (2009), the Department of Health, Social Services and Public Safety in Northern Ireland (2003) and the Scottish Executive (2006), as well as from the General Medical Council (2008).

Obtaining valid consent should be considered a process rather than an event and it is necessary for patients to be given an adequate length of time to consider the benefits and drawbacks of the proposed treatment before making an informed decision. Patients should be informed of the risks and unwanted effects of ECT (Chapters 7–9) and they need to realise that a general anaesthetic is involved. If there are specific anaesthetic risks, the anaesthetist should explain these and obtain the necessary consent.

It is helpful for patients and carers to be provided with information obtained from different sources. Written information sheets may be useful (e.g. Appendix V); these need to be accompanied by the opportunity to discuss issues with members of the therapeutic team, family members, carers, advocates, etc. Some patients may find over-long sheets daunting: provision of information in a variety of ways (e.g. through face-to-face interview, video, audiotape, podcast, interactive DVD) may be more acceptable.

Although UK law makes no distinction between the validity of written, verbal or even implied consent, it is recommended practice to seek the patient's written consent using a standard consent form – designed specifically for ECT – which complies with national guidelines (e.g. Appendix VI). The absence of a written statement of consent may make it very difficult to provide evidence that consent has in fact been given. In Ireland, written consent is required. Since written consent is obtained for the course of treatment and not for each treatment session, it is important to ensure patients clearly understand that they can withdraw consent at any time, despite having signed a consent form. They should also understand how they might inform staff about a change in consent. The continuation of consent should be verbally checked before each treatment, usually by a member of staff in the ECT suite. It is good practice for consent forms to specify the maximum number of treatments to which the patient has agreed to consent. The figure can be agreed with individual patients, although an arbitrary figure of 12 has been suggested as standard. Further treatment beyond the agreed figure would require new written consent, although consent could be withdrawn before the number is reached. It is also good practice to record on the consent form whether the patient has specified consent for bilateral or unilateral electrode placement.

An assessment of capacity is an integral part of obtaining a valid consent. This is particularly the case for ECT, where clinicians are likely to encounter patients who have limitations on their capacity to understand and process information. It is therefore good practice for consent to be obtained by a senior clinician (e.g. the patient's consultant).

It is important that patients are broadly able to understand the implications of refusing a treatment. They must also be informed that a patient who has capacity has a right to refuse treatment for any given reason or none at all. Refusal in these circumstances does not allow for any form of coercion to persuade reluctant patients to accept ECT (e.g. 'If you don't consent then there is nothing more I will do'). The law is clear that any form of coercion would negate the validity of the consent. It would also be unethical. Although it is unacceptable under any circumstances to use the threat of enforced treatment under mental health legislation to obtain consent, patients do need to understand that a possible consequence of their decision to decline ECT might be an assessment for treatment under compulsory powers. As a part of the discussion, alternative therapies to

ECT should be raised and it should be made clear that a refusal of treatment will not prejudice any further care.

Practical issues related to capacity

Since capacity is both time- and task-specific, it is possible that a patient assessed as having capacity when seen by the consultant may have lost that capacity by the time they attend for ECT, even if the time between the two events is very short (e.g. if there is significant diurnal variation of mood). This might arise, for example, in a very anxious patient who becomes so anxious on arrival in the ECT suite that the level of anxiety impairs their capacity at that moment. Clinicians of all disciplines in the ECT clinic will have to make their own assessment of capacity at the time of treatment. Individual suites will need to decide how this will be managed and agree how they will respond to a change in capacity or difference in opinion. If a patient has given written consent to treatment when mentally competent, this gives valuable guidance as to their wishes and feelings if they lack capacity a short period later. Subject to the qualifications above, ECT might proceed on the basis of mental capacity legislation or common law in a patient who had temporarily lost capacity at the time of treatment, particularly if they had previously given valid consent. It will be a matter for the person providing the treatment on that occasion to decide whether they are prepared to proceed on this basis.

England and Wales

Since the publication of the last edition of this handbook, the law in relation to mental health and capacity in England and Wales has changed considerably with the Mental Capacity Act 2005 coming into force and the 2007 amendments of the Mental Health Act 1983 significantly changing legislation with regard to ECT. Both of these acts have implications for the process of consent to ECT. At the time of writing, there is little case law to clarify some of the issues arising from the new legislation and the full impact on clinical practice remains to be seen. It is impossible therefore to give a definitive statement on some of the issues. This chapter gives information on the current position, as well as advice on how clinicians may wish to proceed. It is not intended to be a thorough review of the acts and focuses principally on those parts of the legislation most relevant to ECT.

Mental Capacity Act 2005

The Mental Capacity Act provides safeguards for those who care for people who lack capacity to make decisions for themselves. It also makes provision for proxies to be appointed to make decisions on behalf of other people, who lack capacity themselves at the time when a decision has to be made about their treatment. These proxies may be appointed by the Court of Protection on behalf of the incapacitated person (deputies) or chosen in advance by a person with capacity, who is concerned that there may be a future time when they will lack capacity to make decisions for themselves (attorneys). A person may create a Lasting Power of Attorney for personal finances and/or health and personal welfare matters. The Court of Protection refers to the holders of Lasting Power of Attorney as 'donees'. The Mental Capacity Act also allows people, when they are competent, to make an advance decision to refuse any specified medical treatment (including ECT) on a future occasion when they are incapable. The Court of Protection may make rulings on any matter relating to mental capacity, including whether a person has capacity in respect of a particular decision, or whether a treatment would be in a person's best interests. The Act establishes independent mental capacity advocates, who are professionals whose role is to assist people who have impaired capacity, but who have no family or friends who take an interest in their welfare.

A decision by the donee of a health and welfare Lasting Power of Attorney or a court-appointed deputy to refuse ECT on behalf of a patient who lacks capacity is legally binding, as is a valid and applicable advance decision to refuse ECT made under Section 25 (unless treatment is urgently necessary and can be given under the authority of Section 62(1A) of the Mental Health Act).

Principles

Section 1 states:

(1) The following principles apply for the purposes of this Act.
(2) A person must be assumed to have capacity unless it is established that he lacks capacity.
(3) A person is not to be treated as unable to make a decision unless all practicable steps to help him to do so have been taken without success.
(4) A person is not to be treated as unable to make a decision merely because he makes an unwise decision.
(5) An act done, or decision made, under this Act for or on behalf of a person who lacks capacity must be done, or made, in his best interests.
(6) Before the act is done, or the decision is made, regard must be had to whether the purpose for which it is needed can be as effectively achieved in a way that is less restrictive of the person's rights and freedom of action.

Definition of capacity

The Mental Capacity Act (Section 3) defines incapacity as:

(1) A person is unable to make a decision for himself if he is unable:
  (a) to understand the information relevant to the decision
  (b) to retain that information

(c) to use or weigh that information as part of the process of making the decision, or

(d) to communicate his decision (whether by talking, using sign language or any other means).

(2) A person is not to be regarded as unable to understand the information relevant to a decision if he is able to understand an explanation of it given to him in a way that is appropriate to his circumstances (using simple language, visual aids or any other means).

(3) The fact that a person is able to retain the information relevant to a decision for a short period only does not prevent him from being regarded as able to make the decision.

(4) The information relevant to a decision includes information about the reasonably foreseeable consequences of:

(a) deciding one way or another, or

(b) failing to make the decision.

A person failing on any one of the above criteria lacks the legal capacity to make that decision at that time. Although the Act gives no further guidance on what constitutes 'relevant information' or what length of time is 'a short period', some advice on these matters is given in the Department of Health's guide to consent (Department of Health, 2009).

Best interests

If someone is assessed as lacking capacity to make a particular decision, a decision will need to be made on that patient's behalf by a 'decision maker' to determine whether a proposed decision would be in the patient's 'best interests'. The Mental Capacity Act does not define best interests but it imposes a duty (Section 4) on decision makers to undertake a series of actions:

- they must consider if and when the patient will regain capacity
- they must involve the patient as much as possible in the decision-making process
- they must consider the patient's past and present wishes and feelings (particularly any written statements), their beliefs and values, and any other relevant factors
- they should try to consult with carers, friends, attorneys and deputies and take into account their views.

There is a fuller explanation of the concept of best interests and how they should be assessed in the Act's *Code of Practice* (Department for Constitutional Affairs, 2007). It is important to establish whether any relevant advance decisions have been made, and whether any Lasting Power of Attorney exists. Typically, the decision maker will be expected to consult with the patient and appropriate next of kin, family and carers. They also need to consult with any donee appointed under a Lasting Power of Attorney for health and personal welfare, or court-appointed deputy. There is no register of advance decisions, but the Office of the Public Guardian (see Appendix VII) can provide details of deputies and attorneys where clinicians require this information. Consultation with colleagues may also be appropriate. If the incapacitated person has no friends or relatives who can speak on their behalf, the *Code of Practice* says that an independent mental capacity advocate must be involved (paras 10.42 and 10.45).

Mental Health Act 1983

The Mental Health Act was significantly amended in 2007. Although many of the provisions are unaffected by these amendments, Part IV, which deals with consent to treatment, has been altered considerably so that the law relating to ECT is now substantially different. Practitioners must also have regard to the Mental Health Act *Code of Practice* (Department of Health, 2008) or the Mental Health Act *Code of Practice for Wales* (Welsh Assembly Government, 2008).

The professional in charge of a detained patient in England and Wales is the responsible clinician who need not now be a registered medical practitioner. It is the Royal College of Psychiatrists' view that any detained patient receiving ECT should have a consultant psychiatrist as their responsible clinician. Electroconvulsive therapy is now regulated by Section 58A of the amended Act. Under this section, ECT cannot lawfully be given to a detained patient who has capacity to consent to ECT but refuses. If ECT is immediately necessary to save life or prevent serious deterioration, it could be administered under emergency treatment provisions (Section 62(1A)), but these would not confer authority to complete a course of ECT.

For adult patients detained under Sections 2 or 3 who have capacity to consent to ECT, either the patient's responsible clinician or a second opinion appointed doctor (SOAD) acting on behalf of the Care Quality Commission must provide a certificate of consent to treatment (Form T4). For patients without capacity, a SOAD may authorise a course of ECT if 'it is appropriate for the treatment to be given[...], taking into account the nature and degree of the mental disorder from which he is suffering and all other circumstances of his case' (Section 64(3)). The SOAD is required to speak to the patient and two other people who have been involved in the patient's medical treatment, specifically a nurse and another healthcare professional who is neither a nurse nor a doctor (Section 58A(6)). The Care Quality Commission expects the clinical team making the referral to have checked that there is no conflict with a proxy decision maker or any advance decision to refuse treatment, as a condition of the SOAD visit (Care Quality Commission, 2008). If the SOAD believes that ECT is in the patient's best interests and should be authorised, they will complete Form T6.

For patients on a community treatment order who have not been recalled to hospital it is permissible to give out-patient ECT if the patient wishes; the responsible clinician will need to complete form CTO12 to certify that the patient has capacity and is consenting. The rules for patients without capacity are similar to those for detained in-patients. If a patient on a community treatment order is being given ECT on the basis of a SOAD certificate, a new certificate will be required for ECT if the patient is recalled to hospital, unless the certificate specifically states that ECT may continue to be given on recall (Department of Health, 2008: para. 24.28).

Suggested procedure for consent for people under 18

There are special provisions for ECT for people under the age of 18, whether detained under the Mental Health Act or not (Section 58A). A person aged 16 or 17 is presumed to have capacity to consent unless shown otherwise. If the person under 18 has capacity to consent, ECT may be given only if a SOAD issues a certificate (Form T5) that the young person can and does consent to ECT and that the treatment is appropriate.

If the person under 18 has capacity but refuses to give consent, a SOAD certificate alone does not provide authority to give ECT: there must also be authority from another source. Unlike the situation in those over 18, a court may have authority to overrule this refusal, but it is likely to consider very carefully before doing so. If the young person lacks capacity to consent it is uncertain whether ECT falls within the zone of parental authority of treatments for which a person with parental authority (usually the parents) can give consent (see chapter 36 of the *Code of Practice* for details (Department of Health, 2008) or chapter 33 of the *Code of Practice for Wales* (Welsh Assembly Government, 2008)). Paragraph 36.14 of the *Code of Practice* (Department of Health, 2008) expresses doubt whether ECT is a treatment to which parents can legally consent. The Code recommends seeking legal advice in this situation, and to consider whether authority to give ECT should be sought from a court.

It is possible that the Mental Capacity Act could be used to provide the necessary authority to give ECT to a non-competent person aged 16 or 17. Even though this appears to be a legal possibility, because the law in this area continues to evolve, we suggest that it would be advisable to seek legal advice before doing so. However, if it is considered that giving ECT would involve a deprivation of liberty, then the Mental Capacity Act cannot be used to authorise it for a person under 18, and court approval will be needed (see chapter 36 of the *Code of Practice* for details (Department of Health, 2008)).

Some children under the age of 16 may have sufficient understanding and intelligence to be able to consent to ECT ('Gillick competence'), in which case ECT can be given with their valid consent and SOAD certification. If they are competent but refuse consent, it may be that someone with parental authority could consent for them, but as for people aged 16 or 17, there is doubt whether this falls within the zone of parental authority, and if not, the consent of the court would be required for ECT. The same is true for children under the age of 16 who lack capacity to consent: the Mental Capacity Act cannot authorise treatment, and we suggest that legal advice may be necessary as to whether the consent of the court needs to be obtained.

In cases of emergency when there is insufficient time to obtain parental consent or court authority, the courts have stated that doubt should be resolved in favour of the preservation of life, and it will be acceptable to undertake treatment to preserve life or prevent irreversible serious deterioration of the patient's condition (Department of Health, 2008: para. 36.51).

For further information on the law in England and Wales, see Fennell (2011).

Suggested procedure for consent for people over 18

All patients being considered for ECT will require assessment of their capacity to give their consent specifically to ECT (Table 22.1). Clinicians will also have to consider the patient's legal status under the Mental Health Act and their likely adherence to the proposed treatment plan.

Patient has the capacity to consent and is informal

This remains the most common situation, where the patient is able to give valid consent and is not liable to be detained under the Mental Health Act.

Table 22.1 Assessment of patients over 18 years for ECT in England and Wales

Legal status	Capable of consenting?	Resisting or objecting?	Recommended action
Informal	Yes	No	Treat under normal rules of written consent
	Yes	Yes	Cannot treat with ECT
	No	No	It may be possible to treat under Section 5 of the Mental Capacity Act. Independent opinion (informal) advised
	No	Yes	Not appropriate to use the Mental Capacity Act. If ECT is to proceed, the patient may need to be detained under the Mental Health Act
Detained (where Part IV of the Mental Health Act applies)	Yes	No	Treat with written consent that must be certified on Form T2
	Yes	Yes	Cannot treat with ECT except to save life or prevent serious deterioration (Section 62)
	No	No	Treat if approved by SOAD from CQC on Form T3
	No	Yes	Treat if approved by SOAD from CQC on Form T3

CQC, Care Quality Commission; ECT, electroconvulsive therapy; SOAD, second opinion appointed doctor.

For those patients willing to have ECT, informed consent should be sought. This would include giving appropriate information and an appropriate length of time for consideration. If the patient consents to treatment, a consent form should be completed and the procedure may go ahead. If the patient declines, then ECT cannot be given. If the patient is under 18, in addition to the above, a Form T5 must be completed by a SOAD.

Patient has the capacity to consent and is detained under the Mental Health Act
As above, if the patient is willing to consider ECT, informed consent should be sought, a consent form filled in and the appropriate Section 58A paperwork (Form T4) completed, confirming their capacity to consent. Treatment can then go ahead.

If a detained patient who has capacity refuses ECT, then it can only be given in an emergency under Section 62. It is difficult to foresee a situation where starting treatment under this provision would be helpful.

Patient lacks capacity to consent and is informal
Here the clinician should make a formal assessment of capacity, which should be clearly documented (e.g. Appendix VIII), bearing in mind the guidance in the Mental Capacity Act *Code of Practice* (Department for Constitutional Affairs, 2007). Once incapacity is established, a decision must be made in the patient's best interests, which will require the clinician to consult appropriately (see p. 208). If the patient has no friend or family to speak for him, the Mental Capacity Act *Code* requires that an independent mental capacity advocate should be involved (Department for Constitutional Affairs, 2007: para. 10.45). Following this consultation, if ECT is not considered to be in the patient's best interests, it should not be given. If, however, it is decided that ECT would be appropriate in the patient's best interests, there are two possible legal mechanisms by which this could be lawfully given, either under the provisions of Section 5 of the Mental Capacity Act or by the patient being detained under the Mental Health Act.

There exist differences of opinion among legal professionals as to which route is preferable. Some would argue that as there is explicit provision in Section 58A of the Mental Health Act on administering ECT to people without capacity, the patient should be detained under the Mental Health Act and this route should be followed. It offers explicit legal safeguards, in particular the need for the treatment to be independently assessed by a SOAD. Against this it could be argued that the least restrictive option should be pursued, and that it is wrong to detain a person who is agreeing to be in hospital. The Mental Health Act Commission (2008: p. 222) has stated that 'unnecessary and therefore unlawful detention under the Act may have resulted from a common misunderstanding that ECT may not be given to compliant but incapacitated patients under the common law'. The Department of Health envisaged that it might be possible to use the Mental Capacity Act in these circumstances by referring to ECT in the *Code of Practice* as 'serious medical treatment' (Department for Constitutional Affairs, 2007: para. 10.4.5) for which an independent mental capacity advocate must be instructed.

In making a choice between the different acts, each practitioner will have to make a decision as they think best in each particular situation, seeking legal advice if necessary. The College is not able to give legal advice. The College's Special Committee for ECT and Related Treatments considers that what follows is a reasonable interpretation of the current state of the law, but it cannot be relied on as an authoritative source of legal guidance.

Mental Health Act or Mental Capacity Act?

The incapacitated informal compliant patient

If an informal patient lacks capacity to consent but appears to adhere to treatment, then it may be preferable to give ECT under the Mental Capacity Act (Table 22.2). This is less restrictive of a patient's freedom than detention under the Mental Health Act, although it offers fewer safeguards than the Mental Health Act procedure. This would be in keeping with the least restriction principle (Department of Health, 2008: para. 1.3). Although it is not a legal requirement, it would seem wise to seek a second opinion from a colleague prior to proceeding. If the patient does not adhere to treatment, and it is felt that it is still needed, it will be necessary to consider whether an assessment for detention under the Mental Health Act is necessary to

Table 22.2 Mental Health Act 1983 or Mental Capacity Act 2005?[1]

Is patient detained under Mental Health Act?	Does patient have capacity?	Does patient consent or comply?	Will patient be deprived of liberty?	Procedure required
No	Yes	Yes	No	Standard consent form
No	Yes	No	No	Cannot treat
No	No	Yes/No	Yes	Consider Mental Health Act
No	No	Yes	No	Section 5 of the Mental Capacity Act or possibly Mental Health Act
Yes	Yes	Yes	Yes/No	Responsible clinician or SOAD can certify
Yes	Yes	No	Yes/No	Cannot treat
Yes	No	Yes/No	Yes/No	SOAD can authorise

SOAD, second opinion appointed doctor.

1. This applies to adults over 18 in England and Wales.

allow treatment to be given. It is important to emphasise that capacity will need to be reassessed before every treatment in these circumstances. Once capacity is regained, ECT cannot proceed without informed consent.

If a patient lacks capacity to consent but is well enough to receive ECT as a day patient (and complies with the procedure), then the Mental Capacity Act will usually be preferable. It is doubtful that criteria for detention under the Mental Health Act would be met in this situation, since for Section 3 of the Mental Health Act to be applied it must be demonstrated that appropriate treatment cannot be provided in a less restrictive way. The argument that in such circumstances the patient should be detained under the Mental Health Act and then put on Section 17 leave or a community treatment order so as to receive ECT seems unjustifiable. A patient should not be detained in hospital only in order to allow a community treatment order to be made.

The incapacitated informal non-compliant patient

If it is thought likely that the patient will not adhere to the treatment – or if attempts to give ECT have clearly shown this – then we would recommend that if ECT is necessary, consideration should be given to using the Mental Health Act procedures. Although it may still be argued that treatment could legally be provided under Section 5 of the Mental Capacity Act and that any restraint required would be permitted under this Act as being both proportionate and necessary, the fact that provisions for treatment of incapacitated detained patients have been specifically included in the Mental Health Act suggests that these provisions should be invoked.

Clinicians should again check that there is no valid and applicable advance decision refusing ECT or objection by a deputy or attorney (except in emergency situations). If there is doubt whether an advance decision refusing ECT is valid or applicable, a ruling should be sought from the Court of Protection. Electroconvulsive therapy could proceed if necessary while the Court's decision is awaited (Section 26, Mental Capacity Act).

As with incapacitated informal compliant patients, the capacity of detained patients should be reviewed after each treatment, as once the patient regains capacity, consent will have to be obtained if treatment is to continue.

Emergency treatment

A patient detained under Section 2 or Section 3 of the Mental Health Act may be given ECT in an emergency if it is immediately necessary to save life or prevent serious deterioration in the patient's condition, and if the treatment does not have unfavourable physical or psychological consequences which cannot be reversed (Section 62). This can happen even if there is a contrary advance decision or an objection by a deputy or attorney. If there is concern about the validity or applicability of the advance decision refusing ECT, consideration should be given to referring the matter to the Court of Protection for a ruling on the legality of treatment. Treatment may be continued while the Court's decision is awaited (Section 26(5), Mental Capacity Act). If there is concern that an attorney or deputy is not acting in the patient's best interests, this should be brought to the attention of the Public Guardian.

Some patients who have received ECT as an emergency treatment under Section 62 of the Mental Health Act and recover capacity may refuse further treatment, even though the clinical team feel their recovery is incomplete. There may be concern that relapse in these circumstances is likely; with a possible cycle of emergency treatment/partial recovery/refusal/relapse/ emergency treatment ensuing. Since this scenario may be anticipated, good practice suggests that the consultant should discuss the possibility with the patient once they have capacity, clarifying in detail what the patient's wishes would be should their condition decline. If a patient with capacity is clear that they do not want further ECT – even if this refusal means that they will put their health at grave risk – then this is likely to be determinative.

Scotland

Since the previous edition of *The ECT Handbook* there has been a significant change in the legislative framework following the implementation of the Mental Health (Care and Treatment) (Scotland) Act 2003. This Act came into force on 5 October 2005 and replaced the Mental Health (Scotland) Act 1984, modified the Criminal Procedure (Scotland) Act 1995 and sits alongside the Adults with Incapacity (Scotland) Act 2000. All of these acts are relevant to patients who may require ECT (Table 22.3).

Informal patients capable of giving consent

This description refers to the majority of patients who receive ECT in Scotland. According to the annual report from SEAN (2011), in 2010 61% of patients treated with ECT were informal patients who gave consent, although the proportion of patients receiving ECT who lack capacity to consent is rising.

If a patient has the capacity (see pp. 217–218) to give informed consent, then this decision should be followed by the clinician, provided there is no need to consider the Mental Health (Care and Treatment) (Scotland) Act 2003. In the case of a competent adult who refuses treatment, such treatment cannot be given. Should an adult with capacity decide to have ECT, then both the doctor who has explained the procedure and the patient should sign a consent form to record the consent. The consent form is a record that the consent has been given but it does not confirm that the consent is valid. It is best practice to record the reasons that the consent is valid in the case notes. It is also considered best practice to use a standard consent form and for the consent to be revisited before each treatment to ensure it remains valid. If there is a gap in treatment of greater than

Table 22.3 Assessment of patients over 18 years for ECT in Scotland

Legal status	Capable of consenting?	Resisting or objecting?	Recommended action
Informal	Yes	No	Treat under normal rules of written consent
	Yes	Yes	Cannot treat with ECT
	No	No	Can treat under Section 48 of the 2000 Act with independent opinion. Mental Welfare Commission will organise
	No	Yes	Not appropriate to use the 2000 Act. If ECT is to proceed, the patient should be detained under the 2003 Act
Detained (where Part 16 of the 2003 Act applies)	Yes	No	Treat with written consent that must be certified on Form T2
	Yes	Yes	Cannot treat with ECT, even if it appears urgent to do so
	No	No	Treat with independent designated medical practitioner opinion certified on Form T3 (best interests test). Mental Welfare Commission will organise
	No	Yes	Treat with independent designated medical practitioner opinion certified on Form T3 (but only to save life, prevent serious deterioration or alleviate serious suffering). Mental Welfare Commission will organise

2000 Act, Adults with Incapacity (Scotland) Act 2000; 2003 Act, Mental Health (Care and Treatment) (Scotland) Act 2003; ECT, electroconvulsive therapy.

2 weeks, it is recommended that consent be recorded anew. The patient should be informed that they can withdraw their consent at any point should they wish to.

Patients incapable of giving informed consent

In order to decide whether a patient is capable of giving informed consent, it is necessary to define capacity and the elements contained within it. In Scotland, as with the other legislative areas of the UK, there is a presumption in favour of capacity. Capacity is specific to a particular time and decision and is thus subject to change. In the context of ECT it is hoped that by treating a patient who has lost capacity through their mental disorder, it will be regained as the symptoms of their illness abate. The issue of capacity should be revisited after each ECT treatment to assess whether the patient may be able to consent to further treatment.

Adults with Incapacity (Scotland) Act 2000

The Adults with Incapacity (Scotland) Act 2000 was a major advance in the area of incapacity as it gives legal definitions of the concepts described earlier. This Act, like the later Mental Health (Care and Treatment) (Scotland) Act 2003, is an example of 'principled legislation', as it sets out (in Section 1) a number of principles which must be considered when applying the Act in practice. These principles can be summarised as:

- the intervention must benefit the adult
- any intervention shall be the least restrictive in relation to the freedom of the adult, consistent with the purpose of the intervention
- account must be taken of the past and present wishes of the adult
- where practicable, account should be taken of:
  - the views of relative and carers
  - the views of relevant others (guardians, attorneys, etc.).

Section 1(6) of the Adults with Incapacity (Scotland) Act 2000 also provides definitions of 'adult' as a person who has attained the age of 16 years, and 'incapable', which means incapable of:

(a) acting
(b) making decisions
(c) communicating decisions
(d) understanding decisions
(e) retaining the memory of decisions,
     [...] by reason of mental disorder or of inability to communicate because of physical disability; but a person shall not fall within this definition by reason only of a lack or deficiency in a faculty of communication if that lack or deficiency can be made good by human or mechanical aid (whether of an interpretative nature or otherwise).

This definition is helpful to the clinician in making decisions about whether the patient has capacity, as it sets out very clear criteria and only one of these requires to be fulfilled for the patient to be incapable.

A general authority to treat is given to the medical practitioner primarily responsible for the medical treatment of an incapable adult, under Section 47. Such treatment must safeguard or promote mental or physical health but treatment must not require the use of force or detention (unless immediately necessary and only for so long as is necessary in the circumstances). When Section 47 is used to give treatment, a certificate of incapacity should be completed. It is of note that the use of force or detention is not permitted and thus the psychiatrist should consider the use of the Mental Health (Care and Treatment) (Scotland) Act 2003 where a patient actively resists or opposes treatment.

Of particular interest to the ECT clinician is that Section 48 of the Adults with Incapacity (Scotland) Act 2000 excludes special treatments as defined in the Mental Health (Care and Treatment) (Scotland) Act 2003 (including ECT, transcranial magnetic stimulation and vagus nerve stimulation)

217

from this general authority to treat and sets in place a procedure whereby a designated medical practitioner second opinion must be sought. The designated medical practitioner will be provided by the Mental Welfare Commission for Scotland and will complete a prescribed form, which is lodged with the Commission within 7 days of issue. The Adults with Incapacity (Scotland) Act 2000 has provision for proxy decision makers such as welfare attorneys, welfare guardians and those exercising an intervention order, all of whom can normally consent to treatment on behalf of an incapable adult, but they cannot consent to special treatments under Section 48 (including ECT).

Mental Health (Care and Treatment) (Scotland) Act 2003

This Act sets out, in Section 1, ten principles which are to be used by any person discharging a function under the Act. These are to have regard for the following:

1   The present and past wishes and feelings of the patient.
2   In so far as is practicable, the views of the patient's named person, carer and any guardian or welfare attorney.
3   The importance of the patient participating as fully as possible in the discharge of the function.
4   The importance of providing information and support for the patient, in the form that is most likely to be understood, to enable the patient to participate.
5   The importance of the range of options available in the patient's case.
6   The importance of providing the maximum benefit to the patient.
7   The importance of the patient's abilities, background and characteristics, including age, gender, sexual orientation, religious persuasion, racial origin, cultural and linguistic background and membership of any ethnic group.
8   The importance of providing appropriate services and continuing care to the patient.
9   The needs and circumstances of the patient's carer, providing such information as might be needed to assist in the care of the patient.
10 The function must be discharged in a manner that involves the minimum restriction on the freedom of the patient that appears to be necessary in the circumstances, encourages equal opportunities and if the patient is a child (under 18 years old) best secures his or her welfare.

The Act also defines mental disorder as any mental illness, personality disorder or learning disability, however caused or manifested (Section 328). In addition, a person is considered not to have mental disorder if the following occur on their own:

• sexual orientation
• sexual deviancy

- trans-sexualism
- transvestism
- dependence on, or use of, alcohol or drugs
- behaviour that causes, or is likely to cause, harassment, alarm or distress to any other person or by acting as no prudent person would act.

'Medical treatment' is defined in Section 329 as treatment for mental disorder; for this purpose, 'treatment' includes nursing, care, psychological interventions, habilitation and rehabilitation. Medical treatment includes pharmacological interventions as well as other physical interventions such as ECT.

Short Term Detention Certificate/compulsory treatment order

The gateway order, or initial section, should be a Short Term Detention Certificate (STDC). This is applied by an approved medical practitioner who is usually, but not necessarily, a psychiatrist, and requires the consent of a specially trained social worker called a mental health officer. This section lasts up to 28 days and gives the patient and their named person a number of rights, including that of appeal. This authorises treatment under Part 16 of the Act, as does a compulsory treatment order. Applications for a compulsory treatment order, which lasts up to 6 months, are made by an mental health officer with supporting medical reports from two registered medical practitioners, one of whom must be an approved medical practitioner. A draft care plan is required at the stage of application and this may include ECT (the *Consent to Treatment* guidance from the Mental Welfare Commission (2006) contains information on how to draft a care plan for ECT). All applications for a compulsory treatment order are heard by the Mental Health Tribunal for Scotland. Part 16 also applies to most people subject to mental healthcare and treatment under criminal procedures legislation.

The criteria for detention are similar for each order. They must be met for a compulsory treatment order. They must be 'likely to be met' for an STDC. Criminal procedure orders do not require the patient to have impaired decision-making ability. The criteria are:

- the presence of a mental disorder
- medical treatment which would be likely to prevent the mental disorder worsening, or alleviate the symptoms or effects of the disorder, is available
- there would be significant risk to the health, safety or welfare of the patient or safety of any other person if the patient were not given medical treatment
- because of this mental disorder the patient's ability to make decisions about the provision of medical treatment for mental disorder is significantly impaired
- the making of the order is necessary.

Patients detained by virtue of an STDC or compulsory treatment order may be given medical treatment for mental disorder with or without their consent. Electroconvulsive therapy can only be given to a patient under compulsion if the patient can and does consent or the patient is incapable of consenting and treatment is authorised by a designated medical practitioner.

If a patient does give consent, a written statement to that effect which is witnessed is required and this must be recorded on Form T2. The responsible medical officer is required to certify that this consent has been given and that the treatment is in the patient's best interests, having regard to the likelihood of the treatment alleviating or preventing deterioration in the patient's condition. This is required irrespective of the length of time the patient has been subject to the Act (normally Form T2 is only required after the patient has received treatment for 2 months). In these circumstances the patient can withdraw their consent at any time and no further ECT can be given by virtue of the earlier consent.

If the patient does not consent or is unable to give consent, then ECT can be authorised by a designated medical practitioner using Form T3. The process for this is very similar to that under the Adults with Incapacity (Scotland) Act 2000 in that the designated medical practitioner is provided by the Mental Welfare Commission for Scotland. If the patient is incapable of consenting, the designated medical practitioner must certify that the patient is incapable and that the treatment is in the patient's best interests having regard to the likelihood of the treatment alleviating or preventing deterioration in the patient's condition.

If the patient objects or resists, the designated medical practitioner must certify as such and that the patient is incapable of making the decision and that the treatment is necessary under the urgent medical treatment provisions of Section 243 in order to:

- save the patient's life
- prevent serious deterioration in the patient's condition.
- alleviate serious suffering on the part of the patient.

Should these criteria no longer be met, then no further treatment can be given under these provisions.

There may be a situation, however, whereby the patient urgently requires ECT and it is not possible to arrange a visit from the designated medical practitioner. If emergency treatment is needed under the grounds specified in Section 243 of the Act, it must be reported to the Mental Welfare Commission, stating the type of treatment given and its purpose. Form T4 should be used for this. Although there is no legal requirement for a second opinion for emergency treatment, it is advisable to ask a local colleague for an opinion.

Advance statements

The Act introduced the facility for patients to make advance statements under Section 276. This allows a patient to specify which type of care and treatment they would like to receive or not like to receive should they become mentally ill. If such a statement exists, it is necessary for the clinician to have regard to its content when planning care. This does not necessarily mean that it must be followed and it is possible for the clinician to override an advance statement. In such circumstances Section 276(8) requires the clinician to give the reasons, justified with reference to the principles of the Act, for overriding the advance statement in writing, recorded in the case file and given to the patient, named person, welfare attorney, guardian and the Mental Welfare Commission. The Commission will scrutinise such decisions to override an advance statement.

The Act also gives any person with a mental disorder the right to independent advocacy. Advocacy workers can help patients express their views about medical treatment, including ECT.

Northern Ireland

The law in relation to psychiatric treatment in Northern Ireland is laid down in the Mental Health (Northern Ireland) Order 1986. Part IV of this regulation relates to consent to treatment. Unlike other areas in the UK, there is, at the time of writing, no statute law relating to mental capacity in Northern Ireland. Although there are differences in terminology, the legal principles are very similar to those underlying the Mental Health Act 1983 in England and Wales, apart from the aspects relating to mental capacity.

Electroconvulsive therapy may be given to a patient who is consenting, or to a detained patient who has not consented where a second opinion has been obtained from a psychiatrist appointed by the Regulation and Quality Improvement Authority (Article 63). Emergency treatment may be given under Article 68 where it is necessary to save the patient's life or prevent serious deterioration in their condition.

Mental health law in Northern Ireland has been reviewed and a policy consultation document has been issued (Department of Health, Social Services and Public Safety, 2009).

Ireland

Electroconvulsive therapy in Ireland is regulated by the Mental Health Commission, whose revised *Code of Practice* (2009) and *Rules* (2010) on the use of ECT came into effect in 2010. The *Code of Practice* provides guidance on ECT in general, whereas the *Rules* govern the use of ECT specifically for patients detained under the Irish Mental Health Act 2001, which was not fully implemented until November 2006 (Kelly, 2007).

The Mental Health Commission also inspects ECT clinics and now produces an annual report on the use of ECT in approved centres in Ireland. The *Code of Practice* and the *Rules* specify what information must be given to the patient and what information on the course of treatment is to be sent to the Mental Health Commission. The *Rules* also specify cognitive and physical assessments, conditions for the administration of ECT, staffing levels in the ECT suite and documentation. The standards required are similar to those required by ECTAS and SEAN.

The majority of patients in Ireland are treated voluntarily with ECT and provide valid informed consent, as assessed by the responsible consultant psychiatrist, in line with the *Code of Practice* (Mental Health Commission, 2009). There is no mechanism for a relative, carer or guardian to give consent on behalf of the patient. Capacity to consent to ECT should ensure that the voluntary patient can:

- understand the nature of ECT
- understand why ECT is being proposed
- understand the benefits, risks (including the risk of amnesia) and alternatives to receiving ECT
- understand and believe the broad consequences of not receiving ECT
- retain the information long enough to make a decision to receive or not receive ECT
- make a free choice to receive or refuse ECT
- communicate the decision to consent to ECT.

There were 19 619 admissions to approved centres in 2010, of which 1952 (9.95%) were involuntary (Mental Health Commission, 2012). Part IV of the Act covers consent to treatment and, according to Section 59, ECT may only be administered to detained patients if the patient gives consent in writing or where the consultant in charge of the patient's care has approved the programme of treatment, and the programme has been authorised by another consultant psychiatrist. The referring consultant fills out the first two pages of Form 16 and a second psychiatrist completes the third page. There is no statutory prohibition to a detained patient who has capacity being given ECT contrary to their wishes. However, there are moves to bring in appropriate capacity legislation to address this issue, as some detained patients may well have capacity to make an informed decision to refuse ECT (Dunne *et al*, 2009).

Recommendations

- Obtaining consent for ECT is a process, with a need for regular reassessment of capacity and consent.
- Practitioners need to be familiar with the legal requirements of the country in which they are working, and associated good practice guidance.
- The advice given in this chapter may need to be amended in the light of new statute and case law – clinicians will need to keep up to date with developments.

Acknowledgements

The authors thank Michael Mannion and Michael Sergeant for their assistance with this chapter.

References

Care Quality Commission (2008) *Guidance for SOADS: Consent for Treatment & the SOAD Role under the Revised Mental Health Act*. Care Quality Commission.

Department for Constitutional Affairs (2007) *Mental Capacity Act 2005: Code of Practice*. TSO (The Stationery Office).

Department of Health (2008) *Code of Practice: Mental Health Act 1983*. TSO (The Stationery Office).

Department of Health (2009) *Reference Guide to Consent for Examination or Treatment* (2nd edn). Department of Health.

Department of Health, Social Services and Public Safety (2003) *Reference Guide to Consent for Examination, Treatment or Care*. Department of Health, Social Services and Public Safety.

Department of Health, Social Services and Public Safety (2009) *Legislative Framework for Mental Capacity and Mental Health Legislation in Northern Ireland: A Policy Consultation Document*. Department of Health, Social Services and Public Safety.

Dunne, R., Kavanagh, A. & McLoughlin, D. M. (2009) Electroconvulsive therapy, capacity and the law in Ireland. *Irish Journal of Psychological Medicine*, **26**, 3–5.

Fennell, P. (2011) *Mental Health: Law and Practice* (2nd edn). Jordans.

General Medical Council (2008) *Consent: Patients and Doctors Making Decisions Together*. GMC.

Kelly, B. D. (2007) The Irish Mental Health Act 2001. *Psychiatric Bulletin*, **31**, 21–24.

Mental Health Act Commission (2008) *Risk, Rights, Recovery: The Mental Health Commission Twelfth Biennial Report 2005–2007*. TSO (The Stationery Office).

Mental Health Commission (2009) *Code of Practice: Code of Practice on the Use of Electro-Convulsive Therapy for Voluntary Patients (Version 2)*. Mental Health Commission.

Mental Health Commission (2010) *Rules: Rules Governing the Use of Electro-Convulsive Therapy (Version 2)*. Mental Health Commission.

Mental Health Commission (2012) *The Administration of Electro-Convulsive Therapy in Approved Centres: Activity Report 2010*. Mental Health Commission.

Mental Welfare Commission for Scotland (2006) *Consent to Treatment: A Guide for Mental Health Practitioners*. Mental Welfare Commission for Scotland.

Scottish ECT Accreditation Network (2011) *Scottish ECT Accreditation Network Annual Report 2011: A Summary of ECT in Scotland for 2010*. NHS National Services Scotland.

Scottish Executive (2006) *A Good Practice Guide on Consent for Health Professionals in NHS Scotland*. Scottish Executive (http://www.sehd.scot.nhs.uk/mels/HDL2006_34.pdf).

Welsh Assembly Government (2008) *Mental Health Act 1983: Code of Practice for Wales*. TSO (The Stationery Office).

CHAPTER 23

Patients' and carers' perspectives on ECT

Jonathan Waite

Patients' perspectives

The NICE technology appraisal on ECT (2003) that preceded the last edition of *The ECT Handbook* was informed by two systematic reviews. The group tasked with assessing evidence for efficacy (UK ECT Review Group, 2003) concluded that there was evidence that ECT was an effective treatment for depressive disorders. There was also an review of patients' perspectives on ECT – specifically their views on the benefits of treatment and adverse effects on memory – conducted by the Service User Research Enterprise (SURE) at the Institute of Psychiatry (Rose *et al*, 2003). The NICE Committee's decision of recommending ECT only when illness was life-threatening or resistant to other treatments was significantly influenced by service users' views (National Institute for Clinical Excellence, 2003: para. 4.3.8).

Rose *et al* (2003) reviewed 26 studies carried out by clinicians and 9 studies led by patients or undertaken with their collaboration. It was noted that clinicians asked fewer questions and their research had less complex schedules and was undertaken shortly after treatment. Clinician-led studies were much more likely to find that patients had found ECT helpful (Fig. 23.1). Studies that were undertaken in hospital settings by the treating doctor were more likely to report positive views of ECT. Of the 35 studies, 20 considered memory loss. Reported rates of memory impairment were 29–55%. There was no difference between patient- and clinician-led studies in the frequency of memory complaints.

The service user perspective was again explored in two further publications from the SURE group (Philpot *et al*, 2004; Rose *et al*, 2004). In the first of these (Philpot *et al* 2004), a patient-designed 20-item questionnaire was posted to the home addresses of 108 patients 6 weeks after they had completed a course of bilateral ECT. Of the 43 respondents who answered this question, 41% of all forms were returned, although not all were fully completed: 19 patients would have ECT again, 7 would 'possibly' and 17 would 'never have ECT again'. Patients who had found

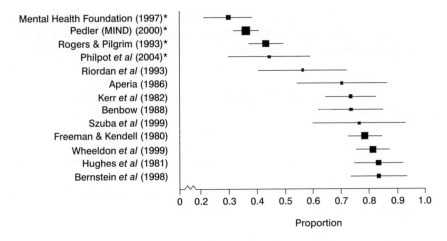

Fig. 23.1 Proportions of patients who would find ECT helpful, by study. Lines indicate approximate 95% confidence intervals; size of box indicates precision. *Patient study.

ECT helpful and those who had received previous courses were more likely to accept the idea of future ECT; out of 19 patients having their first course of ECT, only 4 said they would definitely have ECT again. Thirteen patients felt they had no option to refuse ECT, of which one patient was detained and treated under a section of the Mental Health Act 1983. Thirty-six patients recorded memory disturbance as an adverse effect and eighteen complained of persistent memory loss, but some felt that his was worth putting up with in order to relieve depression.

The other study (Rose et al, 2004) gathered experiences of ECT from three sources: internet websites containing ECT forums, a video archive (the British Library Mental Health Testimony Archive; summaries can be accessed through the British Libarary website) and consumer newsletters, books and other publications known to the authors. From these sources, 139 'testimonies' were collected. Of these, 83 were negative, 43 positive and 13 unclear. Some patients who had experienced ECT felt that the adverse effects were tolerable; others reported that they had tried to minimise symptoms to their psychiatrist in order to avoid receiving further treatment. For several patients, the main concern was about the perceived coercion which lead to them receiving treatment. Of the 139 testimonies, 99 (71%) mentioned memory loss as an adverse effect of treatment: in 86 cases (62%) this was felt to be permanent. There was little variation in complaints of memory loss between people who recently received ECT and those who had been treated 50 years ago. Similar findings are reported by Lawrence (2006).

Several workers have reported findings from in-depth interviews with patients who have received ECT. Johnstone (1999) spoke to 20 people recruited by posters and flyers seeking those who had been distressed by their experiences of ECT. Ten participants had received ECT in the past 10 years and ten respondents spoke of their experiences 10–30 years previously. The responses are largely what would be expected from this group of patients.

Koopowitz *et al* (2003), working in Adelaide, Australia, conducted semi-structured interviews with eight patients who were willing to attend a clinic to discuss their experiences with a medical student. Participants were between 25 and 50 years old: four had unipolar depression and four bipolar affective disorder. Their outcome from treatment varied between full remission and no response.

The four most prevalent and striking themes were: fear of ECT, cognitive decline and memory loss, positive experiences of ECT and suggestions for improving ECT for other patients. Seven of the eight patients complained of memory impairment, although there was some inconsistency in this: 'Some patients complained of large gaps in memory about the actual procedure, yet they were able to describe the procedure in detail' (Koopowitz *et al*, 2003). Suggestions for improving the experience included: reducing waiting time prior to the procedure, improving communication between patients before and during the procedure, reducing the exposure to other patients who are disturbed before or after the procedure, and undertaking further research on the service user experience.

More positive experiences were found by Rayner *et al* (2009) who reported the views of 389 patients who submitted completed questionnaires as part of the ECTAS review process. (Other results from this survey are reported by Kershaw *et al*, 2007.) The median interval between ECT and completing the questionnaire was 90 days (range 0 days to 30 years). Forty-nine respondents referred to memory loss, 21% headaches and 10% feelings of weakness or tiredness. Twelve patients complained of severe and persistent memory loss. Attitudes towards memory loss varied. One patient stated: 'I will never agree to receive ECT again because I have lost so much memory. Many of the memories I have lost are very valuable' (p. 383). Other patients remarked, 'I still suffer from some memory loss, but it is nothing compared to my condition prior to ECT' (p. 384) and 'My memory loss during and after the procedure has been disconcerting to say the least. However, on the whole, my views are positive' (p. 385).

Twelve per cent of patients who were assumed to have consented stated that they felt pressurised or forced to have ECT; others complained that they were rushed into a decision before they were ready. Nineteen patients stated that they were not given sufficient information about the side-effects of treatment. The survey did not include questions on beneficial effects of ECT: of the 109 patients who entered free text comments, 79 reported beneficial effects, 22 had felt ECT had had no effect of their condition, and 7 others had initially experienced benefit but later relapsed. In addition, several patients commented on the reluctance of their psychiatrists to prescribe ECT: 'ECT is the only thing that works for me if I get really ill (suicidal). Some consultants have refused ECT for me and taken a long time to be persuaded' (p. 385).

Similar suggestions about how to improve the patient experience were found in Kershaw *et al*'s (2007) report sent to ECTAS as part of the accreditation process. In total, 1600 questionnaires were sent out to member clinics; 389 were completed by patients. It is gratifying to note that patients generally found that helpful and friendly staff relieved their anxieties. Other surveys conducted by ECT clinic staff (Sienart *et al*, 2005; Rush *et al*, 2007) have had similar results to those reviewed by Rose *et al* (2003).

Bustin *et al* (2008) surveyed attitudes to and knowledge of ECT in patients receiving out-patient treatment for depression who had not experienced ECT. A total of 75 patients were recruited: 30 from Argentina, 30 from England and 15 from Canada. Most patients had a neutral or negative attitude to ECT – those who were more positive had a better level of knowledge about ECT.

Brodarty *et al* (2003) reported on attitudes to ECT in a cohort of 81 elderly patients (mean age 67.2 years) who received ECT for major depression. Prior to treatment, 39.7% expected that their condition would get better, 41.1% thought there would be no change and 19.2% believed they would get worse. Patients with severe depression were most pessimistic about the likelihood of improvement. After treatment, 68.8% felt they had benefited from ECT, 6.5% felt they had become worse, and 24.7% thought their condition was the same. Seven of the patients who responded well to ECT but expected to get worse, changed their opinions of ECT; however, five patients whose post-treatment depression scores indicated remission of their symptoms, did not think that ECT had helped them. The research psychiatrists were more accurate than the patients in predicting treatment outcome, but they overestimated the probability of ECT being successful.

Carers' experiences

Very little research has been published on carers' experiences of ECT. Smith *et al* (2009) report on interviews with 16 people: 9 patients receiving ECT and 7 family members. Each had been involved with a course of ECT during the previous 6 months, with patients receiving between 5 and 100 ECT treatments. The interviews focused on issues about the decision to have ECT, and the aftermath of treatment. Three themes emerged from discussions of the decision-making process:

- the anguish of living with a severe mental disorder
- the feelings that ECT was the last hope
- the blind trust that had to placed in the doctor.

In the aftermath of treatment, further themes emerged: many patients experienced relief with remission of symptoms but there were adverse effects including memory loss (which was more severe than expected), ataxia, mania and confusion. Those who did not improve felt more despondent, and for some who did improve, remission was short lived. Participants felt that they had not been given an adequate explanation about the risks of ECT.

More positive views on ECT were expressed by the parents of young people aged under 19 years who had received ECT. Of the 28 parents interviewed, 17 felt that the treatment had been helpful, 9 thought it had made no difference and 1 believed it had been deleterious (Walter *et al*, 1999). The family members interviewed by Szuba *et al* (1991) also reported positive attitudes to ECT.

Conclusions

Professionals undertaking research into the experiences of patients receiving ECT have generally reported that they have found the procedure helpful and tolerable. Reports coming from service user-led research are less likely to be published in peer-reviewed publications; more individuals reported adverse outcomes.

A consistent theme which emerges from all the studies conducted with service users and carers is the perceived lack of information which they received prior to treatment about the possible adverse effects of ECT, particularly the possibility of adverse effects on memory.

References

Aperia, B. (1986) Hormone pattern and post-treatment attitudes in patients with major depressive disorder given electroconvulsive therapy. *Acta Psychiatrica Scandinavica*, **73**, 271–274.

Benbow, S. M. (1988) Patients views on electroconvulsive therapy on completion of a course of treatment. *Convulsive Therapy*, **4**, 146–152.

Bernstein, H., Beale, M. & Kellner, C. H. (1998) Patient attitudes about ECT after treatment. *Psychiatric Annals*, **28**, 524–527.

Brodarty, H., Berle, D., Hickie, I., *et al* (2003) Perceptions of outcome from electroconvulsive therapy by depressed patients and psychiatrists. *Australian and New Zealand Journal of Psychiatry*, **37**, 196–199.

Bustin, J., Rapoport, M. J., Krishna, M., *et al* (2008) Are patients' attitudes towards and knowledge of electroconvulsive therapy transcultural? A multi-national pilot study. *International Journal of Geriatric Psychiatry*, **23**, 497–503.

Freeman, C. P. & Kendell, R. E. (1980) ECT: 1. Patients' experiences and attitudes. *British Journal of Psychiatry*, **137**, 8–16.

Hughes, J., Barraclough, B. M. & Reeve, W. (1981) Are patients shocked by ECT? *Journal of the Royal Society of Medicine*, **74**, 283–285.

Johnstone, L. (1999) Adverse psychological effects of ECT. *Journal of Mental Health*, **8**, 69–85.

Kerr, R. A., McGrath, J. J., O'Kearney, A., *et al* (1982) ECT: misconceptions and attitudes. *Australian and New Zealand Journal of Psychiatry*, **16**, 43–49.

Kershaw, K., Rayner, L. & Chaplin, R. (2007) Patients' views on the quality of care when receiving electroconvulsive therapy. *Psychiatric Bulletin*, **31**, 414–417.

Koopowitz, L. F., Chur-Hansen, A., Reid, S., *et al* (2003) The subjective experience of patients who received electroconvulsive therapy. *Australian and New Zealand Journal of Psychiatry*, **37**, 49–54.

Lawrence, J. (2006) Voices from within: a study of ECT and patient perceptions. Available online at: http://www.ect.org/voices-from-within-a-study-of-ect-and-patient-perceptions/.

Mental Health Foundation (1997) *Knowing Our Own Minds*. Mental Health Foundation.

National Institute for Clinical Excellence (2003) *Guidance on the Use of Electroconvulsive Therapy* (Technology Appraisal TA59). NICE.

Pedler, M. (2000) Shock treatment: a survey of people's experience of electro-convulsive therapy (ECT). MIND.

Philpot, M., Collins, C., Trivedi, P., *et al* (2004) Eliciting users' views of ECT in two mental health trusts with a user-designed questionnaire. *Journal of Mental Health*, **13**, 403–413.

Rayner, L., Kershaw, K., Hanna, D., *et al* (2009) The patient perspective of the consent process and side effects of electroconvulsive therapy. *Journal of Mental Health*, **18**, 379–388.

Riordan, D. M., Barron, P. & Bowden, M. F. (1993) ECT: a patient-friendly procedure? *Psychiatric Bulletin*, **17**, 531–533.

Rogers, A. & Pilgrim, D. (1993) Service users' views of psychiatric treatments. *Sociology of Health and Illness*, **5**, 612–631.

Rose, D., Wykes, T., Morven, L., *et al* (2003) Patients' perspectives on electroconvulsive therapy: systematic review. *BMJ*, **326**, 1363–1365.

Rose, D., Fleischmann, P., Wykes, T. (2004) Consumers' views of electroconvulsive therapy: a qualitative analysis. *Journal of Mental Health*, **13**, 285–293.

Rush, G., McCarron, S. & Lucey, J. V. (2007) Patient attitudes to electroconvulsive therapy. *Psychiatric Bulletin*, **31**, 212–214.

Sienart, P., de Becker, T., Vansteelandt, K., *et al* (2005) Patient satisfaction after electroconvulsive therapy. *Journal of ECT*, **21**, 227–231.

Smith, M., Vogler, J., Zarrouf, F., *et al* (2009) Electroconvulsive therapy: the struggles in the decision-making process and the aftermath of treatment. *Issues in Mental Health Nursing*, **30**, 554–559.

Szuba, M. P., Baxter, L. R., Liston, E. H., *et al* (1991) Patients and family perspective of electroconvulsive therapy: correlation with outcome. *Convulsive Therapy*, **7**, 175–183.

UK ECT Review Group (2003) Efficacy and safety of electro-convulsive therapy in depressive disorder: a systematic review and meta-analysis. *Lancet*, **361**, 799–808.

Walter, G., Koster, K. & Rey, J. M. (1999) Views about treatment among parents of adolescents who received electroconvulsive therapy. *Psychiatric Services*, **50**, 701–702.

Wheeldon, T. J., Robertson, C., Eagles, J. M., *et al* (1999) The views and outcomes of consenting and non-consenting patients receiving ECT. *Psychological Medicine*, **29**, 221–223.

Out-patient declaration form

If you are receiving ECT as an out-patient your doctor will have explained the procedure to you to ensure that you meet the requirements needed so that you have safe and effective ECT treatments.

You and your carer will both need to sign the form below each time you attend for a treatment to confirm that you have read and understood the following information.

During ECT you will receive a general anaesthetic and therefore the following standard precautions apply.

You must:

- be in the company of a responsible adult for 24 hours following the treatment
- be accompanied home
- not leave the hospital if you are feeling unsteady or confused
- not operate machinery or appliances for 24 hours
- take DVLA advice on driving following an episode of mental illness (your psychiatrist should inform you of this)
- not be left in sole charge of young children until the following morning
- not sign any legal document or make important decisions for 24 hours
- not consume alcohol for 24 hours.

Once you have returned home if you begin to feel unwell please contact:

....

If you are unable to attend for an ECT treatment please contact:

....

I confirm that I have read and understood the following guidelines.

Signed
Patient: ....

Carer: ....

ECT competencies for doctors*

The trainee by year 3 ought to be able to administer ECT without direct supervision, prepare patients for ECT, and explain to patients and relatives about ECT, its indications and broad place within psychiatric treatment. Trainees ought to be able to monitor a patient's mental state and cognitive functioning during a course of ECT.

Consultants and trainees by the end of year 6 ought to have a good understanding of the place of ECT in modern clinical practice sufficient to obtain informed consent from patients to reach level 1 competency. Only consultants responsible for the ECT clinic or specialist trainees (ST4–6) with an interest in the administration of ECT would be expected to have level 1 competency in the practical aspects of the administration of ECT (sufficient to run an ECT clinic).

Name:..

1   Fully conversant (FC)
2   Working knowledge (WK)
3   Awareness (A)

Verbally assessed

1 FC   Is able to explain accurately all the important features to a standard that shows sufficient understanding that would allow them to competently and independently apply the knowledge.

2 WK   Is able to explain the key features to a standard that shows sufficient understanding that would allow them to apply the knowledge in common situations and access further information if necessary.

3 A   Is aware of the topic and knows where to get further information but not to a level that provides a WK.

*Available from: www.rcpsych.ac.uk/college/cecommitteestructure/specialcommitteesofcec/ectandrelatedtreatments/currentworkanddocuments.aspx.

Observed

1 FC Is able to carry out the procedure to a standard that shows sufficient skill and understanding that would allow them to competently and independently carry it out.

2 WK Is able to carry out the procedure to a standard that shows sufficient skill and understanding that would allow them to carry it out in usual situations but to know their limitations and access further help if necessary.

3 A Is aware of the topic and knows where to get further information but not to a level that provides a WK.

Required competencies

Foundation doctors

Theory and background	Awareness	1–6
Practical aspects of ECT	Not required	
Other aspects of ECT practice (a) and (b)	Not required	

ST1–3 and core trainees CT1–3

Theory and background	Working knowledge	1, 3–6
	Awareness	2
Practical aspects of ECT	Fully conversant	1–5, 7
	Working knowledge	6
Other aspects of ECT practice (a)	1–5 to be achieved	
Other aspects of ECT practice (b)	Not required	

ST4–6 and prescribing consultants

Theory and background	Fully conversant	1–6
Practical aspects of ECT	Working knowledge	1–7
Other aspects of ECT practice (a) and (b)	Not required	

ECT consultants

Theory and background	Fully conversant	1–6
Practical aspects of ECT	Fully conversant	1–7
Other aspects of ECT practice (a)	Not required	
Other aspects of ECT practice (b)	1–6 to be achieved	

1 Theory and background

Competency	How evidenced	Level	Date	Signature
1. *NICE guidance*: demonstrate a knowledge of NICE guidance relevant to ECT, including TA59[a] and other relevant guidance	Verbally			
2. *Royal College standards*: demonstrate an awareness of standards, including ECTAS and SEAN	Verbally			
3. *Local protocols*: demonstrate a knowledge of local policies and procedures, including: i. emergency ECT ii. out-patient ECT iii. high-risk patients iv. continuation ECT v. when ECT should be discontinued vi. choice of unilateral or bilateral treatment	Verbally			
4. *Consent process*: demonstrate a knowledge of the consent to treatment requirements, including common law and Mental Health Act and mental Capacity Act documentation/ requirements	Verbally			
5. *ECT process*: able to describe the: i. indications for ECT ii. contraindications to ECT iii. possible side-effects, risks and benefits of ECT iv. pre-treatment preparations required to be undertaken by referring doctor v. procedure for the administration of ECT	Verbally			
6. *Mechanisms of action*: knowledge of: i. current theories of mechanism ii. physiological effects of ECT	Verbally			

a. National Institute for Clinical Excellence (2003) *Guidance on the Use of Electroconvulsive Therapy* (Technology Appraisal TA59). NICE.

2 Practical aspects of ECT

Competency	How evidenced	Level	Date	Signature
1. *Clinic protocol* i. Understand clinic dosing protocol ii. Understand when to restimulate iii. Understand procedure for prolonged seizure	Verbally			
2. *Using the ECT machine* i. Attaching EEG leads ii. Apply electrodes bilateral iii. Apply electrodes unilateral iv. Impedance testing	Observed			
3. *Delivering the dose*: set correct stimulus	Observed			
4. *Monitoring* i. Observe motor seizure ii. Observe EEG monitoring iii. Understand how to interpret EEG	Observed			
5. *Recording*: correct recording of treatment in patient record	Observed			
6. Knowledge of anaesthetics and muscle relaxants used in ECT	Verbally			
7. Basic resuscitation training[a]	Written			
14. Immediate life support training	Written			

a. Fully conversant = training in last year; working knowledge = training in last 5 years.

3(a) Other aspects of ECT practice[a]

Competency	How evidenced	Level	Date	Signature
1. Attended induction to ECT				
2. Observed clinical application of ECT	Observed			
3. Supervised clinical application 1	Observed			
4. Supervised clinical application 2	Observed			
5. Supervised clinical application 3	Observed			
6. Supervised clinical application 4	Observed			
7. Supervised clinical application 5	Observed			
8. Supervised clinical application 6	Observed			
9. Additional clinical application 1	Observed			
10. Additional clinical application 2	Observed			
11. Additional clinical application 3	Observed			
12. Additional clinical application 4	Observed			

a. Trainees are required to be signed off for attending an induction (1), observing another person administer ECT (2), and then being supervised in administering ECT themselves (3–8).

234

3(b) Other aspects of ECT practice

Competency	How evidenced	Level	Date	Signature
1. Participation in audit of ECT	Audit reports			
2. Participation in 1 day of continued professional development relating to ECT each year	Continued professional development returns			
3. Able to advise consultant colleagues on: i. relative merits of bilateral/unilateral treatment ii. suitability of patient for ECT iii. drug treatments during ECT iv. management of side-effects during ECT	Practice			
4. Involved in regular review of policies and procedures in ECT clinic	Practice			
6. Evidence of training and supervising doctors in training in ECT practice	Practice			

Example of a job description for an ECT nurse specialist

Title: Sister/Charge Nurse – ECT clinic
Grade: Band 6/7
Hours: Full-time, 37.5 h per week – flexible to meet needs
Reports to: Modern Matron
Responsible to: Senior Manager, In-patient and Community Services

Minimum qualification: Registered Mental Nurse

Job summary

The post-holder will act as the clinical and functional lead in the ECT clinic, taking responsibility for the day-to-day operation of the clinic. This will include working in partnership with all disciplines involved with ECT across the Trust.

Specific responsibilities

The post-holder will be responsible for the operational management, development and delivery of the above services, ensuring that they meet accepted quality and safety standards, in accordance with national and local guidelines. The post-holder will be required to lead, teach, supervise and support junior colleagues. The post-holder will offer clinical advice to professional colleagues in the services, and take a lead role in evaluation and research activities.

1. Clinical

1.1 To have a thorough understanding of the current national and local operational policies, procedures and guidelines relating to the above services.

1.2 To take the clinical lead in the organisation, operation and delivery of the ECT clinic, in conjunction with medical, nursing and other professional staff involved.

1.3 To ensure that patients attending for ECT treatment (and their relatives/carers where appropriate), receive information relevant to their needs.

1.4 To practice in a manner consistent with the principles and standards of the services, ensuring that national and local policies and guidelines are observed, inclusive of NICE, ECTAS, SEAN, the Nursing and Midwifery Council, Royal College of Nursing, Care Quality Commission, and Quality Improvement Scotland.

1.5 To ensure that the patient is fully informed about the rationale for their treatment, and is involved in the implementation and evaluation of their treatment.

1.6 To provide effective evidence-based interventions.

1.7 To work collaboratively with all disciplines and agencies involved in the ECT service, acting as a resource for staff, patients, carers and relatives in relation to these services.

1.8 To supervise, advise, guide and provide specialist training in ECT recovery, for junior staff as required.

1.9 To actively liaise with user/carer representation groups to enhance the quality and standard of the services.

1.10 To act in accordance with agreed practice placement standards for learner nurses undertaking observational placements with the services, cooperate with the practice placement manager in the evaluation of the learner experience.

1.11 To ensure patients receive accurate, up-to-date information on the following:
  i   their treatment
  ii their mental illness
  iii what they can expect from the service
  iv how they can access user representation.

1.12 Undertake the role of treatment nurse and deputise for the recovery nurse as required, within the ECT department.

2. Management

2.1 To manage the departmental financial budget to accommodate physical and environmental maintenance, repair and replacement cost.

2.2 To deliver cost-effective services, making efficient use of allocated resources.

2.3 To ensure that the ECT service meets the legal obligations appertaining to the detention and treatment of patients under the Mental Health Act 1983 (amended 2007).

2.4 To have an in-depth understanding of the legal issues relating to consent to ECT and the Mental Health Act (including 2007 amendments and Code of Practice).

2.5 To take a lead role in regular reviews of the services, including reviews of the relevant policies, participating in such reviews in the capacity of functional manager.

2.6 To efficiently use staffing resources in the treatment areas, ensuring that staffing levels are safe, appropriate and contain the necessary skill mix on each shift.

2.7 To ensure that appropriate equipment and supplies are available to enable the smooth running of the services.

2.8 To participate in service planning and development.

2.9 To participate in working groups as required.

2.10 To assist in the recruitment and induction of staff as required.

2.11 To participate in appraisal.

2.12 To supervise, guide and advise other nursing staff and disciplines as required.

2.13 To encompass all aspects of managing care, including infection control.

2.14 To ensure that national and local policies and guidelines are adhered to.

2.15 To keep central records of clinics, patient attendance figures and other statistical information, and to produce activity and outcome reports as required.

2.16 To report and participate in the investigation of accidents, complaints and untoward incidents in accordance with Trust policy.

3. Quality

3.1 To participate in service governance initiatives, including audit, evaluation and reviews of the services.

3.2 To ensure that Patients' Charter Standards, Local Service Standards, Purchaser Quality Standards, and Trust Quality Standards are met.

3.3 To ensure that all relevant equipment is regularly serviced and maintained, confirming that servicing contracts are updated and maintained.

3.4 To ensure that clinical areas are maintained to the required standards, liaising with relevant facilities managers as necessary.

4. Professional development

4.1 To act as clinical supervisor and mentor for learner nurses and junior staff as required.

4.2 To participate in the training and education of junior medical staff, in conjunction with the lead ECT consultant.

4.3 To give presentations/talks about the ECT service.

4.4 To maintain and update a professional portfolio.

4.5 To attend statutory and any other relevant training in line with directorate policy.

4.6 To receive regular line management supervision.

4.7 To work without direct supervision in clinical practice.

4.8 To maintain an up-to-date knowledge of current trends, practices and research in mental nursing, in particular those issues relating to the above services.

4.9 To assist in research and development.

4.10 To participate in clinical governance initiatives as required.

4.11 To seek peer group supervision from national and regional ECT special interest groups.

5. Health and safety

All employees have a duty to take reasonable care to avoid injury to themselves and to others and to cooperate with the Trust in meeting statutory responsibility for care of the unconscious patient, post anaesthesia.

6. Confidentiality

All information relating to patients and staff gained through your employment with .... Mental Health Trust is confidential. Disclosures to any unauthorised person may be a disciplinary offence.

7. Other

7.1 To undertake any other general requirements as directed by the Modern Matron/Senior Manager – In-patient and Community Services.

7.2 This job description will be subject to periodic review and amendment in accordance with the needs of the Trust.

Signed: .... Head of Department

Signed: .... Director of Personnel

Date: ....

Personal specification

Job Title: Sister/Charge Nurse – ECT clinic, Band 6/7

Area: ....…....................Mental Health Services

Signed: .... Date: ....

Professional qualifications

Essential: Registered Mental Nurse. Evidence of post-qualification professional training (or equivalent experience) relevant to the delivery of ECT service.

Desirable: Professional degree. Registered General Nurse. D32/33 or ENB998. Clinical supervision training. Further qualifications relevant to severe mental illness.

Knowledge

Essential: In-depth understanding of the principles and practice of ECT, including legal issues relating to the Mental Health Act. Knowledge of the problems and disadvantages associated with these treatment options.
Desirable: Sound knowledge of the issues involved in the treatment of all mental illness and key features of relapse prevention.

Job training/experience

Essential: Two years' post-registration, part of which must be at Band 5, with some experience of working with people with severe mental illness.
Desirable: Extensive experience of working within an ECT treatment clinic. IT literacy. Psychosocial interventions.

Personal qualities

Essential: Team worker. Organisational skills. Determination. Flexibility. Good communication skills. Positive attitude to change.

Interests/motivation

Essential: Strong team player. Self-motivated. Able to use initiative. Committed to developing and improving mental health services.
Desirable: Evidence of a commitment to user involvement.

Sources

Association of Anaesthetists of Great Britain and Ireland (2005) *The Anaesthesia Team: Revised Edition 2005*. AAGBI.

Cresswell, J., Murphy, G. & Hodge, S. (2012) *The ECT Accreditation Service (ECTAS): Standards for the Administration of ECT* (10th edn). Royal College of Psychiatrists' Centre for Quality Improvement.

ECT Clinic, Murray Royal Hospital, Tayside, UK.

Finch, S. (2009) ECT nurse competencies. National Association of Lead Nurses in ECT. Available at: http://www.nalnect.org.uk/ect-nurse-competencies/.

Scottish ECT Accreditation Network (2010) *SEAN Standards, Version V1.0*. SEAN.

Example of a job description for an ECT nurse/ECT coordinator

Scope and range

Sole nursing responsibility for management/supervision of all nursing staff involved in the ECT process, within the department (1 × Band 7, 1 × Band 6, 2 × Band 5). Participate in the ECT Induction training programme for senior house officers, new trained and untrained members of nursing staff and learner nurses. Act as a source of advice/support for medical and nursing staff, patients and relatives. Responsible for coordinating training/ updates for 2 anaesthetic nurses and 3 recovery nurses (Bands 5–7).

Practice population and boundaries – all in- and out-patients within [name of area] aged 16 years and above (Old Age, Adult & Forensic Psychiatry).

Main duties/responsibilities

Engaging in management supervision with line manager and participating in appraisal and a personal development framework as per Trust policy.

- Provide guidance, support and expertise relating to patient care in the psychological and physical preparation for ECT.
- Offer full knowledge and understanding of informed consent and its application to individual patient circumstances/needs.
- Have knowledge of Mental Health Act legislation in relation to ECT, as well as the wider context.
- Ensure effective communication between all disciplines involved in ECT delivery and good customer and public relations within the hospital, the Trust and the community.
- Provide anaesthetic support, practice and knowledge, including:
  - suitable preparation of the environment
  - pre-treatment clinical assessment and workup
  - anaesthetic circuits and other equipment available within the treatment area
  - all related pharmacology, including induction agents, depolarising muscle relaxants and emergency drugs

- identification of a normal ECG and recognition of arrhythmias and their treatment
- identification of the importance of baseline recordings and how anaesthetic agents affect them
- oxygenation needs pre-, during and post-treatment
- care of and protection of the unconscious patient
- identification of monitoring needs and the operation of equipment/ procedures related to this function
- post-anaesthetic care, complete recovery criteria and the principles involved
- basic and advanced life support skills.
- Ensure the smooth implementation of all organisational/operational issues related to this professional service.
- Have full knowledge in contraindications, indications and adverse effects of ECT and be able to effectively communicate this information.
- Assess/evaluate immediate and longer-term response to ECT.
- Develop internal audit mechanisms in liaison with other disciplines.
- Actively participate in research/further study for the improvement of care and ECT delivery, as well as support of other staff involved.
- Provide an annual report for service managers to include statistical details, developmental achievements and future aims of the service.
- Provide ongoing enhancement of training/induction programmes for all staff (e.g. learner nurses, nurses and medical staff).
- Ensure policy development, implementation and systematic review.
- Implement and support clinical development plans for nursing staff within the department.
- Liaise with clinical nurse manager in the identification of staffing requirements and agree appropriate actioning.
- Ensure annual leave is balanced and allocate appropriately and efficiently.
- Adhere to policies and procedures for reporting accidents and incidents and ensure matters are fully discussed with appropriate staff.
- Establish and maintain an effective and facultative communication system, which will maximise the dissemination of information.
- Advise, support and assist with organising ECT to be carried out in the local general hospital.
- Carry out administrative work – statistical data collection (local and national), reviewing protocols, typing, etc. (No dedicated administrative support.)

Communications and relationships

- Communicate and liaise with other professionals (ward staff, consultants, anaesthetists, other colleagues in local general hospital) to ensure a smooth throughput of care.

- Communicate, liaise, educate and support patients and relatives pre-, during and post-treatment, which can include highly sensitive and contentious information/treatment.
- Liaise with clinical governance for audit/report issues.
- Act as source of advice for clinical governance regarding issues concerned with ECT.
- Submit an annual report and attend the clinical governance director's meetings to discuss relevant issues.
- Regularly attend conferences.
- Regularly participate in the North of Scotland ECT Nurses Forum.
- Liaise with other ECT nurses within [name of area].
- Develop a good professional relationship with all members of the multidisciplinary team to ensure safe, effective and efficient provision of service.

Knowledge, training and experience required

- Registered Mental Nurse with minimum of 4 years' post-registration experience.
- Ability to work autonomously and as part of a team.
- Ability to work well under pressure.
- Good communication and interpersonal skills.
- Good IT skills.
- Keep up to date with mandatory and essential training and regular updates to comply with national standards (basic life support, immediate life support, anaesthetic, and recovery and ECT).
- Ability to forward plan.
- Ability to work within the professional governing bodies' code of conduct (Nursing and Midwifery Council).

Systems and equipment

- Using and maintenance[1] of mechanical hoists.
- Using and maintenance of glide sheets.
- Using and maintenance of variable and non-variable height trolleys.
- Maintenance of anaesthetic machine.
- Using and maintenance of monitoring equipment.
- Using and maintenance of ECT machine; involved in interpreting EEG tracings.
- Using and maintenance of portable ECT machine.
- Using and maintenance of tourniquet machine.
- Using and maintenance of automated external defibrillator/manual defibrillator.

---

1. Safety checks, reporting any faults, restocking/replacing additional/disposable equipment, ensuring regular maintenance programme carried out from medical physics, etc.

- Downloading patient data into national database.
- Recording patient information into ECT records.

Physical/mental/emotional demands of the job

Physical skills

- Preparing patient for anaesthesia.
- Assisting the anaesthetist.
- Preparing patient for ECT.
- Assisting the psychiatrist.
- Assessing the patient until fully recovered from the anaesthetic.
- Competent airway management.
- Competent basic life support skills.
- Competent immediate life support skills.
- Competent defibrillation: automated external defibrillator/manual skills.
- Patient and load manual handling skills.
- Regular use of IT skills.
- Patient movement with use of manual handling aids.
- Movement of trolleys.
- Movement of equipment.
- Ensuring ECT is given legally.
- Observant for change in patient's conscious level.
- Observant for early warning signs.
- Developing/updating protocols.
- Dealing with the most severe mentally and physically ill patients.

Working conditions

- Autonomous worker majority of the time.
- Exposure to body fluids (e.g. blood, urine, faeces).
- Manual handling of unconscious patients.
- Exposure to an explosive atmosphere (8–10 oxygen cylinders in department).
- Lengthy spells of exposure to computer.

Sources

Association of Anaesthetists of Great Britain and Ireland (2005) *The Anaesthesia Team: Revised Edition 2005*. AAGBI.

Cresswell, J., Murphy, G. & Hodge, S. (2012) *The ECT Accreditation Service (ECTAS): Standards for the Administration of ECT* (10th edn). Royal College of Psychiatrists' Centre for Quality Improvement.

ECT Clinic, Murray Royal Hospital, Tayside, UK.

Finch, S. (2009) ECT nurse competencies. National Association of Lead Nurses in ECT. Available at: http://www.nalnect.org.uk/ect-nurse-competencies/.

Scottish ECT Accreditation Network (2010) *SEAN Standards, Version V1.0*. SEAN.

Information for patients and carers*

This leaflet is for anyone who wants to know more about electroconvulsive therapy (ECT). It discusses how it works, why it is used, its effects and side-effects, and alternative treatments.

Electroconvulsive therapy remains a controversial treatment and some of the conflicting views about it are described. If your questions are not answered in this leaflet, there are some sources of further information at the end of the leaflet.

Where there are areas of uncertainty, we have listed other sources of information that you can use. Important concerns are the effectiveness and side-effects of ECT and how it compares with other treatments. At the time of writing, these references are available free and in full on the internet.

What is ECT?

Electroconvulsive therapy is a treatment for a small number of severe mental illnesses. It was originally developed in the 1930s and was used widely during the 1950s and 1960s for a variety of conditions. It is now clear that ECT should only be used in a smaller number of more serious conditions.

Electroconvulsive therapy consists of passing an electrical current through the brain to produce an epileptic fit – hence the name, electroconvulsive. On the face of it, this sounds bizarre. Why should anyone ever have thought that this was a sensible way to treat a mental disorder? The idea developed from the observation that, in the days before there was any kind of effective medication, some people with depression or schizophrenia, and who also had epilepsy, seemed to feel better after having a fit. Research suggests that the effect is due to the fit rather than the electrical current.

---

*This leaflet was produced by the Royal College of Psychiatrists' Public Education Editorial Board and can be found at: www.rcpsych.ac.uk/mentalhealthinfoforall/treatments/ect.aspx.

How often is it used?

It is now used less often. Between 1985 and 2002 its use in England more than halved, possibly because of better psychological and drug treatments for depression.

How does ECT work?

No one is certain how ECT works, and there are a number of theories.

It can change patterns of blood flow through the brain, it can change the metabolism of areas of the brain which may be affected by depression.

Many doctors believe that severe depression is caused by problems with certain brain chemicals. It is thought that ECT causes the release of these chemicals and, probably more importantly, makes the chemicals more likely to work and so help recovery.

Recent research has suggested that ECT can stimulate the growth of new cells and nerve pathways in certain areas of the brain.

Does ECT really work?

It has been suggested that ECT works not because of the fit, but because of all the other things – like the extra attention and support and the anaesthetic – that happen to someone having it.

Several studies have compared standard ECT with 'sham' or placebo ECT. In placebo ECT, the patient has exactly the same things done to them – including going to the ECT rooms and having the anaesthetic and muscle relaxant – but no electrical current is passed and there is no fit. In these studies, those patients who had standard ECT were much more likely to recover, and did so more quickly than those who had the placebo treatment. Those who didn't have adequate fits did less well than those who did.

Interestingly, a number of the patients having sham treatment recovered too, even though they were very unwell; it's clear that the extra support does have a benefit as might be expected. However, ECT has been shown to have an extra effect in severe depression – it seems, in the short term, to be more helpful than medication.

Pros and cons of ECT

Who is ECT likely to help?

The National Institute for Health and Clinical Excellence (NICE) have looked in detail at the use of ECT and have said that it should be used only in depression, resistant mania or catatonia.

They say ECT should be considered for acute treatment of severe depression that is life-threatening and when a rapid response is required, or when other treatments have failed.

It should not be used routinely in moderate depression, but should be considered for people with moderate depression if their depression has not responded to multiple drug treatments and psychological treatment.

Who is ECT unlikely to help?

Electroconvulsive therapy is unlikely to help those with mild to moderate depression or most other psychiatric conditions. It has no role in the general treatment of schizophrenia.

Why is it given when there are other treatments available?

Electroconvulsive therapy has been shown to be the most effective treatment for severe depression. It would normally be offered if:

- several different medications have been tried but have not helped
- the side-effects of antidepressants are too severe
- you have found ECT helpful in the past
- your life is in danger because you are not eating or drinking enough
- you are seriously considering suicide.

What are the side-effects of ECT?

Electroconvulsive therapy is a major procedure involving, over a few weeks, several epileptic seizures and several anaesthetics. It is used for people with severe illness who are very unwell and whose life may be in danger. As with any treatment, ECT can cause a number of side-effects. Some of these are mild and some are more severe.

Short-term

Many people complain of a headache immediately after ECT and of aching in their muscles. They may feel muzzy-headed and generally out of sorts, or even a bit sick. Some become distressed after the treatment and may be tearful or frightened during recovery. For most people, however, these effects settle within a few hours, particularly with help and support from nursing staff, simple pain killers and some light refreshment.

There may be some temporary loss of memory for the time immediately before and after the ECT.

Older people may be quite confused for 2 or 3 h after a treatment. This can be reduced by changing the way the ECT is given (such as passing the current over only one side of the brain rather than across the whole brain).

There is a small physical risk from having a general anaesthetic – death or serious injury occurs in about 1 in 80 000 treatments, around the same level of risk in dental anaesthesia. However, as ECT is given in a course of treatments the risk per course of treatment will be around 1 in 10 000 courses.

Long-term

The greatest concern is that of the long-term side-effects, particularly memory problems. Surveys conducted by doctors and clinical staff usually find a low level of severe side-effects, maybe around 1 in 10. User-led surveys have found much more, maybe in half of those having ECT. Some surveys conducted by those strongly against ECT say there are severe side-effects in everyone.

Some difficulties with memory are probably present in everyone receiving ECT. Most people find these memories return when the course of ECT has finished and a few weeks have passed. However, some people do complain that their memory has been permanently affected, that their memories never come back. It is not clear how much of this is due to the ECT and how much is due to the depressive illness or other factors.

Some people have complained of more distressing experiences, such as feeling that their personalities have changed, that they have lost skills or that they are no longer the person they were before ECT. They say that they have never got over the experience and feel permanently harmed.

What seems to be generally agreed is that the more ECT someone is given, the more it is likely to affect their memory.

What if ECT is not given?

- You may take longer to recover.
- If you are very depressed and are not eating or drinking enough, you may become physically ill or die.
- There is an increased risk of suicide if your depression is severe and has not been helped by other treatments.

What are the alternatives?

If someone with severe depression declines ECT, there are a number of possibilities. The medication may be changed, new medication added or intensive psychotherapy offered, although this should already have been tried. Given time, some episodes of severe depression will get better on their own, although being severely depressed carries a significant risk of suicide.

Deciding to have (or not to have) ECT

Giving consent to having ECT

Like any significant treatments in medicine or surgery, you will be asked to give consent or permission for the ECT to be done.

The ECT treatment, the reasons for doing it and the possible benefits and side-effects should be explained in a way that you can understand. If you decide to go ahead, you then sign a consent form. It is a record that ECT has been explained to you, that you understand what is going to happen, and that you give your consent to it. However, you can withdraw your consent at any point, even before the first treatment.

What if I really don't want ECT?

If you have very strong feelings about ECT, you should make them known to the doctors and nurses caring for you, but also friends, family or an advocate who can speak for you.

Doctors must consider these views when they think about what to do.

If you have made it very clear that you do not wish to have ECT then you should not receive it. You could write an 'advance decision to refuse ECT' to make clear how you want to be treated if you become unwell again. Alternatively, you could appoint someone to be your Health and Welfare Attorney to make decisions on your behalf when you are not able to decide for yourself.

Can ECT be given to me without my permission?

Most ECT treatments are given to people who have agreed to it. This means that they have had:

- a full discussion of what ECT involves
- why it is being considered in their case
- the advantages and disadvantages
- a discussion of side-effects.

You cannot be given ECT against your wishes, even if you are detained under the Mental Health Act 1983, if you have the capacity to make a decision on this treatment.

It is the responsibility of the doctors and nurses involved to make sure that this discussion has been had – and to document it.

Sometimes, however, people become so unwell that they are unable to take on board all of the issues – perhaps because they are severely withdrawn or have ideas about themselves that stop them fully understanding their position (e.g. they believe their illness is a punishment they deserve).

In these circumstances, it may be impossible for them to give proper agreement or consent. When this happens, it is still possible to give ECT. The legal provisions for this differ from country to country, even within the UK.

In England and Wales, ECT can be given under the Mental Health Act, which requires the agreement of two doctors and another professional who is usually a social worker. There must then be a second opinion from an independent specialist who is not directly involved in the patient's care. The clinical team should also speak to family and other carers, to consider their views and any views the patient may have expressed before.

Sometimes – if a person doesn't have the capacity to give an informed consent – the team may decide the ECT can be given under the Mental

249

Capacity Act 2005. This is unusual, as in most cases the Mental Health Act provides the most appropriate protection for a patient's rights. The Mental Capacity Act can only be used if the patient lacks capacity and a 'decision maker' (usually the consultant in charge of their care) decides that ECT is in the patient's 'best interests'. It is expected that the decision maker will consult with other people to try to find out what the person's views would have been. This would usually include family members and other people close to them. The decision maker should also make 'all reasonable attempts' to help the patient to regain capacity to consent (if this is possible). An independent specialist is not needed, although the clinical team may request a second opinion from another consultant.

Whether ECT is given under the Mental Health Act or the Mental Capacity Act, regular assessments of the patient's ability to understand their treatment must be made. Once they are able to give consent, the treatment can only continue if they do consent and must stop if they refuse.

In Scotland, the principles above are the same, although the laws involved are the Mental Health (Care and Treatment) (Scotland) Act 2003 and the Adults with Incapacity Act (Scotland) 2000.

How is ECT given?

Electroconvulsive therapy is generally used to treat severe illnesses, so the person having it will often be in hospital. If you do not need to be an in-patient it should be possible for you to attend as a day patient to have ECT. You may need to check whether this is available to you from your local service.

The seizure is produced by passing an electrical current across the person's brain in a carefully controlled way from an ECT machine.

An anaesthetic and muscle relaxant are given so that:

- the patient is not conscious when the ECT is given;
- the muscle spasms that would normally be part of a fit – and which could produce serious injuries – are reduced to small, rhythmic movements in the arms, legs and body.

By adjusting the dose of electricity, the ECT team will try to produce a seizure lasting between 20 and 50 s.

Is there any preparation?

In the days before a course of ECT is started, your doctor will arrange for you to have some tests to make sure it is safe for you to have a general anaesthetic. These may include:

- a chest X-ray
- a tracing of your heart working (ECG)
- blood tests.

You will be asked not to have anything to eat or drink for 6 h before the ECT. This is so that that the anaesthetic can be given safely.

Where is ECT done?

Electroconvulsive therapy should always be done in a special set of rooms that are not used for any other purpose, usually called the 'ECT suite'. There should be separate rooms for people to wait, have their treatment, wake up fully from the anaesthetic and then recover properly before leaving.

There should be enough qualified staff to look after the person all the time they are there so that any confusion or distress can be helped.

What happens during ECT?

- You should arrive at the ECT suite with an experienced nurse who you know and who is able to explain what is happening. Many ECT suites are happy for family members to be there, so you may wish to check with your local team that this is possible, if it is reassuring for you. You should be met by a member of the ECT staff who will do routine physical checks if they have not already been done. The staff member will check that you are still willing to have ECT and if you have any further questions.
- When you are ready you will be accompanied into the treatment area and be helped onto a trolley.
- The ECT team will connect monitoring equipment to check your heart rate, blood pressure, oxygen levels, ECG and EEG during the fit.
- A needle will then be put into your hand, through which the anaesthetist will give the anaesthetic drug and, once you are asleep, a muscle relaxant. While you are going off to sleep, the anaesthetist will also give you oxygen to breathe.
- Once you are asleep and fully relaxed, a doctor will give the ECT treatment; your fit will last between 20 and 50 s. The muscle relaxant wears off quickly (within a couple of minutes) and, as soon as the anaesthetist is happy that you are waking up, you will be taken through to the recovery area where an experienced nurse will monitor you until you are fully awake.
- When you wake up, you will be in the recovery room with a nurse. He or she will take your blood pressure and ask you simple questions to check on how awake you are. There will be a small monitor on your finger to measure the oxygen in your blood and you may wake up with an oxygen mask. You will probably take a while to wake up and may not know quite where you are at first. You may feel a bit sick. After half an hour or so, these effects should have worn off.
- Most ECT units have a second area for light refreshments. You will be free to leave the suite when the staff are happy that your physical state is stable and you feel ready to do so.
- The whole process usually takes about half an hour.

What are bilateral and unilateral ECT?

In bilateral ECT, the electrical current is passed across the whole brain; in unilateral ECT, it is just passed across one side. Both of them cause a seizure in the whole of the brain.

Bilateral ECT seems to work more quickly and effectively and it's probably the most widely used in Britain; however, there has been concern that it may cause more side-effects.

Unilateral ECT is now used less. It had been thought to cause less memory loss, but recent research has shown that it is necessary to use much larger doses of electricity to make unilateral ECT as effective as bilateral ECT. If the dose of electricity is increased to make it equally effective, the risks of memory loss are as great as with bilateral ECT.

Sometimes ECT clinics will start a course of treatment with bilateral ECT and switch to unilateral if the patient experiences side-effects. Alternatively, they may start with unilateral and switch to bilateral if the person isn't getting better.

You may wish to speak to the doctor who is suggesting ECT for you to decide whether unilateral or bilateral ECT is best for you.

How often and how many times is ECT given?

Most units give ECT twice per week, often on a Monday and Thursday, or Tuesday and Friday. It is impossible to predict how many treatments someone will need. However, in general, it will take 2 or 3 treatments before you see any difference, and 4–5 treatments for noticeable improvement.

A course will, on average, be 6–8 treatments, although as many as 12 may be needed, particularly if you have been depressed for a long time. If after 12 treatments you feel no better, it is unlikely that ECT is going to help and the course would usually stop. A member of the mental health team should see you after each treatment, to see how you are responding to treatment and check that you are not experiencing any serious side-effects. Your consultant should see you after every two treatments. Electroconvulsive therapy should be stopped as soon as you have made a recovery or if you say you don't want to have it any more.

What happens after a course of ECT?

Even when someone finds it effective, ECT is only a part of recovering from depression. Like antidepressants, it can help to ease problems so you are able to look at why you became unwell. Hopefully you can then take steps to continue your recovery and perhaps find ways to make sure the situation doesn't happen again. Psychotherapy and counselling can help and many sufferers find their own ways to help themselves. Certainly people who have ECT, and then do not have other forms of help, are likely to quickly become unwell again.

The ECT controversy

There are many areas in which people disagree over ECT, including whether it should even be done at all. People tend to have very strong feelings about ECT, often based on their own experiences. The main areas of disagreement are over whether it works, how it works and what the side-effects are.

Why is ECT still being given?

Electroconvulsive therapy is now used much less and is mostly a treatment for severe depression. This is almost certainly because modern treatments for depression such as psychotherapy (talking treatments), antidepressants and other psychological and social supports are much more effective than they were in the past.

Even so, depression can for some people still be very severe and life-threatening, with extreme withdrawal and reluctance, or inability to eat, drink or communicate properly. Occasionally, people may also develop strange ideas (delusions) about themselves or others. If other treatments have not have worked, it may be worth considering ECT.

What do patients think of ECT?

In 2003 researchers analysed all the work carried out on patients' experiences of ECT. They found that the proportion of people who had had ECT and found it helpful ranged from 30% to 80%. The researchers commented that studies reporting lower satisfaction tended to have been conducted by patients and those reporting higher satisfaction were carried out by doctors. Between 30% and 50% of patients complained of difficulties with memory after ECT.

What do those in favour of ECT say?

Many doctors and nurses will say that they have seen ECT relieve very severe depressive illnesses when other treatments have failed. Bearing in mind that 15% of people with severe depression will kill themselves, they feel that ECT has saved patients' lives, and therefore the overall benefits are greater than the risks. Some people who have had ECT will agree and may ask for it if they find themselves becoming depressed again.

What do those against ECT say?

There are many different views and many different reasons why people object to ECT. Some say that ECT is an inhumane and degrading treatment, which belongs to the past. They say that the side-effects are severe and that psychiatrists have either accidentally or deliberately ignored how severe they can be. They say that ECT permanently damages both the brain and the mind, and if it does work at all, does so in a way that is ultimately harmful for the patient. Many would want to see it banned.

What happens in other countries?

At the moment, ECT is part of standard psychiatric practice in Britain and the majority of countries worldwide. Some countries (and some states in America also) have restricted its use more than in the UK, although only a small number have prohibited its use.

How do I know if ECT is done properly locally?

The Royal College of Psychiatrists has set up the ECT Accreditation Service (ECTAS) to provide an independent assessment of the quality of ECT services. The ECT Accreditation Service sets very high standards for ECT, and visits all the ECT units that have registered with it. The visiting team involves psychiatrists, anaesthetists and nurses. It publishes the results of its findings and also provides a forum for sharing best clinical practice. Membership of ECTAS is not compulsory but every ECT unit should be able to tell you:

- if they have signed up to ECTAS;
- the result of their most recent report;
- who to speak to if you are concerned that your local unit has not been assessed.

A list of accredited sites is available on the Royal College of Psychiatrists' website.

Where can I get more information?

Many ECT suites provide their own information packs and they should be able to give written information to patients or their family/carers before a course starts. The information in these packs is often strongly in favour of ECT.

The internet has many websites discussing ECT that are produced by professionals, organisations, people who have had ECT, or others with particular opinions. There are more negative than positive websites.

Further information

National Institute for Health and Clinical Excellence (NICE)

- *Guidance on the Use of Electroconvulsive Therapy* (Technology Appraisal TA59).
- *Depression: The Treatment and Management of Depression in Adults (Update)* (Clinical Guideline CG90).

Scottish ECT Accreditation Network (SEAN)

A website designed to complement the work of SEAN, by enabling communication of the latest information on ECT in Scotland.

ECT Accreditation Services (ECTAS)

Launched in May 2003, ECTAS aims to assure and improve the quality of the administration of ECT; it awards an accreditation rating to clinics that meet the essential standard.

Sources

Department of Health (2007) *Electro Convulsive Therapy: Survey Covering the Period from January 2002 to March 2002, England*. Department of Health.

Ebmeier, K., Donaghey, C. & Steele, J. D. (2006) Recent development and current controversies in depression. *Lancet*, **367**, 153–167.

Eranti, S. V. & McLoughlin, D. M. (2003) Electroconvulsive therapy – state of the art. *British Journal of Psychiatry*, **182**, 8–9.

Rose, D., Fleischmann, P., Wykes, T., *et al* (2003) Patients' perspectives on electroconvulsive therapy: systematic review. *BMJ*, **326**, 1363–1368.

Scott, A. I. F. (ed.) (2005) *The ECT Handbook: The Third Report of the Royal College of Psychiatrists' Special Committee on ECT* (2nd edn) (Council Report CR128), pp. 9–24. Royal College of Psychiatrists.

UK ECT Review Group (2003) Efficacy and safety of electroconvulsive therapy in depressive disorders: a systematic review and meta-analysis. *Lancet*, **361**, 799–808.

Example of a consent form

Patient agreement to investigation or treatment

Patient's details (or pre-printed label)

Patient's surname/family name: ....

Patient's first names: ....

Date of birth: ....

Responsible health professional: ....

Job title: ....

NHS number (or other identifier): ....

Male ☐   Female ☐

Special requirements: ....
(e.g. other language/communication methods)

To be retained in patient's notes

Name of proposed procedure or course of treatment

Electroconvulsive therapy: Unilateral ☐   Bilateral ☐   Either ☐
(Please tick laterality)

Statement of health professional

(To be filled in by health professional with appropriate knowledge of proposed procedure, as specified in consent policy)

I have explained the procedure to the patient. In particular, I have explained:

☐ The intended benefits and the use of bilateral or unilateral treatment

☐ Serious or frequently occurring risks

☐ What the procedure involves, the benefits and likely risks of any alternative treatments (including no treatment) and discussed any particular concerns of this patient

☐ Which medication to take and not to take on the morning of ECT

I have also explained any procedures which may become necessary during the procedure

☐ No   ☐ Yes (Please specify below)

....

This procedure will involve:

General anaesthesia ☐   Local anaesthesia ☐   Sedation ☐

The following information has been provided:

Understanding Electroconvulsive Thearapy (ECT): An Information Guide ☐

General Advice for the Care of People Who Have Received ECT ☐

Other forms of information: ....

Signed: .... Job title: ....
Name (print): ....
Contact details: ....

Statement of interpreter (where appropriate)

I have interpreted the information above to the patient to the best of my ability and in a way in which I believe they can understand.

Signed: .... Name (print): ....
Date: ....

Top copy accepted by patient: Yes ☐   No ☐

Statement of patient

Please read this form carefully. If your treatment has been planned in advance, you should already have your own copy of page 2 which describes the benefits and risks of the proposed treatment. If not, you will be offered a copy now. If you have any further questions, do ask – we are here to help you. You have the right to change your mind at any time, including after you have signed this form.

I agree to the procedure or course of treatment described on this form.

I understand that you cannot give me a guarantee that a particular person will perform the procedure. The person will, however, have appropriate experience.

I understand that I will have the opportunity to discuss the details of anaesthesia with an anaesthetist before the procedure, unless the urgency of my situation prevents this. (This only applies to patients having general or regional anaesthesia.)

I understand that any procedure in addition to those described on this form will only be carried out if it is necessary to save my life or to prevent serious harm to my health.

I have been told about additional procedures which may become necessary during my treatment. I have listed below any procedures **which I do not wish to be carried out** without further discussion.

....

Patient's consent

Total number of treatments consented to:

Patient's signature: .... Date: ....

Name (print): ....

A witness should sign below if the patient is unable to sign but has indicated his or her consent. Young people/children may also like a parent to sign here (see notes).

Signed: .... Date: ....

Name (print): ....

Confirmation of consent

(To be completed by a health professional when the patient is admitted for the procedure, if the patient has signed the form in advance)

On behalf of the team treating the patient, I have confirmed with the patient that they have no further questions and wish the procedure to go ahead.

Signed: .... Job title: ....

Name: .... Date: ....

Important notes (tick if applicable)

☐   See also advance directive/living will (e.g. Jehovah's Witness form)

Patient has withdrawn consent ☐

Patient signature: ....

Date: ....

Useful contacts

Professional organisations

Committee of Nurses at ECT in Scotland
(CONECTS)
Email: linda.cullen2@nhs.net

ECT Accreditation Service (ECTAS)
4th Floor, Standon House
21 Mansell Street
London E1 8AA
Email: ectas@cru.rcpsych.ac.uk
Website: www.rcpsych.ac.uk/quality/
qualityandaccreditation/ectclinics/ectas.
aspx

National Association of Lead Nurses
in ECT (NALNECT)
Website: www.nalnect.org.uk

Royal College of Psychiatrists
17 Belgrave Square
London SW1X 8PG
Tel: 020 7235 2351
Fax: 020 7245 1231
Email: reception@rcpsych.ac.uk
Website: www.rcpsych.ac.uk

Scottish ECT Accreditation Network (SEAN)
Email: contacts@sean.org.uk
Website: www.sean.org.uk

Manufacturers of ECT machines

Ectron Ltd (Ectron ECT machines do not
have an EEG recording facility)
Anvil Street
Temple Quay
Bristol BS2 0QQ
Tel: 0117 941 3979
Fax: 01462 481463
Email: enquiries@ectron.co.uk
Website: www.ectron.co.uk

Mecta (UK distributor)
Micromed Electronics Ltd.
11 Drakes Way
Mayford
Woking
Surrey GU22 ONX
Tel: 01483 728822
Fax: 01483 755663
Email: mmeduk@aol.com

Thymatron (UK distributor)
Dantec Dynamics
Garonor Way
Royal Portbury
Bristol BS20 7XER
Tel: 01275 375333
Fax: 01275 375336
Website: www.dantecdynamics.co.uk

Statutory bodies

England and Wales

Care Quality Commission (Customer Service Centre)
Citygate
Gallowgate
Newcastle upon Tyne NE1 4PA
Tel: 03000 616161
Fax: 03000 616171
Website: www.cqc.org.uk

Office of the Public Guardian
PO Box 16185
Birmingham B2 2WH
Tel: 0300 456 0300 (Mon–Fri 09.00–17.00h, except Wed 10.00–19.00h)
Fax: 0870 739 5780
Email: customerservices@publicguardian.gsi.gov.uk
Website www.justice.gov.uk/global/contacts/opg.htm

Scotland

Mental Welfare Commission for Scotland
Thistle House
91 Haymarket Terrace
Edinburgh EH12 5HE
Advice line: 0131 313 8777
Freephone for service users and carers: 0800 389 6809
(Telephone service available Mon–Thu 09.00–17.00h and Fri 09.30–16.30h)
Fax: 0131 313 8778
Email: enquiries@mwcscot.org.uk
Website: www.mwcscot.org.uk

Office of the Public Guardian (Scotland)
Hadrian House
Callendar Business Park
Callendar Road
Falkirk FK1 1XR
Tel: 01324 678300
Fax: 01324 678301
DX 550360 FALKIRK 3
LP-17 FALKIRK
Email: opg@scotcourts.gov.uk
Website: www.publicguardian-scotland.gov.uk

Northern Ireland

The Regulation and Quality Improvement Authority
9th floor Riverside Tower
5 Lanyon Place
Belfast BT1 3BT
Tel: 028 9051 7500
Fax: 028 9051 7501
Email: info@rqia.org.uk
Website: www.rqia.org.uk

The Regulation and Quality Improvement Authority
Hilltop
Tyrone and Fermanagh Hospital
Omagh
Co. Tyrone
BT79 0NS
Tel: 028 8224 5828
Fax: 028 8225 2544

Ireland

Mental Health Commission
St Martin's House
Waterloo Road
Dublin 4
Tel: +353 (1) 636 2400
Fax: +353 (1) 636 2440
Email: info@mhcirl.org
Website: www.mhcirl.ie

Example of a certificate of incapacity

For adults who are <u>unable</u> to consent to investigation or treatment

All sections to be completed by the health professional proposing the procedure

Patient's details (or pre-printed label)

Patient's surname/family name: ....

Patient's first names: ....

Date of birth: ....

Responsible health professional: ....

Job title: ....

NHS number (or other identifier): ....

Male ☐   Female ☐

Special requirements: ....
(e.g. other language/communication methods)

Signature of health professional proposing treatment

The procedure, detailed overleaf, is, in my clinical judgement, in the best interests of the patient, who lacks capacity, to consent for himself or herself. Where possible and appropriate I have discussed the patient's condition with those close to them and taken their knowledge of the patient's views and beliefs into account in determining their best interests.

☐ I have/have not sought a non-statutory second opinion (see below). (Delete as appropriate.)

☐ I confirm that I have read the legislation table and have taken account of all the issues governing the administration of ECT as pertaining to the Mental Capacity Act 2005 and where relevant the Mental Health Act 1983.

Signature:.. Date: ....
Name (print): .... Job title: ....

Where second opinion sought, the patient should sign below to confirm agreement:
Signature: .... Date: ....
Name (print): .... Job title: ....

Where the patient is detained under the MHA 1983:
A   Has a Second Opinion been requested from CQC? Yes / No
B   Is a T6 completed and attached? Yes / No Date completed: ....
C   Has a Section 62 Form been completed? Yes / No

(A) *Name of proposed procedure or course of treatment*

Electroconvulsive therapy: Unilateral ☐   Bilateral ☐   Either ☐
(Please tick laterality)

(B) *Assessment of patient's capacity*

I confirm that:

☐ The patient is unable to comprehend and retain information material to the decision; and/or

☐ The patient is unable to use and weigh this information in the decision-making process; or

☐ The patient is unable to communicate their decision (whether by talking, using sign language or any other means)

☐ The patient is unconscious

Please provide details (excluding where patient unconscious): for example of how above judgements were reached; which colleagues consulted; what attempts made to assist the patient make their own decision and why these were not successful.

....

(C) Number of treatments to be given under this authority:

Where Section 58A(5) is applicable, the number of treatments will also be stated on the Form T6)

☐

(D) Assessment of patient's best interests

☐ To the best of my knowledge, the patient has not refused this procedure in a valid advance directive.

☐ Where possible and appropriate, I have consulted with colleagues and those close to the patient, and I believe the procedure to be in the patient's best interests because:

....

(Where incapacity is likely to be temporary, for example if patient unconscious, or where patient has fluctuating capacity)

☐ The treatment cannot wait until the patient recovers capacity because:

....

(E) Change in capacity status

If the patient's condition alters, during the treatment course, such that they are deemed to become capacitous, Consent Form (1) will need to be completed.

Additionally, if Section 58A(3) applies, Form T4 will also need to be completed.

(F) Involvement of the patient's family and others close to patient

The final responsibility, for determining whether a procedure is in an incapacitated patient's best interests, lies with the health professional performing the procedure.

However, it is good practice to consult with those close to the patient (e.g. spouse/partner, family and friends, carer, supporter or advocate) unless you have good reason to believe that the patient would not have wished particular individuals to be consulted, or unless the urgency of their situation prevents this. 'Best interests' go far wider than 'best medical interests', and include factors such as the patient's wishes and beliefs when competent, their current wishes, their general well-being and their spiritual and religious welfare. (To be signed by a person or persons close to the patient, if they wish.)

In addition, where substitute decision-making is in place, i.e. an individual holding Lasting Power of Attorney (LPA) or Deputy appointed by the Court (CAD), then the healthcare professional must take account of their views as to this treatment and this should be recorded below. (See Legislation table for full details.)

I/We have been involved in a discussion with the relevant health professionals over the treatment of [insert patient's name].

I/We understand that the patient is unable to give their own consent, based on the criteria set out in this form.

I/We also understand that treatment can lawfully be provided if it is in the patient's best interests to receive it.

Any other comments (including any concerns about decision):

....

Name: .... Relationship to patient: ....

LPA (Yes/No): .... CAD (Yes/No): ....
(Delete as appropriate)

Address (if not the same as patient): ....
....

Signature: .... Date: ....

If a person close to the patient was not available in person, has this matter been discussed in any other way (e.g. over the telephone?)

☐ Yes   ☐ No

Details: ....
....
....

Index

Compiled by Linda English